Regulatory Disorders in Infants

Manfred Cierpka
Editor

Regulatory Disorders in Infants

Assessment, Diagnosis, and Treatment

Springer

Editor
Manfred Cierpka
Institute for Psychosocial Prevention
University Hospital Heidelberg
Heidelberg, Germany

Translation from German language edition: Regulationsstörungen by Manfred Cierpka

ISBN 978-3-319-43554-1 ISBN 978-3-319-43556-5 (eBook)
DOI 10.1007/978-3-319-43556-5

Library of Congress Control Number: 2016950010

Printed on acid-free paper

This Springer imprint is published by Springer Nature
The registered company is Springer International Publishing AG
The registered company address is: Gewerbestrasse 11, 6330 Cham, Switzerland

Preface

The present book addresses the most important regulatory disorders in infants and toddlers. Disorders of early behavioral regulation, i.e., crying, sleeping, or feeding disorders, are those most commonly encountered in this age group. The symptoms, which can affect a number of functional domains simultaneously, fall under the umbrella term of "regulatory disorders."

Epidemiological studies indicate that early childhood disorders occur in 5–20 % of infants and toddlers. Disorders are mostly transient and resolve in the course of early childhood development, either as a result of the infant's growing maturity or since the parents find a way to compensate for their infant's difficulties.

Infant development depends on communication with significant caregivers, generally the parents. Childhood maturation and development evolve within the natural context of early interaction with parents. Both parents and infant are well prepared for this reciprocal process by virtue of biologically anchored skills. In the first months of their infant's life, parents learn to "read" their baby and understand its signals, enabling them to respond to its needs with sensitivity. Thus, these intuitive parenting skills ensure that expectant mothers and fathers are well prepared for parenthood. By experiencing that its need will be reliably and appropriately satisfied, the infant develops a secure attachment to its parents, who become its "safe haven."

Therefore, any book on regulatory disorders in early childhood must seek to avoid prematurely "pathologizing" the problem in the infant, in the parents, and in the dysfunctional parent–infant interaction. Having said that, possible behavioral disorders in infants need to be taken extremely seriously for the reasons discussed below.

An infant's inconsolable crying, disordered sleep, violent and persistent temper tantrums, or clinginess can put a considerable strain not only on the parents but also on the infant. If the problem becomes entrenched, parents generally turn to their pediatrician, midwife, or other expert qualified to provide support in the context of pregnancy and childbirth. A knowledge of the problems and symptoms that can manifest in infants during early childhood is also relevant to professionals active in the field of "early support," since they will be confronted with these problems in the performance of their profession, e.g., as family midwives or family nurses on their home visits. Youth welfare services now offer far greater support in terms of child protection and relevant help for parents with infants aged 0–3 years. The aim of this book is to sensitize these professional groups to the problem of regulatory disorders and to provide information on the options available to them in terms of intervention.

Excessive and persistent regulatory disorders in early childhood need to be taken very seriously. Immediate help is required for two reasons: Firstly, a regulatory disorder can strain and exhaust parents and their infant so rapidly that an acute crisis situation may emerge within the family. Situations of overload can, in rare cases, result in impulsive actions on the part of the parents, generally toward their infant. Secondly, if left untreated, regulatory disorders that persist over a long period of time can lead to developmental deficits in the infant, as well as to behavioral disorders in the further course. Approximately a third of disorders persist. The greater the burden on parents and family—and the less they provide their infant with the attention and affection it needs—the poorer their ability to compensate their infant's emotional and cognitive developmental deficits.

The individual chapters of the book attempt to illustrate how support for parents and their infant can look. The idea on which our interventional approaches are based is that parents should regain the "fit" they had with their infant as rapidly as possible. In some cases, a "low-dose" intervention is sufficient to achieve this goal. Counseling of this kind attempts to combine different methods and techniques in order to help the family on various levels as rapidly as possible. If parents are motivated to be guided by their infant's needs, they can fulfill the developmental potential all parents have to be good parents. They can achieve this all the better when their interpretation of their infant's behaviors is not superimposed by exaggerated wishes and fears based mostly on difficult experiences in their own childhood. Counseling approaches are inadequate in cases where parental perceptions and interpretations have a lasting dysfunctional effect on parent–infant interaction. Psychotherapy (sometimes long term) is indicated in such cases. Psychodynamic approaches focus above all on the mostly subconscious expectations and attitudes (representations) of the parents and on the relational patterns these give rise to. Over the course of treatment, parents become aware that they contribute to this dysfunctional interaction with their own biographies and, by so doing, maintain a negative interaction cycle. This insight, and the repeated working-through of problems within the protected sphere of psychotherapy, enables them to modify interaction with their infant.

This book, authored by German experts in parent–infant/toddler psychotherapy, aims to illustrate clinical work in Germany. It is the editor's hope that our concept of clinical work will be stimulating and rewarding for experts in other countries.

I would like to thank all the authors involved for their contributions and active collaboration. Springer-Verlag, Heidelberg and New York, has once again provided me expert support for the publication of this book. My special thanks go to Mrs. Christine Schaefer for her excellent translation from German to English and her painstaking copyediting of the manuscript.

It is my sincere hope that readers will find this book both inspiring and informative!

Heidelberg, Germany Manfred Cierpka

Contents

Contributors

Marisa Benz, Dipl.Psych. Florida State University, University Center, Tallahassee, FL, USA

Astrid Cierpka, Dipl.Soz.Arb. Private Practice, Heidelberg, Germany

Manfred Cierpka, M.D. Institute for Psychosocial Prevention, University Hospital Heidelberg, Heidelberg, Germany

Hortense Demant, Dipl.Psych. Department of Child and Youth Medicine, Psychological Service, Hospital of Karlsruhe, Karlsruhe, Germany

Sarah Groß, Dipl.Psych. Psychosoziale Beratungsstelle, Studentenwerk Heidelberg, University of Heidelberg, Heidelberg, Germany

Nikolaus von Hofacker, Dr.med. Private Practice for Infant, Child and Adolescent Psychiatry, August-Exter-Straße, München, Germany

Mechthild Papoušek, M.D. Institute for Social Pediatrics and Youth Medicine, University of Munich, Munich, Germany

Kerstin Scholtes-Spang, Dipl.Psych. Institute for Psychosocial Prevention, University Hospital Heidelberg, Heidelberg, Germany

Michael Stasch, Dipl.Psych. Private Practice, Heidelberg, Germany

Consolata Thiel-Bonney, M.D. Center for Children, Adolescents and Families, Hospital Hochried, Hochried, Murnau, Germany

Eberhard Windaus, Dr.phil. Private Practice, Frankfurt, Germany

About the Editor

Manfred Cierpka is a Senior Professor at the University Hospital of Heidelberg. He is a Medical Doctor of Psychiatry and Psychosomatic Medicine, a Psychoanalyst, and Family Therapist. He completed his doctorate at the University of Ulm, after which he became a Professor of Psychosomatics and Family Therapy at the University of Göttingen. From 1998 to 2015 he was the Medical Director of the Institute for Psychosomatic Cooperation Research and Family Therapy at the University Hospital of Heidelberg. He is the author or editor of many books including the *Handbuch der Familiendiagnostik*, published by Springer. He is also co-editor of the journal *Psychotherapeut*, also published by Springer.

From Normal Development to Developmental Crisis and Regulatory Disorder

1

Marisa Benz and Kerstin Scholtes-Spang

1.1 Early Childhood Development

The development and maturation of an individual spans their entire lifetime. Thus, developmental tasks are encountered throughout life, such as the manifold physical and emotional changes experienced in puberty or during the transition to parenthood (Erikson 1973; Havighurst 1948). During the early years of life, however, an individual develops faster than at any other time. Children undergo approximately 50 % of their entire development during the first 4 years of life (Largo 2010). As a result, humans are confronted with an exceptional number of developmental tasks in their early childhood and have a relatively short time in which to solve these tasks. On the one hand, development generally follows a highly uniform course, with the individual developmental stages occurring as a rule in the same sequence in all children. For example, all children develop the ability first to lift their head, then to sit, and finally to walk upright. On the other hand, child development is also characterized by astounding diversity and marked inter-individual and intraindividual differences. Most notably, the time at which certain developmental phases take place and the extent to which certain behaviors occur are unique to each child.

M. Benz, Dipl.Psych. (✉)
Florida State University, 4600 University Center, Tallahassee, FL 32306, USA
e-mail: mbenz@lsi.fsu.edu

K. Scholtes-Spang, Dipl.Psych.
Institute for Psychosocial Prevention, University Hospital Heidelberg,
Bergheimer Str. 54, Heidelberg 69115, Germany
e-mail: kontakt@psychotherapie-scholtes.de

M. Cierpka (ed.), *Regulatory Disorders in Infants*,
DOI 10.1007/978-3-319-43556-5_1

Case Study 1 At the age of 11 months, Max had already started several months earlier to pull himself up while holding onto furniture, followed by walking while holding a parent's hand, and had just taken his first steps on his own; in contrast, 17-month-old Leo had still been sliding about on the floor of his parent's home on the seat of his trousers. "I hadn't ever really given it a thought, since he's so far ahead in many other areas, but my mother was phoning almost daily to ask whether he was finally walking," the mother reported. "I kept telling her that it would take a bit longer; after all, up to that point, Leo hadn't shown even the slightest urge to stand. But then things changed from one day to the next: suddenly, he was standing in front of me in the middle of the living room. I have no idea how he managed that."

While some infants start walking at as early as 10 months, others can take up to the age of 18 months. Moreover, while one infant follows the classic developmental course of rolling, crawling, sitting up, and standing up, another may skip the crawling stage altogether or slide about instead on the seat of his trousers before taking his first upright steps. This phenomenon is partly explained by inherited movement patterns, as well as by variations in infants' urge to move, which also play a role here. There is no relationship between the speed of motor skill development and development in other areas. Hence, it is not unusual for an infant to be far advanced in its motor skill development compared with its peers, while its first words are a long time in coming, and vice versa.

1.1.1 Self-Regulation as a Central Developmental Task

Self-regulation: self-regulation describes a child's ability to control their behavior according to the cognitive, emotional, and social demands of a particular situation (Posner and Rothbart 2000).

An infant's regulatory capacity plays a central role in early childhood development (Papoušek 2008). For example, in the context of physiological regulation during the first 3 months of life: an infant needs to learn about basic physical processes and adapt to these accordingly. This includes, amongst other things, the regulation of behavioral states (alert wakefulness and quiet sleep, as well as the transition between the two). From the age of 6 months, an infant begins to move about independently (locomotion). He or she is now capable of actively seeking attachment figures, but also of missing these when they are absent. Autonomy is now the big issue. Once able to walk independently, an infant has mastered the skill of unrestricted autonomous locomotion; now they also want to feed themselves, indeed do as much as possible on their own. These major steps toward autonomy are coupled with demands on the infant to tolerate greater levels of frustration and deal with physical and social boundaries. This often results in greater dissatisfaction and, despite their new-found autonomy, an increased need for love and affection (see Chaps. 6 and 7). Thus, again, self-regulation plays a crucial role in addressing the conflicting needs for exploration and closeness and in closeness–distance regulation.

1.2 Parent–Infant Communication

Infants are dependent on the care of their parents or other caregivers for a long period of time. This applies not only in terms of their physical care and welfare, but also in terms of their ability to accomplish the tasks of early development, tasks that an infant is only capable of achieving with the help of its parents. According to Cierpka's family model, this is the core task of the family: to ensure and protect the psychosocial development of its members (Cierpka 2005).

As part of this process, preverbal parent–infant communication takes place on various sensory levels, that is to say, with the help of all observable behavior. Affects and moods, needs and incentives, as well as interests and intentions expressed in behavior are as much a part of this process as specific interactions.

▶ From the outset, infants are capable of perceiving and reacting to their environment. With the help of a diversity of signals, such as gaze behavior, facial expressions, posture and body tension, as well as their movement and voice (crying and noises), they are active interaction partners engaging in contact with their parents in order to communicate their needs via a variety of channels.

To ensure this type of communication, infants are inherently equipped with a particularly strong interest in social interaction. They focus their attention preferably on a human face, as well as on the voice and language of their primary caregiver. This ability for and interest in interaction in infants encourages adults to actively care for them. Thus, infant signals ensure that a baby receives the basic and appropriate care it needs, thereby also making it possible to jointly accomplish the developmental tasks at hand.

1.2.1 Demands on Parents

It is the task of all parents to support the development of their infant. The principal requirement here is to respond as appropriately as possible to the individual needs of an infant and to identify where its self-regulatory abilities are perhaps not yet sufficient and need to be supported by parental co-regulation. To meet this requirement, all parents are inherently equipped with intuitive skills to deal with their infant.

Intuitive skills: the innate, universally valid motivation in human beings to recognize and adequately respond to the needs of an infant.

These intuitive skills enable parents to cater to the individual characteristics of their infant. However, parents differ in the extent of their parental sensitivity. Parental sensitivity is defined as the ability to perceive and correctly interpret an infant's signals and to respond to these signals both promptly and appropriately according to developmental stage and situation (Ainsworth 1977). This can be seen in everyday interactions, e.g., when parents, prompted by their infant's signal, soothe their infant when it is not capable of self-calming, or, guided by their parental sensitivity, recognize and respond to their infant's need for closeness and reassurance. In this way, parents compensate for what their infant cannot yet manage alone. The infant learns that it can depend on its parents' support, as well as learning what the possible responses to inner states may be. A high level of parental sensitivity on the part of the caregiver results in an infant feeling emotionally secure.

Jonas (12 weeks) and his mother were immersed in an intimate exchange. The mother was talking to Jonas in a melodic voice, her eyes wide open. He was watching her facial expressions keenly, all the while moving his arms and legs and making happy cooing sounds. The mother imitated Jonas' sounds. Every now and then, Jonas turned his head to the side and his mother waited while he took a short break before reestablishing eye contact with her. After a while, Jonas started to deflect his gaze ever more frequently and his mother noticed that it was becoming increasingly tiring for him to maintain eye contact. Jonas started to move about restlessly and yawn. His mother recognized his signals of fatigue. She took Jonas in her arms with his head on her shoulder and softly hummed a lullaby while rocking him gently and dimming the light in the room. By the time she placed Jonas in his cot, his eyes were already virtually closed and shortly thereafter he fell asleep.

Thanks to the early recognition of Jonas' signals of fatigue and the ensuing opportunity he is given to sleep, Jonas is increasingly able to identify his initially diffuse discomfort as fatigue due to the maternal "labeling" that takes places, as well as his own cognitive development. For the mother's part, Jonas' positive reaction to the support offered results in her experiencing a sense of competence, which in turn increases her parental confidence ("I know my child; I know what he needs, hence I also know what needs to be done"). In this way, interactions based on positive reciprocity are formed between parent and infant ("virtuous circles" according to Papoušek 2008), which enable both sides to jointly tackle the next interaction sequence with each another. Thus, parents and infants that regularly experience stable and successful communication sequences with each other are able to form a constellation whereby the parents offer the secure foundation and sheltered environment in which an infant can increasingly discover and test its own self-regulatory skills.

Experiencing that they are able to offer their infant appropriate support permits parents in the further course of the infant's development to gain increasing trust in its growing abilities. They are able to distinguish whether and to what extent their infant needs regulatory support and which situations it is potentially already capable of tackling alone.

In turn, infants that are supported with parental sensitivity in the regulation of behavioral states are thus increasingly able to put what they have learned into practice independently and are able to deal with situations in a self-efficacious manner. This sends parents the signal that they can gradually withdraw their support.

Likewise, misunderstandings of the type that occur every now and then as a matter of course in the communication between all parents and infants are coped with well by both sides in constellations in which both sides regularly experience successful interaction.

1.3 "Goodness of Fit"

Reconciling an infant's needs with the demands and support opportunities of their environment (as described in the previous section) can be seen as a matching of—or a "fit" between—the two. The term "goodness of fit" was coined by Chess and Thomas (1984) in the course of their research.

▶ According to Chess and Thomas, infants develop best when there is good congruence between an infant's motivation and temperament on the one hand, and the opportunities, expectations, and demands of their environment on the other. A good fit between these two results in satisfied parents as well as a satisfied infant. A less good fit, in contrast, can lead to perturbation on both sides.

Thus, there are likely to be few problems of fit between the infant that has a particular need for calm and quiet and parents that are by nature calm and quiet themselves, whereas an infant with highly active and lively parents may need to demand their calm and quiet more vigorously. In the latter case, there is a particular demand on the parents to perceive their infant's need for calm and quiet and to create sufficient opportunities in the turbulent family routine for their infant to rest.

An optimal fit, however, is never guaranteed in the long-term. An infant's development is continuous, meaning that parents are constantly required to readapt to their infant. Temporary phases of less good fit in the course of new adaptation processes are, therefore, in the nature of things. Indeed, they can be seen positively, as a sign that a new stage of development is about to begin or has been successfully completed and is now, as in a crisis, placing more demands on those involved.

The processes of need recognition and adaptation may function highly successfully in one developmental phase and possibly be associated with difficulties in another, difficulties which manifest in the form of more frequent expressions of dissatisfaction in the infant, an increased burden on the parents, or difficulties in interaction. Difficult phases such as these are not infrequently the result of misunderstandings in communication.

Exhausted, the parents of 11-week-old Lilly sought advice at a parent–infant outpatient clinic. "Lilly cries nearly all day—I think mostly when she is bored. I now spend almost all of my time keeping Lilly amused and offering her new stimuli" her mother reported. "Although I really love playing with Lilly, I'm often so tired that I simply can't any longer. Lilly needs constant amusement; I can't even make myself a sandwich without her instantly starting to cry. Lilly sleeps around 8 h straight through the night. Of course, that's great, since I'm able to get some rest myself." Lilly's father went on to add: "My mother advised us early on not to let Lilly sleep too much during the day, so that she'd be tired in the evening and would start sleeping through the night as soon as possible. My mother brought up four children herself and knows how tiring the nights can be otherwise." "That's why the nights are so good. It's the daytime that's a problem." Lilly's mother reported: "Lilly usually has three, sometimes only two short naps of 30 min each during the day; she's awake the rest of the time and never really happy. About 2 weeks ago, she cried so much that I took her to the A&E department at the local pediatric hospital. The doctor there advised us to feed Lilly more often, since her crying could be a sign of hunger and she doesn't weigh much for her age. Although we had thought up to then that Lilly was being fed enough, she actually did calm down, usually very quickly, when I put her to the breast. We feel like terrible parents for not recognizing that Lilly was hungry. We both have too little experience with babies and often don't know what Lilly's trying to tell us. The regular breastfeeding is also quite tiring. Lilly often just sucks without really feeding properly and she often falls asleep at the breast. Then I have to wake her so that she carries on feeding; it breaks my heart to do it, because she seems so exhausted." During this conversation, Lilly was at first very interested and looked attentively around the room. Then, after a few minutes, she became restless, started rubbing her eyes, yawning, arching her back, and sucking her fingers. The parents took it in turns to calm and distract Lilly, which worked, but only for short periods at a time. The mother noted in exasperation: "This is exactly the sort of situation we're talking about. What does she want? When she yawns, I think she's tired, but then she sees something and is suddenly all interested and everything seems fine—so maybe she was just bored? Then the next minute she's crying again and trying to eat her own hand—so is she perhaps hungry after all?"

Although the parents recognize their infant's signals, they are unsure how to interpret them. As a result, they respond inappropriately, e.g., by offering stimulation in response to signs of tiredness. Whilst rapid changes in their infant's behavior make the parents feel insecure and diminish their confidence in their intuitive assessment of Lilly's needs on the one hand, Lilly, on the other, has not yet experienced an association: "When this feeling appears (hunger, tiredness, or boredom), certain behaviors (eating, sleeping, or stimulation) help me to resolve it."

In the same way that infants develop in highly distinct ways, they also differ greatly in terms of their temperament traits and, consequently, also in terms of their needs. In addition to their own temperament and personality traits, parents in turn additionally bring notions of what they consider normal in infant development into their interaction with their infant. These expectations may be based on their own (biographical) experience, but also on advice and information from their environment.

As in the case study above, parents have a particular notion about the sleep requirements of an infant. This notion is born of their own sleep requirements, experience with their infant's older siblings, accounts they hear from relatives and friends, as well as what they read in parenting manuals. In actual fact, the sleep requirements of an individual infant vary considerably (between 12.5 and 17.5 h in the first 6 months; Basler et al. 1980). Thus, it is quite possible that the notions and expectations of parents do not correspond with the actual amount of sleep their infant needs, but that these requirements are instead being over- or underestimated. Particularly in the case of underestimated sleep requirements, an overwrought infant may fuss and cry more as a result of their lack of sleep (see Chap. 3). Prolonged misunderstandings of this kind arise when parents either fail to perceive their infant's signal, or perceive it incorrectly. It is possible that parents are unable to recognize their infant's signals in particular due to their own stressors or a lack of parental sensitivity, or that they lack confidence in their intuition as a result of insecurity. It might be that, although parents recognize their infant's signals, they misinterpret them: thus, for example, signs of fatigue, as in Lilly's case, are often interpreted as boredom and responded to as such. Especially infants that are hypersensitive to stimuli can always be temporarily distracted from their fatigue to a certain degree by new stimuli. This short-term pseudo-stability reinforces the parents' impression that their infant is bored; as a result, they tend to offer new stimulation ever faster, ultimately exacerbating their infant's overstimulation. Another common misconception is that breastfeeding serves not only food intake, but also as an effective means of comforting an infant by virtue of the physical closeness and soothing effect that nursing and sucking provide. This often results in a mix-up in the perception of the need for closeness and calming and the perception of hunger signals.

It is essential, when working with parents and infants, to discover not only the needs and signals of the infant, but also the expectations and impressions of the parents: How do parents recognize fatigue? How does your infant signal their hunger? Do you recognize differences in how your infant expresses differing needs? In addition to posing questions to the parents, observations on an infant's signals in the counseling setting are of central importance. An objective log kept by the parents (e.g., in the form of a sleep diary; see Chap. 3) and video recordings can also yield valuable clues to possible misunderstandings in parent–infant communication.

A poor fit between the perception, expectations, attitudes, and life circumstances of parents on the one hand and the individual needs of an infant on the other can cause temporary difficulties in parent–infant communication, difficulties that need to be resolved together in the further course.

1.4 Normal Developmental Crises

The parents of 17-month-old Emma hardly recognized their daughter. Up until that point, Emma had always been a happy and balanced infant; however, over the previous few weeks she had been constantly unhappy, fussing a lot of the time, and occasionally throwing "real tantrums." Emma would go wild, throw herself on the floor kicking and screaming and was impossible to soothe. The parents reported that there had been several changes in Emma's life over the previous few weeks: Emma was now going to a child care provider on weekday mornings. To the parents' surprise, she had settled there without any problems. The mother reported with relief: "The first few days, Emma cried a little when I left her. After only a week, she happily waved goodbye to me. I think Emma's very happy at the child care provider's, who in turn says she has absolutely no problems with Emma. The problems start when I pick her up at lunchtime." The mother reported that she always looked forward to picking Emma up from the child care provider at 12 midday and spending the afternoon with her daughter. However, Emma was often so crotchety that playing together was out of the question. The mother had the impression that Emma was bored at home after her stimulating morning at the child care provider's with the other three children. Although the mother tried to entertain Emma and occupy her with games, nothing seemed to make her happy. Emma's daily routine had also changed as a result of visiting the child care provider: up until that time, Emma had always taken a 1.5-h midday nap at around 1.00 p.m. Although her parents believed that she still urgently needed this sleep, she often refused it vehemently. "If she doesn't have a midday nap, she is so tired by the end of the afternoon that she's impossible to deal with. She's so tired, she's virtually tripping over her own feet; she can't manage anything and gets all the more frustrated." Food had also become a point of conflict. Emma had discovered that she was particularly fond of biscuits and cheese and continually asked for these between meals. Emma's mother was unwilling to give her these snacks, since they had a significant effect on mealtimes. Although both parents had accepted that it would be necessary to set clear and definite boundaries in Emma's development, they were unprepared for how challenging it would be to remain consistent in their approach. In this respect, Emma clearly had the greater stamina and, especially since there were already numerous conflicts, the mother often found it difficult to remain firm. "Sometimes giving in is the lesser of two evils. Since Emma's been going to the child care provider in the mornings, we see much less of each other, so I don't want to spend the whole afternoon fighting with her."

It is clear from their accounts that parents of infants and toddlers are particularly challenged in terms of their ability to adapt in order to keep up with the rapid pace of their infant's development. At the same time, it is their task to offer their infant support and guidance, particularly during phases of change.

> Crisis situations form a natural and integral part of meeting the challenges posed in normal infant development. Coping with these challenges is part of everyday life for parents and infants (Largo and Benz-Castellano 2008).

In the past, development processes have been described on a number of occasions in the context of developmental crises (Erikson 1973) or developmental tasks (Havighurst 1948). Stage models of development, like those proposed by Havighurst and Erikson, assume that each transition from one phase to the next is characterized by problems and conflicts. Coping successfully with a crisis fosters new skills and increases self-confidence.

As in the models of normative developmental crises, problems in early childhood are typically expressed as a function of the developmental phases and tasks at hand. Thus, they generally arise during certain age periods and in those areas of behavior in the foreground of the respective developmental phase (the "touchpoints" concept) (Brazelton 1999). For example, excessive crying is seen most notably in the first months of life in conjunction with physiological adaptation processes (see Chap. 3), as clearly demonstrated by the age distribution of children referred to the parent–infant/toddler outpatient clinic at the Heidelberg University Hospital due to excessive crying (see Fig. 1.1). In their second year of life, toddlers

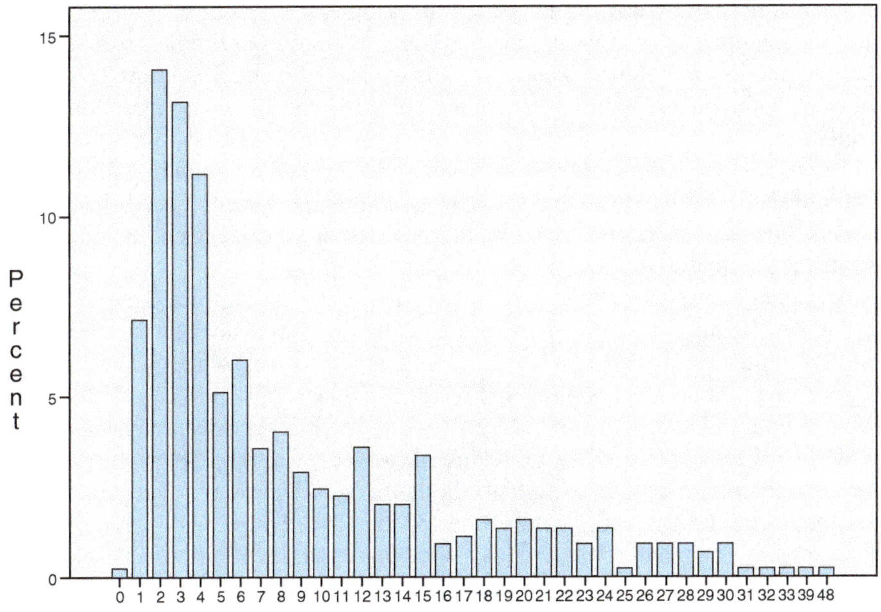

Fig. 1.1 Age distribution of children referred to the parent–infant/toddler outpatient clinic at the Heidelberg University Hospital due to excessive crying (Thiel-Bonney and Erb 2011)

are increasingly required to cope with the frustrations associated with their growing autonomy, on the one hand in relation to the boundaries set by their parents and social rules, on the other due to their still limited own potential, e.g., in terms of motor skills. Against this backdrop, increased acts of defiance and expressions of dissatisfaction are often seen during this phase (see Chap. 7).

The mother of almost 10-month-old Anton recounted to a friend that Anton had started to crawl 2 weeks previously. The mother's pride at her son's new skills was mixed with considerable relief. "The last few weeks with Anton before he learned to crawl were really tiring," she told her friend. "He was constantly in a bad mood and crotchety. He just wanted to be carried the whole time. When he was picked up, he pointed from one place to the other and woe betide anyone who didn't take him where he wanted to go immediately. And before that he used to occupy himself so happily on his play mat; in the end, he didn't want to go on it at all. He was still happiest in his high-chair, but he kept dropping his toys and I kept having to pick them up and give them back to him; but even that didn't seem to make him happy. I think he was frustrated that he couldn't get his things himself and that he couldn't get to where he wanted to go. He's been in a much better mood since he's been able to crawl, even though nowhere is safe from him at home and we've started having to put everything up on shelves out of his reach."

In addition to normative crises, critical life events as described by Filipp and Aymanns (2010) can also trigger normal developmental crises. The birth of a sibling, for example, or changes in the caregiver situation, as in Emma's example, can cause temporary difficulties. Therefore, it is advisable to enquire during counseling about recent changes, both in an infant's behavior and its environment and daily family life.

The shape that an individual crisis takes is determined not only by the task to be accomplished, but also to a crucial extent by the temperament of the infant and its parents, their resources and stressors, the interaction experiences garnered to date, as well as the quality of the relationship.

An infant's ever-advancing development requires parents to constantly readapt to the developmental stage of their infant, as described above (see Sect. 1.3). Parental strategies to support self-regulation that were perhaps highly successful up to a certain point in time are possibly no longer age-appropriate. Thus, whilst swaddling an infant or carrying it in a baby sling can be effective ways to promote sleep in the first weeks of life, these strategies are no longer appropriate to the developmental stage of a 6-month-old infant; therefore, new and more appropriate strategies for promoting sleep need to be found and introduced (see Chap. 4). This process of need recognition and adaptation can work highly efficiently in one developmental phase, while being associated with difficulties in another, difficulties that may manifest in the form of an infant expressing dissatisfaction more often, increased strain on the parents, or intermittent difficulties in interaction.

As a general rule, parents and infants are capable of coping with temporary developmental crises, i.e., of recognizing and resolving a "misfit." Being able to resolve a crisis together strengthens the parent's intuitive skills. Experience has shown them that they are able to respond appropriately to their infant's signals and are thus able to resolve challenging situations. This experience also serves to strengthen their confidence in their intuitive parenting skills in future crisis situations.

Emma's parents observed their daughter carefully over the following weeks. When she came home from the child care provider, she was still fussing, going around the home aimlessly, and throwing her toys around the room in frustration. "If we think about it, that's how Emma behaves when she's tired. Her busy mornings playing with the other children are probably very tiring for her. Up until now, she was usually just at home alone with us." Over the ensuing weeks, the mother refrained from encouraging Emma to play, offering her instead plenty of opportunities for "cuddle time" in Emma's bedroom. "I draw the curtains and then we cuddle up together on Emma's big floor cushion and quietly look at a book together. This gives her the chance to have a rest and, some days, she even falls asleep. Ideally, she should still be taking a midday nap, but we've tried and she just doesn't want to. So this gives us a bit of downtime together, which acts as reinforcement for those situations where she's difficult." After introducing the downtime ritual, the parents found their daughter to be in a better mood and the mother expressed her relief at having recognized how she could best support her daughter. This helped her to hold her ground in boundary-setting situations. "I know what's good for her and I stick by that. It's almost as if Emma feels this and can accept my 'no' better," the mother recounted.

1.5 The Concept of Early Childhood Regulatory Disorders

Early childhood regulatory disorders can be seen as extreme variants in ways of coping with age-typical crises. They are distinct from normal developmental crises in that they last longer in conjunction with existing stressors and may spread to other areas of development. Jointly accomplishing the developmental tasks at hand under such circumstances is not possible, and the result is almost always impairment to infant self-regulation and to the parent–infant relationship (Cierpka et al. 2002).

The following disorders are classed as early childhood regulatory disorders: excessive crying during the first 3 months of life (see "Lilly" Case Report above), disorders of initiating and maintaining sleep, feeding disorders, persistent agitation and dysphoria with disinterest in play, excessive clinginess, social anxiety and persistent separation anxiety, excessive defiance, as well as provocative/oppositional and aggressive behavior.

1.5.1 Triad of Symptoms in Early Childhood Regulatory Disorders

Diagnostic and therapeutic considerations in early childhood regulatory disorders, unlike disorders in later life, include an assessment of both the infant and the primary attachment figures, as well as of parent–infant interaction and relationship regulation between these individuals (Papoušek 2008).

▶ Triad of Symptoms in Early Childhood Regulatory Disorders

1. ***Difficulty(ies) on the part of the infant*** *in one or more area of early childhood adjustment and developmental tasks.*
2. ***Exhaustion Syndrome in the mother/father/both parents*** *in the sense of an adjustment disorder in the transition to parenthood or in dealing with a "difficult" infant.*
3. ***Dysfunctional behavioral pattern*** *specifically when dealing with the infant's abnormal behavior; this pattern in turn perpetuates or worsens the behavior and results in escalation.*

If the infant's ability to self-regulate is limited to an extreme extent, this can put excessive strain on the parents in terms of their intuitive communication skills and the self-regulation aides they have at their disposal. An example here would be infants with a "difficult temperament" that often exhibit irregular sleeping and eating behavior, express their emotions more intensely, and tend toward fussing and crying more than other infants. Particularly when infants are hypersensitive, irritable, and unable to distinguish between external and internal sensations (or react particularly sensitively to these), they are often overchallenged and overstimulated by the flood of incoming information and hence difficult to soothe. However, states of exhaustion that can be expected, e.g., due to illness or fatigue, can also disable self-regulation skills.

In addition to the difficulties experienced by the infant along the way to developing self-regulation skills, the required parental co-regulation may fail. Intuitive parental communication skills can be hindered by physical, psychological, and social factors in the prepartum, peripartum, and postpartum phase. Such factors may include, among others, biographical stressors in the parents, e.g., experiences of loss or violence, maternal depression, substance abuse, social isolation, couples conflicts, previous miscarriages, problematic pregnancies, as well as antenatal stress and anxiety. Persistent self-regulatory problems in an infant, coupled with parents repeatedly experiencing a sense of failure and helplessness in dealing with their infant, further exacerbate parental stressors that were possibly already present before the infant's birth. Dysfunctional communication patterns emerge that contribute to causing escalations, perpetuating the regulatory problem, and extending it to other areas of development.

The interaction of several psychosocial and organic risk factors in the infant and/or parents is typical in the emergence of early childhood regulatory disorders. When talking with parents, it is important to address possible stressors that hamper the joint accomplishment of the current developmental task at hand. It is essential here that the question of whether the regulatory disorder is the cause or the effect of a strained family situation does not form the focus of counseling. The central principle of the triad of symptoms is that the stressors on the infant and those on the parents are mutually determining. Assigning a cause or apportioning blame in one or other direction is therefore futile and contraindicated in the further course. Instead, systemic events within the family should form the focus of counseling.

Permanent overload on parents, combined with failed efforts to help their infant, increases the likelihood of acts of impulsivity, thereby posing a risk for emotional and/or physical abuse in infancy. Therefore, when talking with parents, it is always important to additionally discuss an emergency plan for possible situations of extreme overload and, where necessary, formulate such a plan (e.g., timeout for the parents while the infant is taken to a safe place, their cot, for instance).

Entrenchment of the interaction patterns that underlie interpersonal contact can have a negative impact on overall child development in the long term, since the associated lack of flexibility hinders parents from adequately supporting their infant's developmental steps. For this reason, formulating options together with the family to relieve strain should always be one of the main objectives of providing support and guidance in self-regulatory disorders. Here, the emphasis lies on developing ideas that are both suited to and realistic for the family in question: short breaks that can be easily incorporated into everyday life often promise greater success than extensive modifications that are complicated and time-consuming to implement. This is not to say, however, that one should not seek to make fundamental changes to the extent deemed possible. Whatever the intervention undertaken, the ultimate decision and responsibility lies with the parents—the purpose of counseling is to: consistently reinforce family members in their individual skills as well as the family in their joint skills, identify the family's joint resources, support parent–infant communication, and promote parental sensitivity.

1.5.2 Mixed Regulatory Disorders

The disorders that fall under the umbrella term "regulatory disorders" show considerable similarities in terms of the conditions under which they emerge and their burden of risk, course, and prognosis. Depending on the developmental phase, they often occur successively; however, they frequently also occur simultaneously and sometimes persist largely unabated into toddlerhood or preschool age (Papoušek 2008). In terms of severity, all early childhood regulatory disorders range from crises in isolated areas (e.g., difficulties initiating sleep in the evening) to persistent disorders that affect several, or in some cases all areas of self-regulatory development.

Given the similarities and poor differentiation between the individual regulatory disorders, the shift or spread of disorders from one developmental area to another is unsurprising. For example, 78.8 % of parents presenting with infants aged 0–6 months to the parent–infant/toddler clinic of the Heidelberg University Hospital between 1999 and 2009 also reported problems in sleep–wake regulation or sleeping disorders. The parents of 28.6 % of infants with excessive crying additionally reported problems associated with feeding (Thiel-Bonney 2006). In 66.9 % of infants with feeding problems, parents also spoke of sleeping difficulties. In contrast, isolated cases of these problems were seen in only 2.2 % of infants presenting due to excessive defiance and in 1 % of infants with excessive clinginess. Studies on the sample at the Heidelberg specialist outpatient clinic (Erb et al. 2014) showed that only the probability of feeding disorders is higher in the case of premature birth, and this as a function of falling birth weight.

Whilst difficulties in several areas of self-regulation undoubtedly contribute to increasing exhaustion and an entrenchment of interactional difficulties, a prolonged period of persistent strain on the parents and infant also has the same effect, thereby additionally contributing to the spread of disorders to other areas of development. In the study sample at the parent–infant/toddler clinic at the Heidelberg University Hospital, the interval between the onset of behavioral disorders and presentation at the clinic was 8 months on average (Thiel-Bonney 2006).

These findings underscore the need for early prevention and intervention measures. The increasing extent to which help is sought from parent–infant/toddler counseling centers is a sign of the growing acceptance among perplexed and exhausted parents of this type of support (Cierpka et al. 2007). However, specific, low-threshold forms of support for families with multiple psychosocial stressors are also extremely important in this context, since self-regulatory disorders tend to spread especially in those cases where the intuitive skills of parents are limited or hampered by a variety of stressors. These stressors amplify the effect of recurrent negative feedback loops on parent–infant communication and can contribute to an escalation in dysfunctional communication patterns, as well as to the spread of behavioral disorders to other areas of development. In such cases, support to improve the general living situation is crucial, otherwise stressors in everyday family life can stand in the way of improving parent–infant interaction despite optimal counseling in this area.

With regard to the emergence of externalizing (symptoms of hyperkinesis, aggression, and opposition) and internalizing disorders (symptoms of anxiety and depression) in later childhood and adolescence, prevention and early intervention in the area of self-regulatory disorders is particularly beneficial in those infants in whom multiple areas of self-regulation are affected, parent–infant interaction is impaired, organic factors hamper development, and/or the family environment is subject to psychosocial stressors (Laucht et al. 2008; Sidor et al. 2013).

1.6 Conclusion

In the course of child development, parents and infants are constantly required to jointly accomplish the developmental tasks at hand. Crisis situations in this context are generally seen as normal developmental crises, which parents and infants are capable of accomplishing together. Inability to jointly tackle the developmental task at hand in conjunction with existing stress factors almost always results in impaired infant self-regulation, as well as impaired parent–infant relationships. These extreme variants of normal developmental crises, known as early childhood self-regulatory disorders, can sometimes persist for prolonged periods of time and extend to other areas of development. Targeted family guidance and counseling are indicated in such cases.

References

Ainsworth MDS (1977) Skalen zur Erfassung mütterlichen Verhaltens von Mary D.S. Ainsworth: Feinfühligkeit versus Unempfindlichkeit gegenüber den Signalen des Babys. In: Grossmann, K.E. (Hrsg.): Entwicklung der Lernfähigkeit in der sozialen Umwelt. Kindler. S., München, pp. 98–107

Basler K, Largo RH, Molinari L (1980) Die Entwicklung des Schlafverhaltens in den ersten fünf Lebensjahren. Helv Paediatr Acta 35:211–223

Brazelton TB (1999) How to help parents of young children: the touchpoints model. J Perinatol 19:6–7

Chess S, Thomas A (1984) Origins and evolution of behavior disorders. Bruner and Mazel, New York

Cierpka M (2005) The three-level model of family assessment. In: Cierpka M, Thomas V, Sprenkle D (eds) Family assessment: multiple perspectives. Hogrefe, Seattle, pp 2–15

Cierpka M, Loetz S, Cierpka A (2002) Beratung für Familien mit Säuglingen und Kleinkindern. In: Wirsching M, Scheib P (eds) Paar- und familientherapie. Springer, Heidelberg

Cierpka M, Stasch M, Groß S (2007) Expertise zum Stand der Prävention/Frühintervention in der frühen Kindheit in Deutschland, vol 34. Bundeszentrale für gesundheitliche Aufklärung, (BzgA), Köln

Erikson EH (1973) Identität und lebenszyklus. Suhrkamp, Frankfurt

Erb L, Thiel-Bonney C, Cierpka M (2014) Zum Zusammenhang von Frühgeburtlichkeit und frühkindlichen Fütterstörungen. Ärztliche Psychotherapie 2014(9):19–25

Filipp SH, Aymanns P (2010) Kritische Lebensereignisse und Lebenskrisen: vom Umgang mit den Schattenseiten des Lebens. Kohlhammer, Stuttgart

Havighurst RJ (1948) Developmental tasks and education. David McKay, New York

Largo RH (2010) Babyjahre. Piper, München

Largo RH, Benz-Castellano C (2008) Critical moments in childhood development: the Zurich fit model. In: Papoušek M, Schieche M, Wurmser H (eds) Disorders of behavioral and emotional regulation in the first years of life: Early risks and intervention in the developing parent–infant relationship. Zero to Three, Washington, DC, pp. 1–11 (original work published in 2004)

Laucht M, Schmidt MH, Esser G (2008) Problems of behavioral and emotional regulation: Precursors to psychiatric disorders in later childhood? In: Papoušek M, Schieche M, Wurmser H (eds) Disorders of behavioral and emotional regulation in the first years of life: Early risks and intervention in the developing parent–infant relationship. Zero to Three, Washington, DC, pp. 299–315 (original work published in 2004)

Papoušek M (2008) Disorders of behavioral and emotional regulation: clinical evidence for a new diagnostic concept. In: Papoušek M, Schieche M, Wurmser H (eds) Disorders of behavioral and emotional regulation in the first years of life: Early risks and intervention in the developing parent–infant relationship. Zero to Three, Washington, DC, pp. 53–84 (original work published in 2004)

Posner MI, Rothbart MK (2000) Developing mechanisms of self-regulation. Dev Psychopathol 12:427–441

Sidor A, Fischer C, Cierpka M (2013) Early regulatory problems in infancy and psychopathological symptoms at 24 months: a longitudinal study in a high-risk sample. J Child Adolesc Behav 1:116

Thiel-Bonney C (2006) Deskriptive Daten aus dem Elternfragebogen der interdisziplinären Spezialambulanz für Eltern mit Säuglingen und Kleinkindern. Institut für Psychosomatische Kooperationsforschung und Familientherapie, Universitätsklinikum Heidelberg. Unveröffentlicht

Thiel-Bonney, C, Erb L (2011) Deskriptive Daten aus den Elternfragebogen der Interdisziplinären Sprechstunde für Eltern, Säuglinge und Kleinkinder. Unveröffentlichtes Manuskript. Heidelberg, Institut für Psychosomatische Kooperationsforschung und Familientherapie

Approaches to Diagnosing Regulatory Disorders in Infants

2

Sarah Groß

One of the fundamental problems of diagnosing psychopathology in infancy is summed up in a quote by Stern: "The new, as yet unknown patient is not a person so much as an—albeit asymmetrical—relationship" (Stern 1998, p. 11). Gergely and Watson (1996) also question whether an intrinsic disorder in infancy or young childhood can in fact exist independent of a dysfunctional parent–infant relationship, given the strong dependence of the infant's emotional development on its physical and psychological environment. Focusing on the infant's syndrome goes against the grain of the facts and clinical findings of developmental psychology (Emde 2003), since the infant's psychosomatically organized affect regulation system is inseparable from the co-regulatory function of the primary caregiver. Doing nothing more than coding behavior runs the risk of overly relegating parental psychological strain, as well the information garnered through investigator empathy, to the sidelines.

2.1 Diagnosing Subjective Aspects

The subjective psychological strain on parents is of practical significance insofar as, while a family with good psychosocial resources can cope well with moderate crying, a vulnerable family may require urgent intervention to resolve the problem, which, in the worst case, can lead to abuse.

> When a disorder is found to not be in the child alone, the primary caregiver, usually the mother, quickly develops a sense of guilt that she has done something wrong.

S. Groß, Dipl.Psych. (✉)
Psychosoziale Beratungsstelle, Studentenwerk Heidelberg, University of Heidelberg, Gartenstr. 2, Heidelberg 69115, Germany
e-mail: sarah_gross@gmx.de

M. Cierpka (ed.), *Regulatory Disorders in Infants*,
DOI 10.1007/978-3-319-43556-5_2

Communication requiring particular attention during interviews with parents: Parents can be relieved of the sole responsibility for the emergence of a regulatory disorder, since an infant brings its own temperament traits into the equation; thus, the parent's behavior may have been wholly unproblematic with another child. Due to absent or negative feedback from the infant, interaction often becomes increasingly dysfunctional as parents become increasingly insecure (a "vicious circle" according to Papoušek et al. 2010). In this context, skill appreciation is important as early on as in the diagnostic phase, in order that the diagnostic assessment remains resource-oriented and endows the parents with greater trust in their intuitive skills, despite the required search for symptoms and possible causes.

2.2 Diagnostic Interviews

Also in parent–infant counseling or psychotherapy, the initial interview is of central importance. Where possible, it is conducted with both parents in the presence of the infant. Sufficient time in a child-friendly room should be planned to ask questions about current behavioral problems and their previous history from the perspective of both parents and to experience interaction between family members. Assuming an essentially appreciative and supportive stance takes into account not only the strain on, but also the resources of, an infant and their parents, and serves to build the relationship on which further treatment will be based. Depending on the reason for presentation, a differential, disorder-specific diagnosis is indicated, as discussed in greater detail in later chapters on individual disorders.

Case Study 1 The parents of 25-month-old Katharina presented to the parent–infant/toddler counseling service, reporting loud crying as a symptom. Already in infancy, Katharina had cried excessively; she had now started crying whenever she did not get her own way. The parents had had their daughter examined by a pediatrician and were alarmed that this had resulted in them being sent for "counseling." They had always suspected a physical cause during infancy; however, since this could not be the sole explanation, they feared that their daughter would be given a "psychological diagnosis" or that they as parents had done something wrong.

2.2.1 General Diagnosis

Since somatic (motor and vegetative) functions and reaction patterns in the infant are closely linked with their experience and behavior, a well-coordinated interdisciplinary approach is required. Close collaboration with pediatricians in the identification of organic disease ensures early recognition of somatic disorders. It is important to ascertain and understand current symptoms on the basis of a thorough developmental history-taking. In order to be able to reliably assess abnormal behavior, one effectively needs to be guided by the normal developmental stages and often sudden developmental spurts, as well as their range of variation. It may be necessary to include a variety of other professional groups, such as speech therapists, to evaluate developmental status.

Information, offered either spontaneously or requested in the context of history-taking, is gathered on the following aspects:

- Etiology of the disorder (onset and duration of current symptoms).
- Course of pregnancy and birth.
- Emotional status during pregnancy.
- Developmental stages of the infant.
- Parental attitude toward the infant.
- Current stressors.
- Parental origin and childhood biography.

At the same time, particular attention should be paid to stressful prenatal, perinatal, and postnatal experiences, such as a physically or psychologically difficult pregnancy, serious complications during birth, postpartum disorders in the mother, as well as disease in the child. Previous miscarriages, stillbirths, and prolonged periods of infertility should also be included in the history.

Pitfalls in practice: Even though the cause of the disorder may appear obvious, it is important not to assume one-dimensional cause-and-effect relationships too hastily. It is often the accumulation of several stressors that contributes to the development of a regulatory disorder.

Communication requiring particular attention during interviews with parents: Talking about stressors can bring relief to the parents as early on as in the diagnostic phase and set the initial processing of stressful experiences (e.g., associated with the birth) in motion, processes for which there is little time in the hectic daily routine with an infant or toddler.

Case Study 1 Continued Katharina's mother cried a lot as she spoke of the stressful early days when she felt rejected by her daughter; Katharina had cried constantly when put to the breast and had only stopped when the mother finally gave up her attempts at breastfeeding. During this part of the interview, the father and Katharina were busy playing, and the family's sense of relief at feeling accepted with their difficulties was tangible.

2.2.2 Psychodynamic Diagnosis

The family's openness to transference, which influences relationships within the family, as well as within the family-and-therapist system in the here and now, can also be diagnostically helpful. The interactional intensity of the family also evokes countertransferences in the therapists. The transference–countertransference process in the initial interview primarily helps in understanding the unconscious scene of the parents with their child and in formulating a psychodynamic focus.

When using transference–countertransference dynamics for diagnostic purposes, a distinction can be made between past unconscious and present unconscious (Reich and Cierpka 2005). The past remains active and influences current relational wishes and conflicts without those affected being aware of this association. Impulses originating from the past unconscious (wishes, fears, memories) are distressing and therefore result in two groups of adjustment processes: since the past needs to be reconciled with the present, it is modified to that effect. If this is not achieved, or not fully achieved, a second adjustment takes place, with the result that the actualized impulse also becomes either distorted or completely suppressed by the individual's defense mechanism, e.g., a reversal to the opposite. This second round of censorship creates the present unconscious, since the present wishes that originated in the past are no longer consciously accessible. The present unconscious serves to maintain current inner equilibrium. To this end, psychosocial compromises are made, which become apparent in interpersonal defense processes, a couple's collusive patterns, and in parent–child interaction.

Case Study 1 Continued At the start of the initial interview, the therapists had the impression that the mother, who was clearly eager to find help, saw them as the rescuers she has longed for, while the father expressed himself in more apologetic terms and apparently feared an apportioning of blame (transference). Over the course of the interview, the therapists noticed that, in the context of parent–child interaction, the mother was quick to react by setting verbal boundaries before fully understanding what it actually was that Katharina wanted. The therapists were aware that they assumed a negative stance towards the mother during this phase (countertransference).

Psychodynamic diagnosis focuses in particular on the entanglement of parental interaction and parental fantasies about their child. The parents' primary relational experiences often play a role in the unconscious attribution of significance through parental projections; these experiences are then reenacted with the child.

The ability of parents to respond appropriately hinges on their ability to attribute sense and meaning to their child's signals. This process of mentalization is closely linked with the capacity to reflect and differentiate their own internal states and those of others. A distorted attribution of meaning suggests (suppressed) inner notions and conflicts and opens the way to as yet unprocessed biographical experiences ("ghosts in the nursery"; Fraiberg et al. 1975). A diagnosis is made of the situations in which—and to what extent—the parents are able to cope with feelings of stress, e.g., when their infant cries excessively, without having to react immediately. This ability of the parents was described by Bion (1962), among others, as "containment."

Case Study 1 Continued When Katharina turned once again to her mother with demands during the course of the interview, Katharina's mother was asked by the therapists to pause before reacting. She should not feel that she had to respond immediately, and Katharina should be distracted for long enough by her father to give her time for her mentalization processes, time which was lacking in real interaction due to the mother's prompt boundary-setting. When asked about her feelings, the mother was able to express the considerable distress she felt in such situations. In the search for causes of her great fear of being completely dominated by the demands of her 2-year-old daughter, biographical links to her relationship with her own parents became obvious: her parents had lived in a state of such perpetual conflict that a hostile atmosphere had prevailed as far back as Katharina's mother could remember and her parents had always made heavy emotional demands on their daughter; now she had become a mother herself and felt obliged to "take care of" family members in both generational directions.

Communication requiring particular attention during interviews with parents: Parents need to interpret their infant's signals and, the younger the infant, the more unclear these are. Therefore, it is inevitable that these interpretations will be influenced by the parents' own relational experiences and their psychodynamic processing. When parents admit this to themselves free of guilt, the conscious perception of distorted interpretations based on the parents' own issues becomes far more feasible.

Psychodynamic hypotheses are often derived from the counseling setting with the family; parents sometimes report their own experiences directly. When asking parents about their own experiences, a cautious approach should be adopted, since parents always want to do as good a job, if not better, than their parents and fear passing on negative experiences from the outset, like a family curse.

2.2.3 Interactional and Relational Diagnosis

Diagnosing Intuitive Parenting Skills How good are the parents' intuitive parenting skills?

Parents seem to understand their infant in a very particular way (intuitive parenthood, primary motherliness). They think about their child (reverie), empathize with them, and are particularly attentive to their infant's signals (e.g., hunger, fatigue). How geared up are the parents for communication with their infant?

Behavioral observations and video-supported micro-analysis of preverbal communication between parents and infants have revealed a behavioral willingness on the part of parents to instinctively provide their infant with specially tailored support in its early maturation, adaptation, and learning processes (see Chap. 1). The concept of intuitive parenting skills refers to the adaptive behavioral adjustments that parents and other caregivers typically make intuitively and without conscious control or intention when they communicate with their infant at the preverbal age. As such, they:

- Are based on innate biological predispositions.
- Are universal and largely independent of age, gender, biological parenthood, and culture.

- Serve the phylogenetically older bonding system by providing the infant with protection and a sense of security and promoting the development of a secure bond.
- Are also intended to complement and compensate for the abilities and limitations of early childhood perception, assimilation of experiences, and behavioral regulation, and are tailored according to age and situation.
- Thus serve species-specific forms of human biological adaptation, i.e., the specific ability of man to integrate, symbolically represent, and exchange experiences and pass these on from generation to generation via communication and language.
- Promote the early development of these species-specific abilities in preverbal communication with infants.

How does one recognize good parenting skills?

In the case of strongly manifest intuitive skills, parents wishing to interact with their baby position their face at a distance of at least 20 cm central to their infant's field of vision and, when the infant's gaze turns and fixes them, they respond with an animated eyebrow flash.

They react instinctively, promptly (with latencies in the millisecond range), and contingent on their infant's gaze allocation, facial expression, and sounds.

They speak to their infant in "baby talk" (higher-pitched voice, slower tempo, pronounced/exaggerated melodics). They affirm their infant's facial expressions and sounds, mimic them, and provide models for their infant to mimic in return (as a "biological mirror" or "biological feedback"). They reduce their tempo, repeat themselves, and pause to give their infant the opportunity to respond.

Guided by their infant's signals, parents provide their baby with regulatory support that is tailored to his or her individual competencies by:

- Stimulating, soothing, and consoling their baby.
- Dosing the type and intensity of stimulation to their infant's receptiveness and tolerance limits.
- Providing emotional reassurance, safety, and a secure basis in stressful situations.
- Compensating for what the infant cannot yet accomplish alone, and providing them with a framework within everyday interaction and dialogue in which they can test and practice their maturing skills in self-efficacy and self-regulation.

Case Study 2 A 6-week-old infant, crying due to overfatigue, was initially being rocked on its mother's lap. The mother appeared to be under considerable strain. The infant could not be soothed. After the subject of rocking was raised with the mother, she became pensive and calmer and modified her behavior. Her voice softened and her movements slowed. The infant relaxed, nestled itself to its mother, and fell asleep. The mother also visibly recovered from the strain her infant's crying had been putting on her. She was happy and clearly experienced the sense that her baby felt safe with her. This feedback boosted her confidence in her intuitive skills.

A distinction needs to be made in interactional and communication dynamics between manifest behavior and latent, unconscious background dispositions. If the latent background is filled with tension and conflict, the parents will not have the appropriate resources at their disposal to soothe their infant, or to stimulate it in a manner conducive to development.

Communication requiring attention during interviews with parents: With regard to parents, attention should be paid to their intuitive communicative competence and emotional relatedness, as well as to potentially distorted perceptions in dealing with their infant. If marked impairment is observed here, parents should be asked in particular detail about experiences of separation and loss in their previous history (e.g., miscarriage), motherhood constellation themes (e.g., fear of failure; Stern 1998), and psychological symptoms (e.g., postnatal depression).

Important diagnostic considerations in the infant: These include infant arousability, self-soothing and communication behaviors, response to new phenomena, showing initiative and exploratory behavior, distractibility, and emotional state. The diagnostic session should offer ample time to not only gather information, but also to observe parent–infant interaction during the short pauses automatically occasioned by the infant's needs.

> The therapist should not put themselves under pressure to gather as much information as possible, but should instead allow periods during the diagnostic phase to "endure" the infant's negative states, such as crying or need for attention, and use these periods for observation. When the diagnostician interacts with the infant themselves, they should take care that the parents do not experience a sense of inferiority should the infant respond positively to the investigator, while they themselves receive only scant positive feedback in deadlocked interaction situations that have the nature of a vicious circle.

2.2.4 Diagnosing Couple and Family Dynamics

The initial interview usually involves at least one parent and the affected infant, but can often involve an entire family system. Numerous interactions between parents, as well as grandparents and siblings that may also be present, can be observed in the sense of a scenic understanding of important indicators of family dynamics. The development in quality of parenting, i.e., coping with the transition from couple to family, should be included in the diagnostic process while taking parental biography and associated unconscious conflicts into consideration. Attention should also be paid to the family's cultural and social background (Cierpka 2005).

> **Case Study 1 Continued**
> The father attempted to prevent Katharina's cries of protest at his wife's boundary-setting by explaining the restrictions in long sentences. Katharina already started crying after the first sentence, which prompted the father to make his explanations even longer and more forceful.

2.3 Diagnostic Systems

In the course of the diagnostic process, one gathers copious information that influences the therapeutic approach. In order to structure this information, diagnostic systems much like those used in other age groups have been developed.

The diagnostic systems for infant developmental stage, infant–parent interaction, and family diagnosis are described in Cierpka (2012). Only classification systems for the standardized description and summarization of the various symptoms of regulatory disorders are presented below.

The fundamental principle of independence from etiological assumptions supported in the ICD-10 (*Deutsches Institut für Medizinische Dokumentation u. Information* 2010) and the DSM-V (American Psychiatric Association 2013) becomes all the more problematic the younger the diagnosed patients are (Wiefel et al. 2007). The exclusion of parental behavior is the main point of criticism leveled at the use of the classical systems and their adaptation for early childhood. Dimensional, relationship-based models reflect the dynamic process of multiple influencing factors in early childhood better than categorical systems. A perspective on the prevention of and early intervention in psychological disorders should be adopted more vigorously at this young age rather than in later childhood and adolescence. Therefore, it is more important to identify factors that expose an infant to increased developmental risk—including the risk of developing psychopathologies—than to detect the presence of intrapsychic disorders, particularly since the classification of categorical diagnoses, most notably in infants under the age of 2 years, is not supported by sufficient empirical evidence (von Gonthard 2010; Schmidt and Poustka 2007).

Classification System Criteria

According to Egger and Emde (2011), classification systems for the first year of life should, at best, fulfill the following criteria stipulating that they ought to:

- Include the full spectrum of early behavioral, emotional, developmental, and relational symptoms, disorders, and impairments.
- Reflect a multidisciplinary, behavior-based orientation aimed at early intervention and prevention.
- Provide links as to how psychopathology and psychiatric impairments are characterized in later life.

Despite all their shortcomings, objective classification instruments are indispensable to early detection, scientifically sound treatment planning, and evaluation, as well as to forming a basis for the submission of claims to health insurance bodies.

2.3.1 ICD-10 and DSM-V

Regulatory disorders in early childhood, with the exception of feeding disorder (F98.2; see also Chap. 5), have not as yet been included in the ICD-10 (International Classification of Diseases 2010) as stand-alone disorders. The developmental dynamics during the first 3 years of life have also not been taken sufficiently into consideration in multiaxial classification schemes (MAS; Remschmidt et al. 2006) for psychological disorders in childhood and adolescence according to ICD-10 (von Gontard 2010). Likewise, "restrictive eating and feeding disorders" were the only regulatory disorders to be included in the *Diagnostic and Statistical Manual of Mental Disorders* (DSM-V, APA) published in 2013 (see Chap. 5).

Due to the lack of alternatives in ICD-10, early childhood regulatory disorders are generally coded as an adjustment disorder (F43.2; von Hofacker et al. 2007), despite the fact that the age criteria for this disorder are inappropriate.

2.3.2 Zero To Three

Zero To Three (DC:0–3R) (2005) was developed for the classification of disorders in infants and young children up to the age of 3 years. In addition to the infant's diagnostic profile, factors that contribute to the occurrence or perpetuation of their problems and areas in which intervention is required are categorized on five axes. Depending on the axis, severity is also dimensionally rated.

Dimensions and Categories of the Zero To Three Classification (2005)

Axis I: Clinical disorders

Categorical assignment to the following diagnoses:

100 Post-traumatic stress disorder
150 Deprivation/maltreatment disorder
200 Disorders of affect: prolonged bereavement, four specific anxiety disorders, depressive disorders, and mixed disorder of emotional expressiveness
300 Adjustment disorder
400 Regulation disorders of sensory processing
Subgroups: hypersensitive type (fearful/cautious type and negative defiant type), hyposensitive/under-responsive type and sensory stimulation seeking/impulsive type
500 Sleep behavior disorder
600 Feeding behavior disorder

(continued)

(continued)

700 Disorders of relating and communicating, including developmental disorders
800 Other disorders according to DSM IV or TR ICD-10

Information-gathering: History-taking interview; questionnaires and behavioral diaries can be used as a complement

Axis II: Relationship classification

Parent–infant relationship global assessment scale (PIR-GAS): Ratings between 0 (abusive) and 100 (well adapted) to achieve a global evaluation of the functionality of the parent–infant relationship on the basis of the following criteria:

- General functional level in the parent/infant
- Distress level in the parent/infant
- Flexibility to adaptation in the parent/infant
- Level of conflict and conflict-solving in the parent/infant
- Effect of relationship quality on the infant's developmental progress

Relationship problems checklist (RPCL) designed to assign the type of relationship problem to the following categories:

- Over-involved or under-involved
- Anxious/tense, angry/hostile
- Verbally abusive
- Physically abusive
- Sexually abusive

Information-gathering: Both are instruments designed to help the diagnostician formulate an external evaluation on the basis of observed behavior between the parent and infant (play interaction and other interaction in the interview setting), as well as on the basis of the parent's subjectively reported experiences.

Axis III: Medical and developmental disorders and conditions

Information-gathering: The diagnosis is established by pediatricians and disease-specific specialist physicians. The following information should be gathered in the history-taking interview: disease type/frequency/duration, age at onset, hospitalizations, and further treatment of current symptoms.

Axis IV: Psychosocial stressors

Psychosocial stressor score, three-tiered scale (no, mild, or severe risk) to evaluate the effect of the risk on the child, again using a three-tiered scale (mild, moderate, or severe effects)

Information-gathering: Both ratings are evaluated by the diagnostician on the basis of information provided on stressors in the history-taking interview.

(continued)

(continued)

Axis V: Emotional and environmental functioning

A six-tiered scale to rate the extent of emotional and social functioning in the following developmental areas:

- Attention/regulation (from 0 to 3 months)
- Relationship formation and mutual engagement (from 3 to 6 months)
- Interactive intentionality and reciprocity (from 4 to 10 months)
- Complex gestures and problem-solving (from 10 to 18 months)

Information-gathering: Ratings are based on the observed behavior between parents and the infant (play interaction and other interaction), as well as the parents' subjective reports on their infant's abilities in relation to the expected stage of development.

With the help of the DC:0-3R Revision Task Force, Zero to Three is once again tackling an update and revision of the DC:0-3R. The DC:0-3R Revision Task Force will consider changes to DC:0-3R, making content-related decisions with input from the clinical and research literature, users worldwide, and feedback from recognized experts in particular areas.

The term "regulation disorder" is more narrowly defined in Zero to Three than in the German-language literature and refers to constitutional difficulties in the appropriate regulation of emotions and behavior in response to sensory stimuli. Excessive crying in the first 3 months of life is not classified as a disorder, but rather as a stress syndrome. One can diagnose this behavior under regulatory disorders of sensory processing, since it is associated with difficulties in the regulation of physiological, sensory, motor, and affective processes. On the other hand, excessive crying cannot be classified as a distinct diagnosis like isolated sleep disorder and isolated feeding disorder, where no disorder of sensory processing is present. Likewise, a sleep disorder can only be diagnosed as a stand-alone disorder from the age of 12 months.

Case Study 1 Continued Using axis 1, Katharina could be diagnosed with a regulatory disorder (negative/defiant type). This implicitly assumed that her crying was associated with a difficulty to remain calm in the presence of multiple or strong environmental stimuli, as well as internal stimuli such as physical arousal or sensations, i.e., she was not able to regulate her arousal level well on her own. Axis II on relationship classification was used to evaluate the aspect of co-regulation or soothing by her parents. According to axis III, closer attention needed to be paid to Katharina's verbal development. Katharina was possibly still finding it difficult to express herself and reacted with frustration when her mother failed to take sufficient time to understand her wishes before forbidding them; moreover, she was unable to understand the long explanations provided by her father.

2.3.3 Guidelines of the German Society for Child and Adolescent Psychiatry and Psychotherapy

Likewise in Germany, a working group set up under the auspices of the German Association of Scientific Medical Societies (*Arbeitsgemeinschaft der Wissenschaftlichen Medizinischen Fachgesellschaft*, AWMF) and the German Society for Child and Adolescent Psychiatry and Psychotherapy (*Deutsche Gesellschaft für Kinder- und Jugendpsychiatrie und Psychotherapie*) has been tasked with drawing up guidelines for the diagnosis of regulatory disorders in infancy and young childhood (Schmidt and Poustka 2007; von Hofacker et al. 2007). These guidelines are based on the principles of evidence-based medicine and provide guidance in the areas of classification, disorder-specific diagnosis, multiaxial assessment, and subsequent intervention. Somatic, behavioral, and relational aspects should be taken into consideration at all levels of the diagnostic processes.

Some regulatory disorders are not interpreted as specific disorders as such, but rather as varying manifestations of an underlying generalized problem of infant behavioral regulation within the context of the parent–infant relationship.

Although based on a dimensional rather than a categorical understanding of disease, the guidelines permit classification according to the main symptoms listed in the box.

Classification Dimensions and Categories of the German Society for Child and Adolescent Psychiatry and Psychotherapy Guidelines (According to von Hofacker et al. 2007)

- **I Regulatory disorders**

Excessive crying up to the age of 6 months: Phases of crying and fussing are defined as excessive primarily on the basis of parental distress and the infant's failure to respond to soothing strategies. The severity of excessive crying is classified according to whether it fulfills, or not, the "rule of threes" (Wessel et al. 1954): crying/fussing lasts on average more than 3 h per day on averagely more than 3 days a weeks for at least 3 weeks.

Sleep disorders: In addition to the parent's subjective perception of the sleep disturbance as a problem, the following objective criteria are applied—Sleep-onset disorder: falling asleep only with parental help past the age of 6 months, sleep-onset time averagely in excess of 30 min. Sleep maintenance disorder: waking more than three times a night on average at least four times a week, combined with the inability to fall asleep again without parental help, and/or nighttime waking periods lasting more than 20 min on average.

(continued)

(continued)

Feeding disorders with/without failure to thrive: Feeding interaction perceived by the parents as problematic over an extended period of time (>1 month). Criteria beyond the age of 3 months include: average duration of individual feeding sessions >45 min and/or intervals of <2 h between meals.

Disinterest in play, chronic fussiness.

Persistent and excessive shyness, excessive clinginess, pronounced anxiety, possibly also a tendency toward social withdrawal in the developmental course, elective mutism.

Excessive defiance.

Aggressive/oppositional behavior.

Anhedonia (joylessness) and lack of interest, distress, depressed mood, passivity, and apathy.

- **II Impaired parent–infant relationship**: A distinction is made between an uncomplicated regulatory disorder in the absence of a relational disorder, an isolated regulatory disorder accompanied by a relational disorder, and a generalized regulatory disorder accompanied by a relational disorder.

III Comorbid disorders accompanying a regulatory disorder: Comorbid disorders may include organic disease, suspected attachment disorder, or post-traumatic stress disorder in infancy and early childhood.

In order for a diagnosis to be established, infant behavioral regulation needs to have been impaired in one or more areas for at least 1 month in a way that is grossly inappropriate in terms of the current developmental phase. Several diagnoses may be established. The guidelines have recently been revised and published in a significantly more detailed form.

Case Study 1 Continued In the further course, Katharina's excessive crying was followed by excessive defiance. As a result of these persisting difficulties, dysfunctional interaction patterns (the mother's hasty setting of boundaries, the father's overly long verbal explanations) had crept in and, in the long run, were straining the relationships between father, mother, and infant. Alone the diagnostic process was able to bring relief to the parents, since they were able to express in words what they had been feeling anyway and were better able understand their own feelings of unease, as well as those of Katharina, due to the greater "insight" they gained into themselves.

The severity of a regulatory disorder is measured according to its duration (persistence), the number of areas of dysregulated interaction (pervasiveness), the extent to which the child and parent are impaired in their accomplishment of infant developmental tasks, as well as the degree of strain on the parent–child relationship.

2.4 Behavior Diaries

There are many different types of behavior diaries to record an infant or young child's varying states. Chapter 4, "Sleep Disorders," provides an example of a crying/sleeping/feeding diary to illustrate the diagnosis of sleep disorders. The diary is given in table format: the lines are intended for infant behavior, while the columns break the day down into 24 h and then again into 15-min intervals. Over a period of several days, the parents record the duration of breastfeeding/feeding, agitation/fussing, crying, and sleep by marking the box for the relevant 15-min interval. There are several questions to answer at the bottom of the table relating to, e.g., how long the infant needed to fall asleep and how often it woke up during the night.

Case Study 1 Continued Prior to the initial interview, Katharina's parents had recorded her behavior over a 4-day period in a diary they had been sent for this purpose. As they were filling in the diary, they themselves noticed that crying phases were more frequent directly after picking Katharina up from the day care center in the early afternoon and again around dinner time. The personnel at the day care center had marked numerous crying phases particularly when Katharina had had only a short midday nap due to being easily woken by the noises of the other children in the sleeping area. These diagnostic findings suggested the need to adjust Katharina's daily structure to her needs, such as quiet periods of undivided attention from a parent during the critical phases of her day, or a somewhat earlier bedtime.

2.5 Questionnaires and Interviews to Gather Data on Behavioral Abnormalities and Regulatory Disorders

As part of a multimodal approach, parent questionnaires are intended as another way to gather data on regulatory skills in early childhood, or as a screening instrument to diagnose an impairment to these skills.

The **Child Behavior Checklist CBCL** 1.5–5 (Achenbach and Rescorla 2000b), a questionnaire intended for use with children aged 1.5–5 years, measures emotional difficulties as well as internalizing and externalizing behavioral problems with the aid of 99 items (Achenbach and Rescorla 2000a). By using a cutoff value for the overall problem score, the questionnaire is able to screen for clinical abnormality in a child. The German-language version of the forerunner to this, the CBCL 2–3 (Achenbach et al. 1987) for children aged 2–3 years, tests the factor structure of the factor analytically derived syndrome scales for behavioral dimensions (Fegert 1996). The **Questionnaire to measure early childhood temperament traits as judged by the parents** (Pauli-Pott et al. 2003)—a translation of the English-language Infant Behavior Questionnaire IBQ (Rothbart 1981)—is often used to measure temperament as an aspect of early childhood regulatory disorders. The parent that spends more time with the child (usually the mother) answers questions on the following areas of temperament:

- Positive emotionality
- Inclination toward introversion and anxiety
- Inclination toward temper tantrums
- Irritability
- Motor activity
- Soothability

The German-language crying, feeding, sleep questionnaire (Groß et al. 2013) covers 53 items altogether: three to gather data on the "rule of threes" (Wessel et al. 1954), 24 on crying, fussing, and sleeping, 13 on feeding, 12 items relating to co-regulation, i.e., soothing strategies used by parents when their infant cries, when it should sleep, and when it wakes up at night, as well as whether medical advice relating to the infant has already been sought. The questionnaire also includes questions on the triad (von Hofacker et al. 2007; Papoušek 2010) of: (1) problems of behavioral regulation in early childhood (e.g., duration of crying, time to sleep onset), (2) dysfunctional communication patterns in contexts relevant to the behavioral problems (soothing strategies, bedtime rituals), and (3) stress syndrome in the primary caregiver (interpretations and explanatory approaches for the child's problematic behavior by the parents, strain due to the child's problematic behavior). The three scales were developed in a factor-analytic manner and yielded high internal consistency. Using these scales, it is possible to calculate an overall score enabling a general evaluation of self-regulatory skills. Evaluation results from 704 infants aged up to 1 year indicate that this diagnostic approach has good validity (Groß et al. 2013).

Conclusion

The present chapter deals with a number of perspectives that approach the diagnosis of regulatory disorders from different angles, including: diagnosis of the infant; the intuitive skills of the parents; interaction; transference and countertransference; factors in the parental biographies; as well as family diagnosis.

The use of standardized diagnostic instruments in the area of regulatory disorders is not yet well established. The guidelines and classification systems are also undergoing constant further development in interaction with their English-language counterparts. Future developments need to be not only individual-centered (infant or primary caregiver) but also interaction-centered (parent–infant relationship).

References

Achenbach TM, Edelbrock CS, Howell DT (1987) Empirically based assessment of the behavioral/emotional problems of 2- and 3-year-old children. J Abnorm Child Psychol 15:629–650

Achenbach TM, Rescorla LA (2000a) CBCL/1,5–5 & C-TRF/1,5-5 profiles. University of Vermont, Research Center for Children, Youth & Families, Burlington, VT

Achenbach TM, Rescorla LA (2000b) Manual for the ASEBA preschool forms and profiles: an integrated system of multi-informant assessment. Department of Psychiatry, University of Vermont, Burlington, VT

American Psychiatric Association (2013) Diagnostic and statistical manual of mental disorders (DSM-V). Arlington, VA

Bion WR (1962/1984) A theory of thinking. Second thoughts: selected papers on psychoanalysis. Karnac, London

Cierpka M (2005) The three-level model of family assessment. In: Cierpka M, Thomas V, Sprenkle D (eds) Family assessment—multiple perspectives. Hogrefe, Seattle, pp 2–15

Cierpka M (ed) (2012) Frühe Kindheit 0–3 Jahre. Beratung und Psychotherapie für Eltern mit Säuglingen und Kleinkindern. Springer, Heidelberg

Deutsches Institut für Medizinische Dokumentation und Information (DIMDI) (2010) International Classification of Diseases ICD-10-GM 2010. http://www.dimdi.de/static/de/klassi/diagnosen/icd10/ls-icdhtml.htm [Accessed 12.01.2010]

Egger HL, Emde RN (2011) Developmentally-sensitive diagnostic criteria for mental health disorders in early childhood: the Diagnostic and Statistical Manual of Mental Disorders IV, the Research Diagnostic Criteria—Preschool Age, and the Diagnostic Classification of Mental Health and Developmental Disorders of Infancy and Early Childhood—Revised. American Psychologist 66(2):95–106

Emde RN (2003) RDC-PA: a major step forward and some issues. Journal of American Academic Child and Adolescent Psychiatry 42:1513–1516

Fegert JM (1996) Verhaltensdimensionen und Verhaltensprobleme bei zweieinhalbjährigen Kindern. Praxis der Kinderpsychologie und Kinderpsychiatrie 45:83–94

Fraiberg S, Adelson E, Shapiro V (1975) Ghosts in the nursery. A psychoanalytic approach to the problems of impaired infant-mother relationships. J Am Acad Child Psychiatry 14(3):387–421

Gergely G, Watson, JS (1996) The social biofeedback theory of parental affect-mirroring: the development of emotional self-awareness and selfcontrol in infancy. International Journal of Psycho-Analysis 77:1181–1212

Gontard A von (2010) Säuglings- und Kleinkindpsychiatrie. Ein Lehrbuch. Kohlhammer, Stuttgart

Groß S, Reck C, Thiel-Bonney C, Cierpka M (2013) Empirische Grundlagen des Fragebogens zum Schreien, Füttern und Schlafen (SFS). Prax Kinderpsychol Kinderpsychiatr 62:327–347

von Hofacker N, Lehmkuhl U, Resch F et al. (2007) Regulationsstörungen im Säuglings- und Kleinkindalter. In: Deutsche Gesellschaft für Kinder- und Jugendpsychiatrie und -psychotherapie (Hrsg) Leitlinien zur Diagnostik und Therapie von psychischen Störungen im Säuglings-, Kindes- und Jugendalter. AWMF Online: http://www.awmf.org/leitlinien/detail/ll/028-041.html<https://mail.med.uni-heidelberg.de/leitlinien/detail/ll/,DanaInfo=www.awmf.org+028-041.html

Papoušek M, Schieche M, Wurmser H (2010) Regulationsstörungen der frühen Kindheit. Frühe Risiken und Hilfen im Entwicklungskontext der Eltern-Kind-Beziehungen. Verlag Hans Huber, Bern

Reich G, Cierpka M (2005) Psychodynamic assessment. In: Cierpka M, Thomas V, Sprenkle D (eds) Family assessment—multiple perspectives. Hogrefe, Seattle, pp 231–256

Remschmidt H, Schmidt MH, Poustka F (2006) Multiaxiales Klassifikationsschema für psychische Störungen des Kindes- und Jugendalters nach ICD-10 der WHO. Mit einem synoptischen Vergleich von ICD-10 und DSM-IV. Hans Huber, Bern

Rothbart MK (1981) Measurement of temperament in infancy. Child Development 52(2):569–578

Pauli-Pott U, Mertesacker B, Beckmann D (2003) Ein Fragebogen zur Erfassung des "frühkindlichen Temperaments" im Elternurteil. Z Kinder Jugendpsychiatr Psychother 31(2):99–110

Schmidt MH, Poustka F (2007) Leitlinien zur Diagnostik und Therapie von psychischen Störungen im Säuglings-, Kindes- und Jugendalter. Deutscher Ärzte Verlag, Köln

Stern DN (1998) Die Mutterschaftskonstellation: Eine vergleichende Darstellung verschiedener Formen der Mutter-Kind-Psychotherapie. Klett-Cotta, Stuttgart

Wessel MA, Cobb JC, Jackson EB, Harris GS, Detwiler AC (1954) Paroxysmal fussing in infancy, sometimes called "colic". Pediatrics 14:421–435

Wiefel A, Titze K, Kuntze L, Winter M, Seither C, Witte B et al (2007) Diagnostik und Klassifikation von Verhaltensauffälligkeiten bei Säuglingen und Kleinkindern von 0–5 Jahren. Prax Kinderpsychol Kinderpsychiatr 56:59–81

Zero To Three (2005) Diagnostic classification: 0–3. Zero To Three: National Center for Infants, Toddlers, and Families, Washington, DC

Excessive Crying in Infancy

3

Consolata Thiel-Bonney and Manfred Cierpka

3.1 Case Study

Mrs. A, together with her daughter, attended an initial interview and reported the following problems to the therapist:

Mother (M): Should I just tell you about the problems?
Therapist (T): Yes, please.
M: She's 6-weeks-old now; everything was fine at first, then after a few days she started crying a lot. When we put her down, she stays calm for a few minutes on her own, then starts crying, so I pick her up. Now I seem to be carrying her around the whole day, either in my arms or in her baby sling. She's quiet and sleeps in the baby sling. Apart from that, she doesn't sleep during the day at all. She can't fall asleep spontaneously, apart from in the baby sling. Thank God the nights are okay.

I often have the feeling that she's completely exhausted and is crying from tiredness, but she just can't manage to fall asleep on her own. In the evenings, she cries for an hour, then often stops crying at 20:45 on the dot and then we can leave her on her own in her bed. Sometimes she starts moaning a bit after a couple of minutes, but then she falls asleep and stays asleep until she wakes up hungry. She's alone in her bed or in our bed. If she's in her bed, I take her in bed with me, since I find it easier to breastfeed in bed and she falls asleep again more easily than if I put her back in her bed. What also strikes me is the fact that she cries

C. Thiel-Bonney, M.D. (✉)
Center for Children, Adolescents and Families, Hospital Hochried, Hochried 1-12, Murnau 82418, Germany
e-mail: cthiel-bonney@gmx.de

M. Cierpka, M.D.
Institute for Psychosocial Prevention, University Hospital Heidelberg, Bergheimer Str. 54, Heidelberg 69115, Germany

M. Cierpka (ed.), *Regulatory Disorders in Infants*,
DOI 10.1007/978-3-319-43556-5_3

extremely loudly. As soon as she starts crying, she really screams; I mean, she doesn't just whine a bit, she really screams. My husband and I try to accept this as it is. It's very important for us that there is no aggression or anything, although it's already there. And I try to tell myself that that's just how my baby is, and when I see other babies that are much, much quieter, I sometimes wish she were more like them, but then I tell myself: that's just how my baby is.

T: Have you noticed that you're rocking your baby at the moment?

M: Yes.

T: Why are you rocking your baby?

M: Because I have the feeling it soothes her.

T: Because you have the feeling it soothes her… does your experience tell you that?

M: Yes, in my experience, she calms down more when I stand up and walk around than when I stay seated with her.

T: Do you think she's agitated? Even at the moment?

M: Yes.

T: Do you consider that agitated, to the point that you need to rock her to calm her down?

M: Well, I'm expecting her to start crying any minute and this is the first sign of that for me.

T: So those are the first signs for you: when she fusses like that, or what's your word for how she is right now?

M: Actually, my word is agitated and fidgety, you know, fidgeting. I find this quite fidgety.

T: Right now as well?

M: Not really; it's usually worse. The fidgeting's okay at the moment. I'd say she was sort of moaning as well, a minute or so ago.

T: So rocking back then would have been preventive.

M: Yes.

T: Is it possible that you do that regularly?

M: Preventively?

T: Now already, because you think it's going to start again.

M: Yes. I noticed it the night before last; she was quite agitated and I got extremely agitated and I noticed it myself, so I wondered to myself: she isn't actually crying yet, but I react already, even though she's just fidgeting about. I'm just not very good at coping when I think she's not okay.

T: It has to do with the fact that you try to prevent it, so that it doesn't get to the point where she's not okay.

M: Yes.

T: But that must be quite a strain on you?

M: Yes.

T: Do you find it tiring?

M: Yes, very tiring. I sort of imagined a calm, relaxed, happy, and balanced baby. That's what I would like. But that's certainly not how things are at the moment—not how I'd like them to be. I also think I project myself onto her quite a lot. I'm often tense; yesterday I even told my husband that I'm never relaxed. He's always telling me that I should be more relaxed about things or take things easier, but I'm always thinking about what's right and what's wrong. And when I do something, is it too much or is it too little?

T: Meaning that you're always agitated. Always thinking, always doing.

M: Yes.

T: But why? What's driving you to do that?

M: It's because I always want to do the right thing for others; I always want to do the right thing for my husband. And we're staying at my parents at the moment, because it's so hot in our apartment, and I have the feeling that I have to help my mother as well. If I concentrate only on my baby, my mother will get the short end of the stick.

3.2 Definition and Symptom Triad of Excessive Crying

3.2.1 Disorder of Behavioral Regulation in Infancy

The crying of an infant is an elemental signal to its environment and is highly motivational in nature: it expresses, in an as yet untargeted manner, a state of physiological arousal (Papoušek 2009) and indicates the infant's state and its needs. Parents generally respond promptly and with intuitive paternal sensitivity by offering the support appropriate to their infant's alarm signal. In this way, the baby and its parents experience themselves in a context of positive mutual efficacy: the infant is soothed and its needs are met, while the parents experience a sense of competence in caring for their infant.

The tendency to fussiness often encountered in the first 3 months of life points to age-specific adjustment and maturational processes. In a cyclical alternation, an infant learns to organize sleep and waking states, as well as hunger and satiety, etc. Infants that are particularly wakeful, hyperresponsive, and eager for stimulation require a considerable amount of regulatory support from their parents for this task.

However, every 5th infant (Wurmser et al. 2001; Wurmser 2009) cries or fusses "excessively" for no apparent reason and to an extent that exceeds the normal level, beginning around the second week of life, peaking in the sixth week of life, and then abating toward the end of the third month, i.e., for more than 3 h per day at least 3 days per week over a period of more than 3 weeks ["rule of threes" according to Wessel et al. (1954)]. There is considerable variation in terms of the intensity and duration of crying and fussing phases in the first months of life. Episodes of inconsolable crying are more problematic than the duration of crying and fussing. Due to the paroxysmal nature of infant crying, involving reddened face, shrill hyperphonic crying, abdominal distension, and muscle hypertonia, infant gastrointestinal symptoms (abdominal pain and cramping, so-called 3-month colic) were initially assumed to be the cause (see also Sect. 3.5.1). The crying has no apparent cause and generally tends to occur in the late afternoon and early evening. What is striking in the infant is its cumulative hyperarousal/overfatigue, having had only short sleep phases during the day (usually between 10 and 30 min), marked difficulties falling asleep, and a diminished total sleep time in the sleep diary (von Hofacker et al. 2007; White et al. 2000; Ziegler et al. 2004). In cases where the infant is inconsolable and unable to self-soothe (Barr 1998), normal soothing strategies on the part of the parents are ineffective; it becomes barely possible to console the infant, particularly in the late afternoon and the child finally falls asleep for the night late in the evening.

During wake phases, infants often appear to be hyperexcitable, more irritable, more susceptible to sensory stimulation, subject to motor restlessness, and are only seldom in a behavioral state of calm attentiveness. Parents describe their baby as highly alert and attentive as in the first weeks of life. Infants exhibit a strong urge to be in a vertical position and appear to literally seek visual and acoustic environmental stimuli. The infant's hyperreactivity to environmental stimuli renders it barely able to "switch off," soothe itself and, in the absence of considerable support from their parents, fall asleep.

3.2.2 Dysfunctional Interaction

The introductory case study illustrates how the parents attempt, in an escalating vicious circle of dysfunctional interaction, to soothe their infant or help it fall asleep. Under conditions of increased stimulation (being carried around for hours on end, vigorous vestibular stimulation, frequent changes in attempts to soothe and distract the infant, the use of "white noise" on car drives or from a vacuum cleaner, etc.), the infant is calmed, yet only in the short term, and fails to achieve a sufficiently long or restorative quiet phase. Tensions and agitation on the part of both the infant and the parents become mutually exacerbating. With the pervasive onset of further disorders in infant behavioral regulation (e.g., in breastfeeding/feeding) and persistent symptoms in the infant, dysregulated infant behavioral states prevail; interaction and relationships decompensate in a predominantly negative reciprocity, which can lead to endangering the infant's welfare.

The risk of abuse is high in excessive crying: in a broad study conducted in The Netherlands ($N=3259$), 5.6 % of the parents with infants aged under 6 months questioned in an anonymous questionnaire stated that they had already struck or shaken their infant at least once due to his crying or had attempted to stifle the crying (Reijneveld et al. 2004). The risk was highest among those parents who considered their infant's crying as excessive. Of 27 cases of shaken-baby syndrome in infants aged up to 1 year (with and without lethal outcome), 88.5 % of parents had sought advice from their pediatrician or another specialist due to their infant's excessive crying or irritability prior to the incident (Talvik et al. 2008). Inconsolable crying is considered the most relevant trigger for early abuse (Lee et al. 2007; Barr et al. 2006).

3.2.3 Parental Overload Syndrome

Due to the acute stress reaction it elicits, inconsolable crying inevitably leads to maternal/parental overload syndrome. This is characterized by profound exhaustion in the presence of a persistent sleep deficit and significant insecurity about one's own competence, ranging from self-doubt, feelings of failure, and overload to isolation accompanied by depressive mood or angry conflicts of ambivalence (see also Levitzky and Cooper 2000). Parents feel rejected by their infant in their efforts and receive no reward despite all their endeavors to soothe the child. They neglect their own needs and relaxed moments or moments of happy playful interaction with their baby are few and far between. Some parents respond increasingly inappropriately or ineffectively to their infant's crying, or with delayed latency, ultimately ignoring their signals. The relationship is under extreme strain.

If parents succeed in activating their own or familial resources, it is possible to compensate for these stressors. However, in cases where there are preexisting stressors in the parental biography (e.g., mental illness, own experiences of separation/loss/violence), cumulative psychosocial stressors and insufficient support within the family (e.g., conflicts in the parental family of origin, massive partnership conflicts), as well as an unviable social network, can derail the system: highly overloaded themselves, the parents have no access to their own intuitive and co-regulatory skills in dealing with their infant.

3.3 Prevalence and Prognosis

Prevalence studies show a significant variation in the frequency of excessive crying from around 5 to 19 % depending on case definition criteria, evaluation tools, and methodology (Lucassen et al. 2001). In the only German epidemiological study to date on the prevalence of excessive crying, Wurmser et al. (2001) found a prevalence of 21 % in their retrospective telephone survey. In 40 % of cases (i.e., in approximately 8 % of the total population), crying persisted after the age of 3 months. Wake and colleagues (2006) found that crying/fussing and sleeping problems persisted in approximately 6 % of infants aged 2–24 months.

It would appear that, in order to assess the developmental prognosis of the infant that cries excessively, it is not the extent of excessive crying or fussing that is of crucial importance, but rather its persistence beyond the age of 3–4 months. In 77 and 55 %, respectively, of infants referred to the Munich Program for Fussy Babies after the age of 6 months with sleeping or feeding disorders, the symptoms existing at the time of presentation had in each case been preceded by excessive crying in infancy (Wurmser and Papoušek 2004; Schieche et al. 2004). Von Kries et al. (2006) investigated persistent significant sleeping and feeding/eating disorders in infants aged between 6 months and 4 years. These symptoms were not more commonly found among those infants that had cried excessively only up to the age of 3 months. However, in infants in whom excessive crying had persisted up to the age of 6 months, symptoms were increased by a factor of 6–9 (see also von Kries 2006).

The persistence and "spread" of infant problems in behavioral regulation to other areas of behavior contribute to an increased risk for emotional problems or behavioral disorders in later life. Psychosocial stressors in the family carry the greatest prognostic significance: the greatest number of mental disorders in children in the Mannheim children-at-risk study was seen in children with earlier regulatory disorders in infancy and that were at the same time heavily burdened with psychosocial risk factors (for a more detailed discussion, see Cierpka 2012, Chap. 13, p. 176 et seq.).

In summary, while transient crying up to the age of 3 months—assuming there are no further disorders of behavioral regulation and that the family has good psychosocial resources—may be stressful for infants and parents, it would appear that, overall, it primarily represents a set of benign symptoms (von Gontard 2010). ***However, persistent problems of crying that pervade other regulatory areas and interactional contexts, combined with existing psychosocial stressors in the family, represent a particular risk in terms of accomplishing the further developmental tasks in infancy.*** Children on the outer end of the crying spectrum with strained parent–infant relationships bear an increased risk of impaired socioemotional development and mental health at school age (see also Brown et al. 2009).

3.4 Development of Behavioral Regulation in the First Months of Life

For the first 3 months of life, an infant is dependent on the intuitive and sensitive parental support of their primary caregiver in all areas of adjustment to their environment and their maturation. Only in this way can the infant accomplish the developmental tasks at hand: the regulation of hunger, food intake, and satiety; the regulation of physiological adjustment (e.g., thermoregulation, energy balance, metabolism, digestion, reaction to visual, acoustic, and sensory stimuli); and the alternation from quiet alert wake phases, emerging fatigue, and sleep. Adjustment to the environment takes place in the interplay between, and balancing of, activating/arousing and inhibitory/soothing processes (Papoušek 2009). The initiatives and skills of the infant and its parents combine in everyday parent–child interactions to promote co-regulation and "affective attunement" (Papousek 1999; Stern 1985) and are determined by an "interpersonal interpretive mechanism" (Fonagy and Target 2002): parents understand the inner state of their infant and adjust their own behavior to the needs of their infant in such a way that it increasingly recognizes and "understands" itself therein in the further developmental course (Fonagy and Target 1997). In this way, the primary caregivers also contribute to "downregulating" a potential state of stress in their infant and promote infant self-regulatory skills; the infant becomes increasingly successful at maintaining a quiet attentive waking state, "switching off" when tired, and falling asleep quietly. Already early on, the infant itself has the ability to display its own inner state and, in primary intersubjectivity, share experiences in interactions with its counterparts; social referencing, sharing, and signaling affects are also observed in triangular interactions (Stern 1985; Fivaz-Depeursinge and Corboz-Warnery 2001; Fivaz-Depeursinge 2009). Successful joint behavioral regulation between mother/father and infant likely forms the basis for an implicit relational knowledge that is stored on a procedural level.

Infants that cry excessively in the first weeks of life often exhibit greater reactivity, irritability, and sensory hyperarousal, leaving them barely able to withdraw from stimulation when tired. They are easily distracted and remain in a quiet alert waking state for only short periods of time; they appear hyperexcitable and quickly overstimulated, are difficult to console, have difficulties settling, show little or no self-soothing behavior (e.g., finger sucking, gaze aversion when stressed), and are unable to achieve restorative and sufficiently long daytime naps. Other infants demonstrate excessive arousal-inhibiting behavior, including gaze avoidance, social inaccessibility, and defensive behaviors (Papoušek 2009), which can impair the structure of interaction between parent and infant, e.g., during attempts to soothe the infant. Thus, greater demands in terms of interaction and co-regulation are placed on the parents of these infants.

With the second spurt of biopsychosocial development, the "social awakening" seen at the age of 3 months, a new and more mature level of behavioral regulation and communication between parents and infant is formed. The crying that was previously of a more nonspecific nature becomes a signal that can also be intentionally targeted in the case of frustration, seeking physical closeness, or when renouncing up habits (Papoušek 2009). Enabled by their greater social, motor, and sensory skills, many infants are now capable of: organizing longer quiet alert wakeful phases involving positive relatedness and an enjoyment of exploration, better integrating environmental stimuli, and "using" their improved communication skills in interaction with and positive relatedness to their parents; the excessive crying of the past ceases. In the case of crying problems that persist beyond the age of 3 months combined with continued parental psychosocial stressors and limited resources and intuitive skills, the infant's symptoms can extend to other areas of parent–child interaction. For example, sleeping problems that manifest in the form of scant daytime sleep, as well as difficulties going (back) to sleep in the evening and at night, now develop. The parents complain of long phases of dysregulation, dysphoric agitation, disinterest in play, and hyperarousal involving crying and fussing in their infant. Parents and their infant fail to achieve a shared rhythm and pleasant dialogue; they enter an escalating cycle of negative reciprocity and strained relationships (Papoušek 2009).

3.5 Factors Affecting the Development of Excessive Crying

3.5.1 Organic Stressors and Risk Factors

Excessive infant crying should always undergo pediatric examination and, where appropriate, also treatment. However, an investigation by Freedman et al. (2009) found that medical causes were responsible for infant crying in only 5 % of cases. Once a thorough history taking and physical examination has been performed, further examinations should be undertaken sparingly, since these contribute to establishing a diagnosis in only 1 % of cases.

Organic factors (see also Sect. 3.7) such as infections, gastrointestinal disorders, atopy, injury, or neuropediatric diseases (Savino 2007; Roberts et al. 2004) can cause crying in infancy; however, these factors are generally embedded in multiple prenatal, perinatal, and antenatal organic and psychosocial stressors (Ziegler et al. 2004).

3.5.1.1 Prenatal and Postnatal Organic Stressors and Risk Factors

Infants whose mother/parents smoked during pregnancy have a twofold higher risk of developing excessive crying (Sondergaard et al. 2001; Reijneveld et al. 2005); infants exhibited significantly greater levels of irritability and muscular hypertension (Stroud et al. 2009). According to Shenassa and Brown (2004), there is evidence to suggest a link between nicotine exposure in infants and increased plasma and intestinal motilin levels, which could increase the risk of crying. A low birth weight of less than 2500 g also increases the risk of excessive crying in infancy by more than twofold (Sondergaard et al. 2000). A clinical sample at the Munich Program for Fussy Babies (Ziegler et al. 2004) revealed prenatal organic risk factors to be present in 73 % of infants. Thus, this particular sample differed significantly from the control group, e.g., in terms of the occurrence of preterm labor treated with tocolytic agents. St. James-Roberts and Conroy (2005) found varying results on prenatal and perinatal factors influencing crying in infancy in two birth cohorts and emphasize the fact that there is as yet insufficient evidence.

In a sample of infants at the parent–infant/toddler outpatient clinic of the Heidelberg University Hospital (see Chap. 1), more than 30 % of infants that attended the clinic had been previously treated on an inpatient basis (Thiel-Bonney 2006). In addition to possible medical risk factors, this finding could also point to a stressful start to life in the family and to early insecurity on the part of the young parents in dealing with their baby.

3.5.2 Sleep–Wake Organization

In their study on sleep–wake organization, Ziegler et al. (2004) showed that the extent of infant crying and fussing is associated with the extent of relative sleep deficit. Infants that cried excessively according to the Wessel rule slept for 90 min less compared with the control group (see also White et al. 2000). They needed approximately 20 min longer to fall asleep, and evening settling-to-sleep phases could be protracted over several hours. Excessively crying infants woke up at night more frequently and remained awake for 1 h on average. In addition, these infants were carried around by their parents for significantly longer. Sleep phases overall, as well as the longest daytime sleep phase, were shorter. In infants that cried persistently beyond the age of 3–4 months, sleeping problems increasingly shifted to the second half of the night, involving crying and regular waking. From own clinical observations, sleep diaries show long daytime waking phases of up to 8 h, punctuated by between one and two naps lasting 15–20 min. With a physiologically increased proportion of rapid eye movement (REM) sleep of approximately 50 % in the first months of life, infants wake in the transition between active and quiet sleep from the indeterminate sleep (T-sleep) characteristic of the first weeks of life approximately 20 min after falling asleep, and do not manage to resume sufficiently long and restful sleep.

In contrast to the abovementioned results (Ziegler et al. 2004; White et al. 2000), a Finnish study (Kirjavainen et al. 2004) found no evidence of reduced total sleep times or an early impairment to sleep structure.

Jenni et al. (2008) and Jenni (2009) provide a physiological explanatory model for circadian and homeostatic sleep–wake regulation and excessive crying in the first 12 weeks of life. The increasing circadian alertness over the course of the day, which peaks at around 6 p.m., is not yet opposed by compensatory and counteractive homeostatic sleep pressure. Only with the slow onset of sleep homeostasis at the age of 2 months do early-evening alertness and excessive crying abate. Jenni postulated that, in infants that cry excessively, the development of sleep homeostasis is delayed and, in addition, misaligned with their diurnal processes. The signs of immaturity in excessively crying infants already mentioned above (von Hofacker et al. 1999), together with impaired sleep homeostasis, could point to delayed maturation of neurotransmitter and synaptic functions. White et al. (2000) suspect delayed maturation in the diurnal rhythm of the hypothalamic–pituitary–adrenal (HPA) axis, involving elevated evening cortisol levels that affect sleep–wake activity and crying behavior. Bensel and Haug-Schnabel (2003) postulate that fussy babies capable of maintaining long wake phases are a group of infants with already advanced maturation of the neocortex. Thus, while "precocious" in sub-areas of their behavior, they are overchallenged by the extended phases of wakefulness and activation; they do not yet have sufficient skills at their disposal to use and regulate these long phases of arousal.

3.5.3 Reduced Capacity to Self-Regulate

Administering a few drops of sugar (sucrose) solution to the tongue in 6-week-old crying infants has a soothing effect on all infants; however, this effect only persists beyond the initial taste stimulus in infants that cry "normally." In the case of excessively crying infants, this soothing effect was only brief and did not outlast the initial reaction to the taste stimulus (Barr et al. 1991). Barr and colleagues (1999) interpreted this as an indication of reduced efficacy in regulatory and relational processes, as well as a delayed or diminished response in the central endorphin-dependent soothing and reward mechanism in excessively crying infants. These study results are consistent with parental observations that their crying-prone infants can be soothed only temporarily by breastfeeding and vestibular and visual stimulation, showing renewed signs of fussing as soon as the stimulus ceases.

Barr (1998) points to a "transient increased responsivity" in the excessively crying infant: its readiness to respond (responsivity) and excitability (reactivity) to an environmental stimulus are heightened, while its capacity for self-regulation is reduced and it requires more time to soothe itself and recover.

From our own observations, the apparently stimulus-seeking behavior in the excessively crying infant could be interpreted as an "attempt at stabilization" on the infant's part. Parent and infant "use" the latter's strong reactivity and responsivity to achieve at least a temporary soothing effect.

3.5.4 Temperament Factors

The impact of temperament factors is the subject of controversy. In the Munich catamnesis study (Wurmser et al. 2004; see also Sect. 3.3), the parents of infants meanwhile aged 30 months received a modified version of the ICQ questionnaire (Bates et al. 1979) aimed at gathering data on the following temperament dimensions: fussiness/difficulty, persistence, ability to adjust, irregular rhythm, and dependence. The formerly excessive crying infants differed significantly from the control group infants only on the "fussiness/difficulty" and "persistence" dimensions. The correlation between values from the first examination at the age of 0–6 months and those from the subsequent data collection showed "insufficient capacity to adjust" and "fussiness/difficulty" to be poorly to moderately stable. Bensel and Haug-Schnabel (2003) postulate an unstable temperament construct beyond time and context. Physiological measurements in fussy and normal infants (heart rate, heart rate variability, vagal tone) made in the context of a number of investigations showed no significant differences in the physical response to stress (e.g., White et al. 2000; Kirjavainen et al. 2001), as well as no differences in temperament in the time following excessive crying. It is possible that temperament factors only take on greater relevance when additional factors, e.g., diminished "fit" between parents and infant, a "mis-fit" between infant and environment (Largo and Benz-Castellano 2004) involving perturbations in parent–child interaction and relationship, or psychosocial stressors impair the infant's ability to self-regulate.

3.5.5 Familial and Psychosocial Stressors

The clinical group of excessively crying infants is highly exposed to prenatal and postnatal psychosocial risk factors. Prenatal stressors in the form of maternal stress of long-standing and abnormal anxiety during pregnancy, depression in mothers and fathers, unresolved partnership conflicts and conflicts with families of origin, a sense of hopelessness, a sense of too many insurmountable external demands, stress at work, and adverse/critical life events were associated with increased crying in infancy (Papousek and von Hofacker 1998; Ziegler et al. 2004; Sondergaard et al. 2003; Wurmser 2007; van der Wal et al. 2007; van den Berg et al. 2009). Prenatal stress can impair the physical and constitutional development of the fetus via stress-induced activation of the autonomous nervous system and the HPA axis (Kinsella and Monk 2009) and reduce the parents' emotional resources/access to their intuitive skills in interaction with their (since born) child. In a clinical population investigated by Ziegler et al. (2004), 64 % of subjects were affected by prenatal psychosocial risks. However, a review of studies aimed at predicting infant crying on the basis of pregnancy and course of delivery (St. James-Roberts and Conroy 2005) yielded inconsistent results.

Postnatal stressors, such as partnership conflicts, conflicts in the families of origin, socioeconomic problems, scant support and social isolation, single-parent status (Ziegler et al. 2004), heightened state of anxiety (particularly in young mothers and mothers with low education levels), as well as previous experiences of birth on the part of the parents subjectively perceived as stressful (overview in Thiel-Bonney and Cierpka 2004) were associated with the risk of increased crying in infancy and/or increased the risk for excessive crying. In a Turkish sample of postpartum depressive symptoms and insecure maternal attachment style, Akman and colleagues (2006) observed a link with excessive crying.

Parents of an excessively crying infant generally have a sense of impaired self-esteem (Stifter and Bono 1998), are more likely to suffer symptoms of depression (Vik et al. 2009; see also Wake et al. 2006), experience anxiety, anger, a sense of rejection, guilt, hopelessness, powerlessness, and rage (Ellett and Swenson 2005). Papousek and von Hofacker (1998) found an increased number of impaired or perturbed mother–infant relationships, as well as a dysregulated pattern of dialogue between mother and child in 40 % of clinical dyads (compared with 19 % in the control group). Interaction between fathers and their infants can also be subject to greater dysfunction (Räihä et al. 2002). In a study conducted in the USA (Levitzky and Cooper 2000), more than 90 % of mothers reported considerable tension in their partnerships and a reduction in their social contacts. All mothers in the 23 mother–child pairs investigated exhibited physical and psychological symptoms in response to their infant's excessive crying; 70 % reported having aggressive thoughts and fantasies in relation to their infant, while 26 % had even thought of infanticide.

Räihä et al. (1995) investigated the family context in excessive crying. They observed significant differences in terms of family structure between families with and without colic-related crying. Families affected by infant crying appeared to be less organized, experienced less closeness, and had a less close-knit family union. The hierarchical organization of the family was "chaotic," with indistinct individual and intergenerational boundaries. Families had difficulties accomplishing daily activities and demonstrated little energy, vitality, or flexibility. The family atmosphere appeared to be less optimistic and the level of family conflict high. At 1 year (Räihä et al. 1996), a high level of unresolved conflicts remained in the families under strain, combined with greater dissatisfaction, less mutual empathy, and more difficulties in family communication. However, the overall mood had improved in all groups investigated. At 3 years (Räihä et al. 1997), significant differences could no longer be seen between families. On the other hand, Rautava et al. (1995) found even greater family dissatisfaction with the distribution of responsibility in daily family life and with the amount of leisure time and joint activities also at 3 years after excessive infant crying. The infants that had previously cried excessively in the "colic families" exhibited more sleeping problems and temper tantrums at the age of 3 years. In a qualitative study, Ellett et al. (2005) explored parental perspectives on the lasting impact of infant crying on infant development and on family relationships. Most parents stated that, following the period of "colicky crying," they had not observed any lasting problems in their infant. However, a number of the parents questioned reported their impression that relationships, communication, and mutual support within the family were still impaired due to the earlier period of excessive crying.

Nevertheless, many parents succeeded in developing a well-aligned and intuitively sustained togetherness within the family despite these burdens. A longitudinal

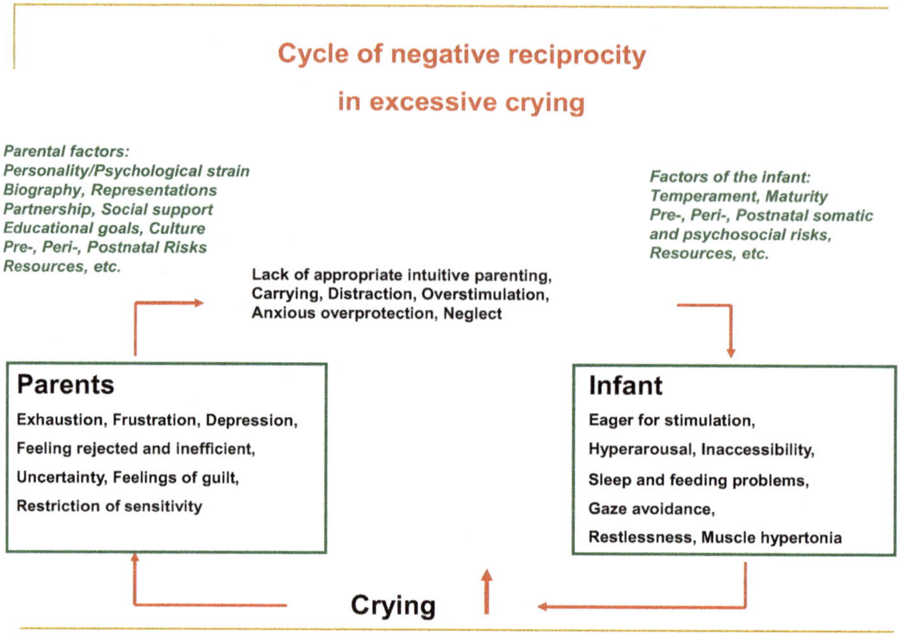

Fig. 3.1 Cycle of negative reciprocity in excessive crying (Thiel-Bonney, adapted from Papoušek 2004)

sample on temperament development conducted by Stifter and Bono (1998) found no differences in attachment classifications between colicky and non-colicky infants at the age of 18 months. A prospective study by St. James-Roberts et al. (1998) on an unselected sample from a maternity hospital showed that most mothers of persistently crying infants cared for their infants with affection and sensitivity despite the crying. The authors stress the need to distinguish between cases from unselected samples of the normal population and cases with high psychosocial and medical risks (see also Sect. 3.3).

Thus, there are close and complex interactions between psychosocial stressors and an infant's propensity toward fussing that need to be taken into consideration in the diagnosis and counseling of affected families. Neither the infant's persistent crying nor the strain on the parents in isolation, but rather an escalating cycle of infant and parental factors, contributes to a deterioration in interaction, particularly in the context of soothing (see Fig. 3.1).

3.6 Diagnostic Methods

The diagnosis of excessive crying is guided by the "Regulatory disorders in infancy and childhood" guidelines (von Hofacker et al. 2007) (see Fig. 3.2) and takes medical, interactional, and psychodynamic aspects into consideration in equal measure. The US multiaxial diagnostic classification manual of the "Zero To Three"

- Episodes of fussiness/agitation and paroxysmal crying for no apparent reason
- Failure to respond to soothing strategies
- Onset is generally at the age of 2 weeks, peaking in intensity and frequency at the age of 6 weeks, and abating toward the age of 3 months, occasionally persisting to the age of 6 months
- Frequent occurrence in the early evening
- Impaired sleepwake regulation, cumulative hyperarousal/overfatigue due to inability to "switch off," marked difficulties falling a sleep, short sleep phases during the day, and diminished total sleep time

Fig. 3.2 Definition of excessive crying (von Hofacker et al. 2007)

working group [DC: 0–3 R; Zero To (2005)] is the subject of controversy. In the manual, the diagnosis "regulation disorder" is codified in axis I as a "regulation disorder of sensory processing" localized primarily in the infant and associated with motor and socioemotional problems. Subgroups of regulatory disorders are described as: hypersensitive type (type I), hyposensitive/unresponsive type (type II), and stimulus seeking/impulsive type (type III). However, findings are inconsistent; the investigated samples are small, and reliable and valid diagnostic instruments for infants that guarantee sufficient discriminatory power between the individual subgroups are lacking. Thus, the DC 0-3R's and Gontards' (2010) call to exclude parental behavior in the diagnostic criteria for this infant disorder, as well as to favor categorical over dimensional diagnoses, does not make sufficient provision for the primarily multidimensional clinical picture and the close interactions between infant and parental factors (see also von Hofacker et al. 2007; Papoušek and Wollwerth 2006).

A diagnostic classification of excessive crying and early childhood regulatory disorder according to the ICD-10 (Dilling et al. 1993) is not as yet possible. Due to the etiological similarity of the clinical picture to early childhood adjustment and maturational processes, it should most likely be classified as an "adjustment disorder (F 43.2) in the form of an early childhood regulatory disorder accompanied by excessive crying."

In order to make a diagnostic assessment, parents are asked about previous and current aspects of the existing symptoms in a detailed history-taking interview (according to von Hofacker et al. 2007):

- **Infant-related aspects:** Description of pregnancy, delivery, medical complications/disease, development to date, the infant's biological and psychosocial risk factors and resources, infant regulatory problems (onset, duration, context).
- **Interactional and relational aspects:** Dysfunctional and successful interactional contexts: What have the parents already tried? Which attempts were successful, which not? To which causes/explanatory models do they attribute the crying and how do they interpret it? On the basis of which experiences with their

infant to date do they attribute the crying to this cause? Relational history since the infant's birth: how do the parents currently see their infant/the relationship to their infant? What expectations do the parents have of their infant and its development? Which interactional contexts are unstrained and which moments in everyday life do the parents enjoy with their infant? How is everyday childcare organized? How are siblings included?

- **Parental aspects:** Parental state of health, subjective experience of stress, biological and psychosocial stressors and resources.
- **Couple- and family-related aspects:** History of the couple's relationship and family situation (e.g., quality of the relationship, transition to parenthood; occupation of the parents; mutual support and social network; individual freedoms). Childhood memories relevant to the relationship (e.g., experiencing socioemotional support; experiences of separation, loss, or trauma). Family of origin (resources, stressors, diseases, and transgenerational relationship conflicts). How have stress situations been dealt with so far in the family?

In order to be able to assess the extent and possible pervasiveness of regulatory symptoms, as well as the infant's strengths and the resources in parent–infant communication, observations should be made of scenes of dyadic or triadic exchange of dialogue or while playing, diapering, and feeding, i.e., outside the disorder-relevant contexts of infant overload and parental attempts at soothing. To this end, resources and stressors can be made "visible" for counselors and parents in a video recording [e.g., dialogue, still-face paradigm, triadic play (Lausanne trilogue play, LTP); see also Cierpka (2012), Chaps. 30, 34, and 35] to assist the therapeutic pathway. The use of protocols and diaries on crying/fussing, sleeping, and feeding (see also, e.g., Papoušek et al. 2004) are extremely helpful in understanding the infant and family situation. (Parental) Questionnaires and scales (e.g., "questionnaire on crying, feeding, and sleeping"; Groß et al. 2007) can contribute to developing a diagnostic approach.

3.7 Counseling and Therapy

Counseling and therapy concepts in early childhood regulatory disorders are guided by the symptom triad (see Chap. 1) and need to cater to a broad spectrum of infant disorders of varying severity and with different organic and psychosocial risk factors (Thiel-Bonney et al. 2005; Wollwerth de Chuquisengo and Papoušek 2004). The principle aims are to reduce or eliminate the infant regulatory disorder as rapidly as possible, enable positive and developmentally appropriate interactional and relational experiences, and ensure an easing of the burden on the parents and the family. The therapeutic spectrum covers four levels, ranging from a developmental crisis in the presence of sufficient parental and infant resources, to severe impairments to relationships and attachments between parents and infants and psychological strain on the parents.

3.7.1 Somatic Level

Acute diseases, such as infections (e.g., middle ear infections, urinary tract infections, bronchitis) gastrointestinal disorders, atopy/allergies, injury, or neuropediatric diseases (Savino 2007; Roberts et al. 2004) need to be excluded or co-treated.

"3-Month Colic"

- Parents of excessively crying infants are still consoled today with references to "colic" and gastrointestinal causes up to the age of 3 months. Visible abdominal distension, however, is usually the result of increased crying and swallowing air, not its cause (Sferra and Heitlinger 1996). Interventions to reduce intestinal gas have no effect on infant crying behavior: Simethicon for the reduction of bloating shows no significant effect on infant crying compared with placebo and has therefore been deemed ineffective in meta-analyses and reviews (Garrison and Christakis 2000). Adding fiber to an infant's diet shows no effect on its crying behavior. The characterization of excessive infant crying as a primary disorder or the intestinal tract ("3-month colic") should be abandoned.
- While herbal tea (a mixture of chamomile, verbena, fennel, and lemon balm) is able to significantly reduce excessive crying, it needs to be administered in a quantity of 150 ml 3× daily. This is not recommended due to its potential to interfere with the volume of milk an infant requires (Garrison and Christakis 2000; Roberts et al. 2004).

Gastroesophageal Reflux (GER)

- GER with/without reflux esophagitis can be a secondary (co-)cause of excessive crying. However, in the absence of frequent vomiting or feeding difficulties, pathological GER is unlikely to be the cause of infant crying (Heine et al. 2006). No evidence has been found of a causal link between the duration of infant crying and GER.

Inflammation of the Gastrointestinal Tract

- A US team (Rhoads et al. 2009) investigated whether inflammation of the gastrointestinal tract and altered colonic flora in excessively crying infants could be causally linked to symptoms. Elevated nonspecific inflammatory markers (fecal calprotectin) were found in stools, suggesting bacterial or allergy-related inflammation in the intestinal mucosa. In addition, significant differences in terms of intestinal bacterial composition were seen between the clinical group of infants compared with the control population. These differences could be responsible for pathophysiological changes such as inflammation, bloating, and altered intestinal motility (see also Savino et al. 2004; Pärtty et al. 2012; Sung et al. 2013).
- A broad meta-analysis conducted in Australia (Sung et al. 2013) investigated the efficacy of the preventive or therapeutic use of probiotics in breastfed and non-breastfed infants. Of the 1180 studies identified, 12 investigations including 1825 infants aged up to 3 months were selected for analysis. In three out of five investigations in breastfed infants with "colic-related" crying, the administration of Lactobacillus reuteri reduced the duration of crying from the age of 21 days

onwards. Two out of seven investigations into prevention revealed a "possible benefit" from the prophylactic use of probiotics. The authors concluded that evidence to support the use of probiotics for the reduction of excessive crying is as yet insufficient and that further clarification is required.

Food Intolerance

- Lactose intolerance
- One can assume a possible lactose intolerance when osmotic diarrhea and acidic stool occur due to carbohydrate malabsorption in lactose deficiency. Only in such cases does lactose-free nutrition result in a significant reduction in infant crying (Hiscock and Jordan 2004). There is no evidence to support feeding with lactose-free foods as a general principle or using lactase as a supplement to breast milk (see reviews: Lucassen et al. 1998; Garrison and Christakis 2000; Leung and Lemay 2004).
- Cow's milk protein intolerance:
- Food allergy to cow's milk or soy protein can be the cause of excessive crying in some infants. However, as with lactose intolerance, other organic symptoms, such as vomiting, mucous bloody diarrhea, poor weight gain, signs of atopy with eczematous skin lesions, and bronchitis are seen in such cases. Cow's milk intolerance also occurs in breastfed infants. In the case of suspected cow's milk allergy (particularly in infants with bloody diarrhea and poor weight gain, as well as mothers that exhibit signs of atopy), an attempt at hypoallergenic infant feeding should be made for an initial period of 1 week (Roberts et al. 2004; Hill et al. 2005): breastfeeding mothers should adhere to a dietary regimen (avoidance of milk and milk products, eggs, cereal and nuts, possibly also citrus fruits, soy, and fish). Infant formula can be temporarily substituted with hydrolyzed (Lucassen et al. 2000) or amino acid-based formula, e.g., Neocate® (Estep and Kulczycki 2000; Savino 2007). Soy-based formulas can have a positive effect on cow's milk allergy (Garrison and Christakis 2000; Leung and Lemay 2004); however, some infants are allergic to soy protein in addition to cow's milk protein (Hiscock and Jordan 2004).
- Nevertheless, ***dietary changes*** should be considered with great care: results from a number of studies appear disparate and an improvement in crying symptoms was seen in only 5–10 % of infants (Ziegler et al. 2004). Zwart et al. (2007) investigated 104 infants referred to their hospital to exclude medical causes of excessive crying or for treatment due to lack of improvement following outpatient care. A change in diet had been undertaken in 77 % of these infants; in none of these cases was a medical cause identified.
- Dietary changes can shorten the duration of breastfeeding as a result of insecurity on the part of both the mother and the infant. In addition, these mothers see their infant as "sick" and allergy-prone to a greater extent; Forsyth and Canny (1991) see the risk here of an "allergy-child syndrome," whereby parents perceive their infant as more vulnerable, which can in turn affect the child's psychosocial development. Moreover, highly hydrolyzed formula can elicit an adverse reaction in infants due to its bitter taste, thereby causing secondary feeding problems.

Functional Neurological Abnormalities/Manual Therapy

- A sample from the Munich Program for Fussy Babies (von Hofacker et al. 1999) revealed 51 % of infants to have mild to moderate functional neurological abnormalities (moderate truncal hypotonia and mild extremity hypotonia/tone regulation disorder, postural asymmetry, and mild central coordination disorders with postural deficit). In the majority of cases, abnormalities improved spontaneously after parents received instruction in occupational therapeutic intervention, as well as short-term physiotherapy or manual therapy.
- head-joint-induced funtional asymmetrie (KISS syndrome; in ca. 3–6 % of infants)—which cause blockage or dysfunction of the upper two vertebrae, increased sensitivity to touch around the nape of the neck, restricted head mobility/tilting or turning of the head to one side, asymmetrical movement (of extremities), and increased overstretching—are also discussed as a possible cause of excessive crying. Following correct prediagnosis and careful indication, Biedermann (2009) described manual KISS therapy as successful in 60 % of infants prone to crying.

A double-blind study on manual therapy/chiropractic interventions in the absence of clear clinical symptoms (Olafsdottir et al. 2001) showed no improvement in infant crying symptoms compared with placebo. A UK study (Hayden and Mullinger 2006), however, revealed a positive effect for cranial osteopathic treatment in terms of a reduction in crying duration and increased sleep time in excessively crying infants. In their questionnaire-based survey of parents in a group of 2- to -3-year-olds referred for chiropractic/manual therapy due to excessive crying (up to 3 months of age), Miller and Phillips (2009) found a reduction in defiant behaviors and sleeping problems compared with a group of former excessively crying infants that had not received manual therapy. However, the specific effect of intervention remained unclear.

Infant massage and the use of a crib vibrator showed no specific effect on the reduction of excessive crying in a Finnish study (Huhtala et al. 2000). Infant massage, however, significantly improved mother–infant interaction in a group of mothers with postnatal depression (Onozawa et al. 2001).

Carrying an excessively crying infant to an increased extent is often extolled as having a beneficial effect of symptoms. Although Hunziker and Barr (1986) indeed found an initial reduction in crying duration, this was seen only in non-excessively crying infants. A subsequent study (Barr et al. 1991) on colic-related crying involving prolonged duration of crying revealed increased carrying of the infant to be ineffective, a result interpreted as an indication of difficulties in infant regulatory processes.

3.7.2 Developmental Level: Developmental Psychological Counseling

Although 3-month colic is popularly recognized as a transient problem, many parents seek pediatric advice. They perceive the excessive crying of their infant as a considerable strain. For this reason, Reijneveld et al. (2001) recommended taking not only the duration of crying, but also the level of parental stress caused into consideration in the definition of "excessive crying."

Counseling geared toward infant development helps parents: (a) achieve a better understanding of their infant/young child's development and their signals in a variety of everyday contexts, and (b) find developmentally appropriate responses to the current needs of their infant (sleep initiation, feeding, etc.).

Working on the assumption that excessive crying is a manifestation of dysregulated sleep–wake organization with cumulative sleep deficit and hyperarousal, parent counseling is based on 24-h diaries kept over the preceding few days (on feeding times, times of successful interaction, phases of crying and fussing, and sleep phases). Possible strategies to soothe the infant that is having difficulty "switching off" and falling asleep due to its increased excitability and reactivity are discussed with the parents (see Info Box 1 for concrete recommendations).

Studies confirm the efficacy of parent counseling and instruction and describe a significant reduction in infant crying duration following counseling. Interventions concentrate primarily on establishing a daily routine, reducing stimulation, and avoiding overstimulation, and focus on giving the infant appropriate support in its development of self-regulatory skills (McKenzie 1991; Wollwerth de Chiquisengo and Papoušek 2004; Garrison and Christakis 2000). The regularity of daily routine, which functions as a social clock, has a significant influence on the infant's inner clock and how it synchronizes its sleep–wake behavior with day–night alternation (Jenni et al. 2008).

A study conducted in The Netherlands (van Sleuwen et al. 2006) recruited 398 healthy excessively crying infants aged up to 3 weeks + 6 days. Parents received behavior-oriented counseling/intervention that specified a regular daily routine and a reduction in stimulation: regular sleep sequence, feeding directly after sleeping, positive playful interaction with the infant and brief playtime alone, observing signs of fatigue followed by prompt settling of the infant to sleep. The regularity of daily structure took into account differences in temperament (see Sect. 3.5.4) between excessively crying infants and their normal age mates. Swaddling prior to sleep was additionally used in 50 % of the infants. A 42 % reduction in crying was seen in both groups at the end of the first week of the intervention. Infants aged under 8 weeks benefited significantly more from swaddling, showing a greater reduction in crying duration over the intervention period. Swaddling brought no additional benefit for older infants. However, in addition to a number of positive effects of swaddling, recent studies warn of an increased possibility of sudden infant death, particularly when swaddling is combined with a prone position (Richardson et al. 2010; van Sleuwen et al. 2007).

3.7.3 Interactional and Communication Level

It is of crucial importance that physicians and therapists take the significant strain on parents seriously, treat them in a manner that reinforces their self-esteem, and offer appropriate help without apportioning blame. Affected parents feel extraordinarily stressed by their infant's inconsolable crying.

Interaction and communication guidance for parents is aimed at sensitizing parents to the needs of their infant. Guided "reading-your-baby lessons" (Barth 2000) encourage parents to respond to their infant's signals with sensitivity, in a developmentally appropriate way, and contingent on the signal (Cierpka 2004). The sessions can take place at particularly stressful points in the daily routine, i.e., feeding, soothing, or settling the infant to sleep. At the same time, it is also important to consider stress-free moments of interaction (e.g., during play) in order to identify resources and positively reinforce parental skills. These dyadic or triadic moments between mother/father and infant can be observed during history taking and counseling, dressing and undressing of the infant/toddler, diaper changing, and feeding; the father should be included in observations and counseling.

3.7.3.1 Extract from a Parent Interview

In their initial interview, the parents of the almost 3-month-old Carla complained of their infant's inconsolable crying, which began around midday and lasted into the night. The parents carried Carla around virtually all day in an upright position to soothe her, looked out of the window with her, or continually offered new visual and acoustic stimulation. Right from the outset, Carla had been highly alert and looking around with wide-open eyes; her sleep requirements appeared to be very low, since she positively fought against going to sleep and slept very little during the day. In order to keep Carla happy, she needed to be "at the breast or kept in constant motion." She frequently got bored and would appear unhappy and fussy. She was generally happy and smiley early in the mornings and started off making little noises to attract her parents' attention. Later on, however, she would increasingly avoid eye contact. The parents wondered whether Carla was perhaps unhappy in their family and whether they were "not doing a good job" as parents, since Carla cried so much and was barely consolable in the evening despite all their efforts.

The sleep diary was presented in the session (see Fig. 3.3).

In order to reinforce parents' trust in their skills while at the same time sensitizing them to their infant's signals and their responses to these, interviews can be, e.g., briefly interrupted with comments such as: "Oh, your baby's looking at you very intensely right now—she's really trying to get your attention! Now she's looking at her daddy—she likes having both parents there. You spotted it straight away and you were able to respond directly to your baby's glance with great sensitivity. Do you see how happy that makes her?" Or one of the infant's signals is discussed directly with the parents, e.g., "Carla seems to be getting more and more agitated. I get the impression you've got to know your baby pretty well in the few months since her birth: What do you think Carla needs now? What is she trying to say with her fussing? What would you do in this situation at home?" Their answer to this question, e.g., that their infant is bored and that in moments like these they would carry her around and show her new things, could be followed by another question aimed at moving their focus to other/new possible explanations: "Yes, boredom is one possible explanation. What else could Carla's fussing mean?" The father and mother may now reply "Well, she can't be hungry at the moment; in fact, she looks a bit tired—but she's only been awake for 3 h!?" The therapist could at this point ask

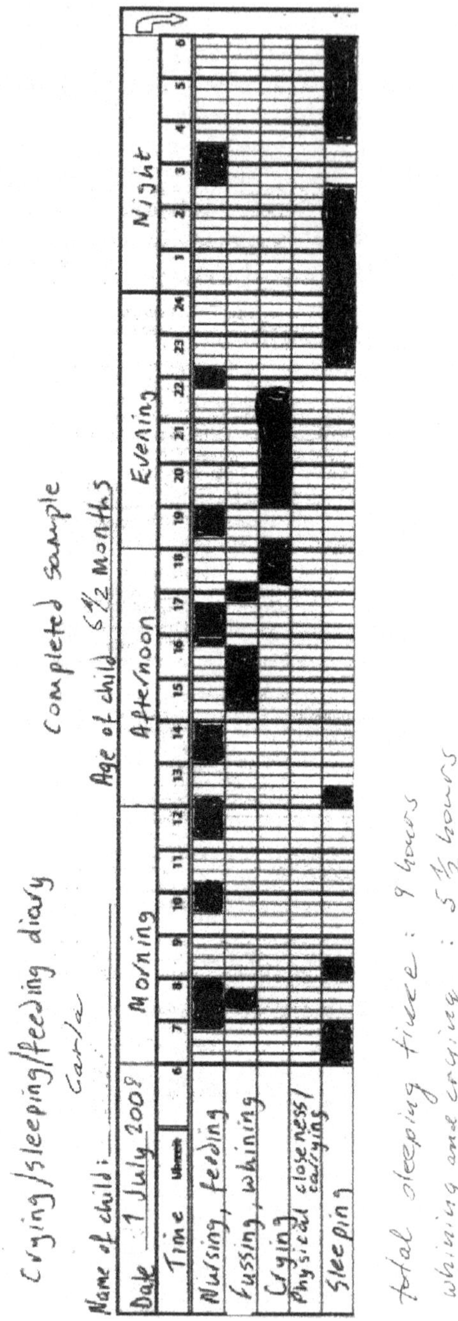

Fig. 3.3 Carla's sleep diary: initial interview

about signs to support this hypothesis: "Yes, that's the impression I'm getting: your baby actually seems tired. How does Carla usually show you she's tired? Have you been able to identify her signals of fatigue? How long are her cheerful and content phases after a sleep? Is Carla already able to make it clear to you when she's hungry or tired, when she's in pain, or when she seeks physical closeness? Or does your baby still make it a bit difficult to recognize and understand these signals? Does she perhaps signal that, despite being tired, she'd rather be carried around and look at things, instead of having a nap? In what situations does Carla want to be breastfed? Is she always hungry in these cases or does she also need the breast as a soothing aid? How successful are you at settling Carla to sleep at home and what would help her "switch off" better?"

Later on, as an observation task for home, the parents can watch out for their infant's first signs of tiredness, that is to say before a crying bout starts: for example, the parents may notice that their infant deflects their gaze during interaction, does not want to "talk" or play with them any longer, shows motor restlessness and becomes "agitated," and starts fussing. When parents recognize these signals, they can, with instruction, attempt to offer their infant the opportunity to sleep as early on as at the first signs of fatigue by using appropriate aids and routines. These attempts are usually more successful when the infant is not yet overstimulated and has not yet started to cry inconsolably.

At the second interview, the parents were happy to report that their daughter was having more frequent and longer sleep periods during the day. To the parents' surprise, the crying and fussing phases in the evening had become shorter and Carla was settling for the night earlier. The parents described with delight many happy moments they enjoyed in everyday interaction with their little daughter. Every now and then, Carla would even play briefly on her own on her blanket; she no longer needed to be carried constantly. They had misinterpreted Carla's signals of fatigue as signs of boredom, and had been prompted to offer her environmental stimulation or to breastfeed her as a soothing strategy.

In the second interview the sleep diary of the last week was presented (see Fig. 3.4).

The parents already received positive feedback on successful interactions in dyadic and triadic exchange during the counseling session. This served to reinforce their sense of parental self-esteem and their intuitive skills. Video-assisted counseling of young families (Papoušek 2000; Thiel-Bonney 2002; Cierpka 2012, Chap. 29) can also make an important contribution to this end.

Developmental and interactional counseling is successful when the caregivers:

- (Still) Have sufficient resources and access to their own intuitive skills and the infant regulatory disorder:
  - Has not extended to other contexts.
  - Is of not more than 3 months' standing.
- The relationship between parents and infant has not undergone any significant impairment (see also von Hofacker et al. 2007).

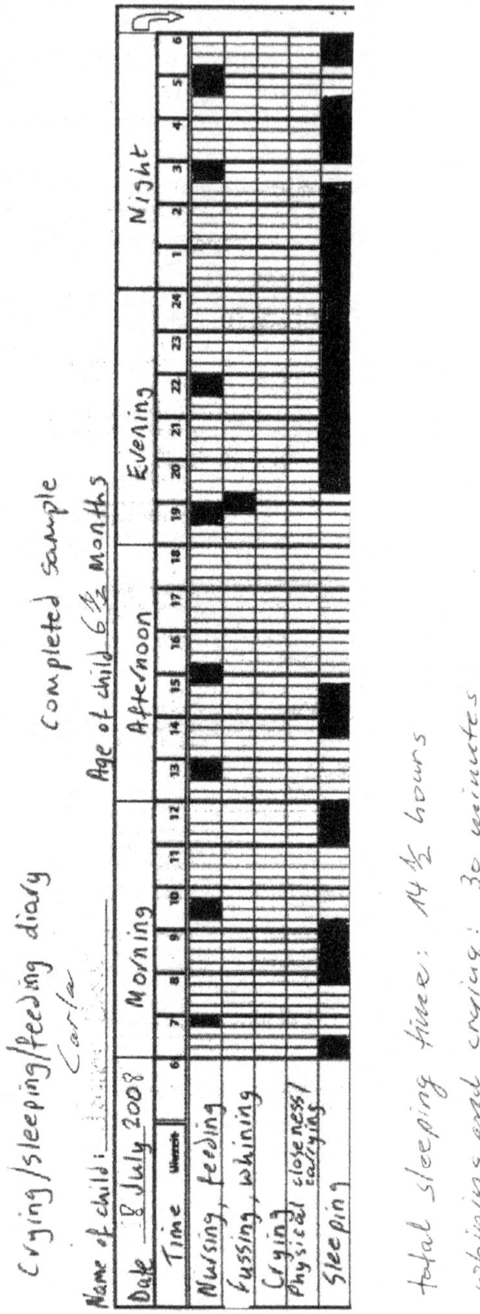

Fig. 3.4 Carla's sleep diary/second session

- Establish a structured daily routine, regular sleep–wake cycles and a sleep-feeding-wake phase-sleep sequence, begin anew every day after waking.
- Recognize and (learn to) understand infant signals: need for physical closeness, willingness to interact, hunger, fatigue, and overstimulation.
- In interaction with the infant: physical contact should serve to convey stability, closeness, and security. Take advantage of the infant's alert wakeful phases for positive dialogue together; short phases of playing alone to encourage self-regulation.
- Use suitable, developmentally appropriate responses to infant signals and avoid overstimulatory soothing strategies (e.g., continually carrying around, offering constant vestibular, visual, and acoustic stimulation). Choose and maintain a soothing strategy that suits both infant and parents.
- "Swaddle" infants aged under 8 weeks in the case of motor restlessness/hyperexcitability, ensuring that a supine position is used.
- Avoid overfatigue by settling infant to sleep at the first signs of tiredness (generally after a 1- to 1.5-h waking period) and reducing stimulation.
- In the case of heightened irritability/hyperreactivity to sensory stimulation: instruction on handling, occupational therapy, sensory integration.
- In the case of overload, possibly with indications of a risk of abuse: timeout for the primary caregivers, provide information on the risk of shaken-baby syndrome. Ease the burden by involving partner, family, and friends. "Prescribe" relaxation periods for the mother/parents.
- If family resources are no longer sufficient and there is a risk of decompensation: possibly apply for household/family assistance (health insurance/social services) or instigate (partial) inpatient care.

Fig. 3.5 Recommended content of counseling in excessive crying (from Zwart et al. 2007; von Hofacker et al. 2007; Papoušek et al. 2004)

Parents often feel reassured to discover that they do not need to be "perfect," but rather that, by simply being "good enough" parents (Winnicott 1990) in the transition to parenthood, they can rest assured that a positive reciprocity will develop; they are entitled to take their own needs seriously and can trust that, with their guidance and appropriate support, their infant's regulatory powers will grow. Infant symptoms generally improve or resolve within two to four counseling sessions (Fig. 3.5).

3.7.4 Psychodynamic-Relational Level: Parent–Infant/Toddler Psychotherapy

Parent–infant/toddler psychotherapy (see also Cierpka 2012, Chap. 30, and Cierpka and Windaus 2007) focuses on parental representations, biographical experiences and stressors in the family of origin, aspects of couple and family systems, and includes the psychosocial family situation, their possibly limited resources, as well as the processing of parental feelings and perceptions (e.g., own experiences of separation, loss, abuse, violence, trauma, etc.).

Parental recollections, experiences, and fantasies from their own biography, as well as unresolved multigenerational relational conflicts in the family of origin can form "ghosts" from the parents' past and interfere in their interaction with their infant (Fraiberg et al. 1975), cause them to misinterpret their infant's signals, and hamper them in providing their child with developmentally appropriate support. Treatment approaches are based on altering the "unrealistic," non-developmentally appropriate parental view of their infant on the basis of which they interpret its behavior. With the help of a therapist while observing their infant, the parents discover new "interpretations" for their child's behavior and are able to distinguish between their own biographically colored perceptions and the developmental and age-appropriate expressions of their "real baby." Once the transition to parenthood is successful, both mother and father become emotionally available and "sensitive," their skills and self-esteem are reinforced, and they are able to deploy their own, as well as the family resources at their disposal (see Lieberman et al. 2005; Papoušek 2011). It is essential that the contribution the infant makes itself—with its difficulties and resources—to the clinical picture always be considered with sensitivity during therapy (see Smart and Hiscock 2007).

3.7.4.1 Case Report

The exhausted parents of the 5-month-old Selina reported how their daughter had started to "cry terribly" at the age of 2 weeks and had had awful "3-month colic." She used to sleep little and would already be barely soothable by the early afternoon. Her fussiness had not improved even after the age of 3 months. Selina was generally fussy, could not occupy herself on her own even for a minute, was continually seeking physical contact, and was only "more or less happy" when she was being carried around. During the day, it was often impossible to settle her to sleep, or she would wake from a short nap tired and unhappy. She also woke up frequently at night; during long crying bouts, her parents would carry her about until she calmed down. Selina would not give her mother a moment's peace and her demanding and at times aggressive crying behavior was difficult to cope with, especially since Selina's 5-year-older brother, Felix, who was more of a quiet type, "had needs as well." The mother was no longer able to endure the situation when Selina cried persistently, "sometimes upset, sometimes angry." A state of such exhausted tension would come over her that she would have to leave the room in order to "calm down a bit herself," which she was finding increasingly difficult to do. A few days previously, she had found herself in front of her daughter with a cushion and suddenly felt the urge to use the cushion to stifle the crying. This development had shocked her deeply.

The father, who was very caring and attentive to his wife and children, spoke of his concerns about his family, as well as the considerable professional pressure he was under. Massive conflicts with the maternal grandparents, with whom the young family was living in the family home, only served to exacerbate the situation. The mother described her own parents' treatment of her as extremely disparaging and hurtful: "Nothing I do is ever good enough! Now they're even using my children against me!" Felix was finding himself increasingly caught in a conflict of loyalty, from which the mother could not protect him due to the close proximity to the grandparents—"but I'm his mother, after all!" She was now starting to have concerns about her son, who had recently started showing sudden bouts of anxious behavior at regular intervals. Although the parents had often thought about moving out of the family home, they had not actually been able to take this step.

In a first step, the family mobilized aids for the mother's daily routine. Once she had been able to improve her relationship with Selina through moments of undivided attention and closeness, and Selina's self-regulatory abilities had improved, e.g., by introducing routines and looking out for early signals of fatigue combined with appropriate help to fall asleep, Selina's sleeping pattern had stabilized. Crying and fussing had abated and the atmosphere in the family was significantly more relaxed. During the course of several psychodynamic and family therapy-oriented sessions, the extent of family stressors had become apparent: the mother had been the victim of a serious sexual assault at the age of 15. The perpetrator, an acquaintance of her parents, had since been released from prison and was now living locally again. Her infant's crying had constantly evoked "memories of that terrible time," during which she had received no emotional support whatsoever from her parents and had oscillated between feelings of loss, distress, and anger. She had seen herself in her daughter as that young girl crying for help, whose parents had not heard her, who had been unprotected, and for whom no relief could be found. In addition, her daughter appeared "to cling to her aggressively," even though she was utterly exhausted. She had tried to be there for her daughter day and night by mobilizing all her strength, but felt overwhelmed and unable to be truly emotionally present for Selina. Confronted with her own neediness, she felt very alone when faced with the demands of everyday life and the conflict with her parents; under no circumstances, however, should Selina feel left alone.

In a fierce conflict of ambivalence between her desire for closeness, care, and a feeling of security and her desire for distance from her family of origin, the mother had (furiously) tried to fulfill the wishes and aspirations of her parents and "done everything to please them." Mutual disappointment about her failure had led more than once to weeks of strained "silence" in the house, interrupted only be the grandmother's attacks on the daughter and her husband, which was extremely stressful for the young son.

In the further course of therapy, the parents reported a discussion they had finally had with Selina's grandparents: with her husband present to support her, the mother had told her parents how she had felt following her assault and how she had needed their support. Following this conversation, her father had cried and hugged her. This was the reaction she had "longed for" since her trauma at the age of 15; instead, her father had withdrawn from her completely and never embraced her, as though the trauma she had experienced had made her no longer worthy of his love. Their announcement to the grandparents that they planned to find an apartment in another town had led to an "eerie but not unfriendly quiet in the house." The escalation in conflict between the generations anticipated by the parents had not materialized; they suspected that their calm resolve and mutual support of one another had contributed to this. The mother expressed pride in herself as a woman at managing—despite the trauma in her youth—to develop her own strength, look after herself, and start "such a wonderful family." Already at the young age of 15, she had had to sort out psychotherapeutic treatment for herself and now wanted, once again, to take advantage of somc thcrapy/counseling sessions.

Selina was presented to us again by her mother at the age of 14 months. Early limit-setting conflicts with the child, in which the mother had not always responded appropriately, were discussed. Once again, she was concerned not to leave her daughter alone in her defiant behavior and "in her desperation," but to give her comfort instead. The mother was once again quickly able to make a connection to her earlier biographical experiences and support Selina in a developmentally appropriate manner in her anger and desire for isolation and autonomy. She was also able to trust her daughter to cope with short moments of frustration and support her in affect regulation.

When based on sound developmental psychology, the psychotherapeutic approach to dysfunctional interactional and relational patterns can follow a variety of pathways (overview in Stern 1998; Lieberman et al. 2000; Cierpka 2012, Chaps. 29–31), which do not differ essentially in terms of their proven efficacy in infant behavioral problems, the mental state of the mother, and relational development (Robert-Tissot et al. 1996; Cohen et al. 1999). Counseling and psychotherapy should not be considered as two essentially separate processes: relational and psychodynamic aspects are also taken into consideration in counseling. Conversely, developmental and interactional aspects form integral parts of parent–infant/toddler psychotherapy.

Parent–infant/toddler psychotherapy in the case of excessive crying is indicated (see also von Hofacker et al. 2007) when crying:

- Persists beyond the age of 3 months and no significant improvement is seen in symptoms following developmental counseling.
- Spreads pervasively to other interactional contexts (e.g., absence of positive interaction, onset of feeding problems).
- Is associated with dysfunctional, maladaptive interaction patterns and a risk of neglect and abuse.
- Marked strains/impairments in parent–child relationships become manifest (e.g., as observed in a hostile, aggressive attitude, distorted perception of the infant's needs, attribution of guilt, and limited emotional access to the infant due to postpartum depression, etc.).

In the presence of organic and/or mental/psychiatric illness [e.g., severe overload syndrome, (postpartum) depression, anxiety disorders, psychosis] in the parents or major partnership conflicts, the mother/father should be referred for individual, e.g., psychotherapeutic/psychiatric treatment or couples counseling/therapy.

The indication for partial or full inpatient mother–infant therapy becomes necessary in the case of severe impairment to the parental behavioral repertoire in dealing with their infant and marked interactional and relational perturbation, in marked organic/constitutional risk factors (e.g., due to premature birth, organic disease, severe failure to thrive), as well as in the case of an immediate threat to the infant's welfare, e.g., due to severe maternal psychopathology.

3.8 Conclusion

Excessive crying, with its persistence and pervasiveness, either as a possible manifestation or result of strained parent–infant relationships and where it threatens an infant's further socioemotional development in particular, should under no circumstances be trivialized.

The scientifically proven diagnostic and therapeutic options available for excessive crying offer counselors the opportunity to intervene in a primary/secondary preventive or therapeutic capacity. The first point of contact for parents (usually the pediatrician), by taking parents' concerns and strains seriously, by offering counseling themselves, or by referring families to a specialist outpatient department should risks be identified, is well placed to set an infant and its family on the right path toward further positive development.

References

Akman I, Kuscu K, Ozdemir N et al (2006) Mother's postpartum psychological adjustment and infantile colic. Arch Dis Child 91(5):417–419

Barr RG (1998) Colic and crying syndromes in infants. Pediatrics 102(5 Suppl E):1282–1286

Barr RG, Mc Mullan SJ, Spiess H et al (1991) Carrying as colic <therapy>: a randomised controlled trial. Pediatrics 87:623–630

Barr RG, Young SN, Wright JH et al (1999) Differential calming responses to sucrose taste in crying infants with and without colic. Pediatrics 103(5):1–9

Barr RG, Trent RB, Cross J (2006) Age-related incidence curve of hospitalized shaken baby syndrome cases: convergent evidence for crying as a trigger to shaking. Child Abuse Neglect 30(1):7–16

Barth R (2000) "Baby-Lese-Stunden" für Eltern mit exzessiv schreienden Säuglingen. Prax Kinderpsychol Kinderpsychiat 49:537–549

Bates JE, Freeland CA, Lounsbury ML (1979) Measurement of infant difficultness. Child Dev 50:794–803

Bensel J, Haug-Schnabel G (2003) Exzessives Schreien. In: Keller H (Hrsg) Handbuch der Kleinkindforschung. Hans Huber, Bern, S1195–1242

Biedermann H (2009) Kopfgelenk-induzierte Symmetrie-Störung beim Neugeborenen. European Workgroup for Manual Medicine. http://www.manmed.de/seiten/themen/manual/kinder/kiss-syndrom/kisskinder.html

Brown M, Heine RG, Jordan B (2009) Health and well-being in school-age children following persistent crying in infancy. J Paediatr Child Health 45:254–262

Canivet C, Jakobsson I, Hagander B (2000) Infantile colic. Follow-up at four years of age: still more "emotional". Acta Pediatr 89(1):13–17
Cierpka M (Hrsg) (2004) Elternkurs "Das Baby verstehen". www.focus-familie.de
Cierpka M, Windaus E (eds) (2007) Psychoanalytische Säuglings-Kleinkind-Eltern-Psychotherapie. Konzepte-Leitlinien-Manual. Verlag Brandes & Apsel, Frankfurt
Cierpka M (2012) Kindheit 0 - 3 Jahre. Beratung und Psychotherapie für Eltern mit Säuglingen und Kleinkindern. Springer Verlag, Berlin Heidelberg
Cohen NJ, Muir E, Parker CJ et al (1999) Watch, wait, and wonder: testing the effectiveness of a new approach to mother-infant psychotherapy. Infant Mental Health J 20(4):429–451
Dilling H, Mombour W, Schmidt MH (eds) (1993) Internationale Klassifikation psychischer Störungen ICD-10. Weltgesundheitsorganisation. Hans Huber, Bern
Ellett ML, Swenson M (2005) Living with a colicky infant. Gastroenterol Nurs 28(1):19–25
Ellett ML, Schuff E, Davis JB (2005) Parental perceptions of the lasting effects of infant colic. MCN Am J Matern Child Nurs 2:127–132
Estep DC, Kulczycki A (2000) Colic in breast-milk-fed infants: treatment by temporary substitution of Neocate infant formula. Acta Pediatr 89(7):795–802
Fivaz-Depeursinge E (2009) Trianguläre Kommunikation von Babys in "Zwei-für-einen"- versus "Zwei-gegen-einen"-Dreiecken. Familiendynamik 34(2):136–145
Fivaz-Depeursinge E, Corboz-Warnery A (2001) Das primäre Dreieck. Carl-Auer-Systeme Verlag, Heidelberg
Fonagy P, Target M (1997) Attachment and reflective function. Dev Psychopathol 9:679–700
Fonagy P, Target M (2002) Early intervention and the development of self-regulation. Psychoanalytic Inq 22:307–335
Forsyth BWC, Canny PF (1991) Perceptions of vulnerability 3½ years after problems of feeding and crying behaviour in early infancy. Pediatrics 88(4):757–763
Fraiberg S, Adelson E, Shapiro V (1975) Ghosts in the nursery. J Am Acad Child Adolesc Psychiatry 14:387–422
Freedman SB, Al-Harthy N, Thull-Freeman J (2009) The crying infant: diagnostic testing and frequency of serious underlying diseases. Pediatrics 123(3):841–848
Garrison MM, Christakis DY (2000) Early childhood: colic, child development, and poisoning prevention. A systematic review of treatments for infant colic. Pediatrics 106:184–190
Groß S, Reck C, Thiel-Bonney C, Cierpka M (2007) Fragebogen zum Schreien, Füttern und Schlafen. Unveröffentlichtes Manuskript, Universitätsklinikum Heidelberg
Hayden C, Mullinger B (2006) A preliminary assessment of the impact of cranial osteopathy for the relief of infantile colic. Complement Ther Clin Pract 12(2):83–90
Heine RG, Jordan B, Lubitz L et al (2006) Clinical predictors of pathological gastro-oesphageal reflux in infants with persistant distress. J Pediatr Child Health 42:134–139
Hill DJ, Roy N, Heine RG et al (2005) Effect of a low-allergen maternal diet on colic among breastfed infants: a randomised, controlled trial. Pediatrics 116:709–715
Hiscock H, Jordan B (2004) Problem crying in infancy. Med J Aust 181(9):507–512
Huhtala V, Lehtonen L, Heinonen R, Korvenranta H (2000) Infant massage compared with crib vibrator in the treatment of colicky infants. Pediatrics 105(6), E84
Hunziker UA, Barr RG (1986) Increased carrying reduces infant crying: a randomized controlled trial. Pediatrics 77(5):641–648
Jenni O (2009) Säuglingsschreien und Schlaf-Wach-Organisation. Monatsschr Kinderheilkd 157:551–557
Jenni OG, Benz C, Largo RH (2008) Schlafstörungen in den ersten Lebensjahren. In: Borke J, Eickhorst A (eds) Systemische Entwicklungsberatung in der frühen Kindheit. Facultas, Wien
Kinsella MT, Monk C (2009) Impact of maternal stress depression and anxiety on fetal neurobehavioural development. Clin Obstet Gynecol 52(3):425–440
Kirjavainen J, Kirjavainen T, Huhtala V, Lehtonen L, Korvenranta H, Kero P (2001) Infants with colic have a normal sleep structure at 2 and 7 months of age. J Pediatr 138(2):218–223
Kirjavainen J, Lehtonen L, Kirjavainen T, Kero P (2004) Sleep of excessively crying infants: a 24-hour ambulatory sleep polygraphy study. Pediatrics 114(3):592–600

Largo RH, Benz-Castellano C (2004) Die ganz normalen Krisen—Fit und Misfit im Kleinkindalter. In: Papoušek M, Schieche M, Wurmser H (eds) Regulationsstörungen der frühen Kindheit. Hans Huber, Bern, pp S17–S30
Leung AKC, Lemay JF (2004) Infantile colic: a review. JRSH 124(4):162–166
Lee C, Barr RG, Catherine N, Wicks A (2007) Age-related incidence of publicly reported shaken baby syndrome cases: is crying a trigger for shaking? J Dev Behav Pediatr 28(4):288–293
Levitzky S, Cooper R (2000) Infant colic syndrome—maternal fantasies of aggression and infanticide. Clin Pediatr (Phila) 39(7):395–400
Lieberman AF, Silverman R, Pawl JH (2000) Infant-parent psychotherapy: core concepts and current approaches. In: Zeanah CH (ed) Handbook of infant mental health, vol 2. Guilford Press, New York, pp 472–484
Lieberman AF, Padrón E, van Horn P et al (2005) Angels in the nursery: intergenerational transmission of benevolent parental influences. Infant Mental Health J 26:504–520
Lucassen PL, Assendelft WJJ, Gubbels JW et al (1998) Effectiveness of treatments for infantile colic: systematic review. BMJ 316:1563–1569
Lucassen PL, Assendelft WJ, Gubbels JW et al (2000) Infantile colic: crying time reduction with a whey hydrolysate: a double-blind, randomized, placebo-controlled trial. Pediatrics 106(6):1349–1354
Lucassen PL, Assendelft WJ, van Eijk JT et al (2001) Systematic review of the occurrence of infantile colic in the community. Arch Dis Child 84(5):398–403
McKenzie S (1991) Troublesome crying in infants: effect of advice to reduce stimulation. Arch Dis Child 66:1416–1420
Miller JE, Phillips HL (2009) Long-term effects of infant colic: a survey comparison of chiropractic treatment and nontreatment groups. J Manipulative Physiol Ther 32(8):635–638
Olafsdottir E, Forshei S, Fluge G et al (2001) Randomised controlled trial of infantile colic treated with chiropractic spinal manipulation. Arch Dis Child 84:138–141
Onozawa K, Glover V, Adams D et al (2001) Infant massage improves mother-infant interaction for mothers with postnatal depression. J Affect Disord 63:201–207
Pärtty AK, Kalliomäki M, Endo A, Salminen S, Isolauri E (2012) Compositional development of Bifidobacterium and Lactobacillus microbiotica is linked with crying and fussing in early infancy. PLoS One 7(3), e32495
Papousek M (1999) Regulationsstörungen der frühen Kindheit: Entstehungsbedingungen im Kontext der Eltern-Kind-Beziehungen. In: Oerter R, von Hagen C, Röper G, Noam G (Hrsg) Klinische Entwicklungspsychologie. Belz Psychologie Verlags Union, Weinheim, S148–169
Papoušek M (2000) Einsatz von Video in der Eltern-Säuglingsberatung und –psychotherapie. Prax Kinderpsychol Kinderpsychiat 49:611–627
Papoušek M (2004) Regulationsstörungen der frühen Kindheit: Klinische Evidenz für ein neues diagnostisches Konzept. In: Papoušek M, Schieche M, Wurmser H (Hrsg) Regulationsstörungen der frühen Kindheit. Frühe Risiken und Hilfen im Entwicklungskontext der Eltern-Kind-Beziehungen. Hans Huber, Bern, S77–110
Papoušek M (2009) Persistierendes Schreien. Schreiprobleme im Entwicklungskontext von Eltern-Kind-Kommunikation und -Beziehung. Monatsschr Kinderheilkd 157:558–566
Papoušek M (2011) Resilience, strengths, and regulatory capacities: hidden resources in developmental disorders of infant mental health. Infant Mental Health J 32(1):29–46
Papousek M, von Hofacker N (1998) Persistent crying in early infancy: a non-trivial condition of risk for the developing mother-infant relationship. Child Care Health Dev 24:395–424
Papoušek M, Wollwerth de Chuquisengo R (2006) Integrative kommunikationszentrierte Eltern-Kleinkind-Psychotherapie bei frühkindlichen Regulationsstörungen. Praxis für Kinderpsychologie und Kinderpsychiatrie 55:235–254
Papoušek M, Schieche M, Wurmser H (eds) (2004) Regulationsstörungen der frühen Kindheit. Frühe Risiken und Hilfen im Entwicklungskontext der Eltern-Kind-Beziehungen. Hans Huber, Bern
Räihä H, Lehtonen L, Korventranta H (1995) Family context of infantile colic. Infant Mental Health J 16(3):206–217

Räihä H, Lehtonen L, Korhonen T, Korventranta H (1996) Family life 1 year after infantile colic. Arch Pediatr Adolesc Med 150(10):1032–1036
Räihä H, Lehtonen L, Korhonen T, Korventrant H (1997) Family functioning 3 years after infantile colic. J Dev Behav Pediatr 18(5):290–294
Räihä H, Lehtonen L, Huhtala V, Saleva K, Korvenranta H (2002) Excessively crying infant in the family: mother-infant, father-infant and mother-father interaction. Child Care Health Dev 28(5):419–429
Rautava P, Lehtonen L, Helenius H, Sillanpaa M (1995) Infantile colic: child and family three years later. Pediatrics 96(1 Pt 1):43–47
Reijneveld SA, Brugman E, Hirasing RA (2001) Excessive infant crying: the impact of varying definitions. Pediatrics 108:893–897
Reijneveld SA, van der Wal MF, Brugman E et al (2004) Infant crying and abuse. Lancet 364:1340–1342
Reijneveld SA, Lanting CI, Crone MR, Von Wouwe JP (2005) Exposure to tobacco smoke and infant crying. Acta Paediatr 94(2):217–221
Rhoads JM et al (2009) Alterded microflora and increased fecal calprotectin in infants with colic. J Pediatr 155:823–828
Richardson HL, Walker AM, Horne SC (2010) Influence of swaddling experience on spontaneous arousal patterns and autonomic control in sleeping infants. J Pediatr 157(1):85–91
Roberts DM, Ostapchuk M, O'Brian JG (2004) Infantile colic. Am Fam Phys 70:735–739, www.aafp.org/afp
Robert-Tissot C, Cramer B, Stern D, Serpa SR et al (1996) Outcomeevaluation in brief mother-infant psychotherapies: report on 75 cases. Infant Mental Health J 17(2):97–114
Savino F (2007) Focus on infantile colic. Acta Paediatr 96:1259–1264
Savino F, Cresi F, Pautasso S et al (2004) Intestinal microflora in breastfed colicky and noncolicky infants. Acta Paediatr 93(6):825–829
Schieche M, Rupprecht C, Papoušek M (2004) Schlafstörungen: Aktuelle Ergebnisse und klinische Erfahrungen. In: Papoušek M, Schieche M, Wurmser H (eds) Regulationsstörungen der frühen Kindheit. Hans Huber, Bern, pp S145–S170
Sferra TJ, Heitlinger LA (1996) Gastrointestinal gas formation and infantile colic. Pediatr Clin North Am 43(2):489–510
Smart J, Hiscock H (2007) Early infant crying and sleeping problems: a pilot study of impact on parental well-being and parent-endorse strategies for management. J Paediatr Child Health 43:284–290
Shenassa ED, Brown MJ (2004) Maternal smoking and infantile gastrointestinal dysregulation: the case of colic. Pediatrics 114:497–505
Sondergaard C, Skajaa E, Henriksen TB (2000) Fetal growth and infantile colic. Arch Dis Child Fetal Neonatal Ed 83:44–47
Sondergaard C, Henriksen TB, Obel C, Wisborg K (2001) Smoking during pregnancy and infantile colic. Pediatrics 108(2):342–346
Sondergaard C, Olsen J, Friis-Hasche E et al (2003) Psychosocial distress during pregnancy and the risk of infantile colic: a follow-up study. Acta Paediatr 92:811–816
Stern DN (1985) Die Lebenserfahrung des Säuglings. Klett-Cotta, Stuttgart
Stern DN (1998) Die Mutterschaftskonstellation. Klett-Cotta, Stuttgart
Stifter CA, Bono MA (1998) The effect of infant colic on maternal self-perceptions and mother-infant attachment. Child Care Health Dev 24:339–351
St. James-Roberts I, Conroy S, Wilsher K (1998) Links between maternal care and persistent infant crying in the early months. Child Care Health Dev 24(5):353–376
St. James-Roberts I, Conroy S (2005) Do pregnancy and childbirth adversities predict infant crying and colic? Findings and recommendations. Neurosci Boibehav Rev 29:313–320
Stroud LR, Paster RL, Goodwin MS et al (2009) Maternal smoking during pregnancy and neonatal behaviour: a large-scale community study. Pediatrics 123:842–848
Sung V, Collett S, de Gooyer T et al (2013) Probiotics and excessive infant crying. JAMA Pediatr 167(12):1150–1157

Talvik I, Alexander RC, Talvik T (2008) Shaken baby syndrome and a baby's cry. Acta Paediatr 97(6):782–785

Thiel-Bonney C (2002) Beratung von Eltern mit Säuglingen und Kleinkindern. Videogestützte Verhaltensbeobachtung und Videomikroanalyse als Interventionsmöglichkeit. Psychotherapeut 47:381–384

Thiel-Bonney C (2006) Deskriptive Daten aus dem Elternfragebogen der interdisziplinären Spezialambulanz für Eltern mit Säuglingen und Kleinkindern. Institut für Psychosomatische Kooperationsforschung und Familientherapie, Universitätsklinikum Heidelberg. Unveröffentlicht

Thiel-Bonney C, Cierpka M (2004) Die Geburt als Belastungserfahrung bei Eltern von Säuglingen mit Selbstregulationsstörungen. Prax Kinderpsychol Kinderpsychiatr 53:601–622

Thiel-Bonney C, Cierpka M, Cierpka A (2005) Präventives Beratungsmodell für Familien mit Säuglingen und Kleinkindern. In: Cierpka M (Hrsg) Möglichkeiten der Gewaltprävention. Vandenhoeck und Ruprecht, Göttingen, S110–138

van den Berg MP, van der Ende J, Crijen AM et al (2009) Paternal depressive symptoms during pregnancy are related to excessive infant crying. Pediatrics 124:96–103

van der Wal MF, van Eijsden M, Bonsel GJ (2007) Stress and emotional problems during pregnancy and excessive infant crying. J Dev Behav Pediatr 28:431–437

van Sleuwen BE, Engelberts AC, Boere-Boonekamp MM et al (2007) Swaddling: a systematik review. Pediatrics 120(4):1097–1106

van Sleuwen BE, L'Hoir MP, Engelberts AC et al (2006) Comparison of behaviour modification with and without swaddling as interventions for excessive crying. J Pediatr 149:512–517

Vik T, Grote V, Escribano J et al (2009) Infantile colic, prolonged crying and maternal postnatal depression. Acta Paediatr 98(8):1344–1348

von Gontard A (2010) Säuglings- und Kleinkindpsychiatrie. Ein Lehrbuch, Kohlhammer, Stuttgart

von Hofacker N, Papoušek M, Jacubeit T, Malinowski M (1999) Rätsel der Säuglingskoliken. Ergebnisse, Erfahrungen und therapeutische Interventionen aus der "Münchner Sprechstunde für Schreibabies". Monatsschr Kinderheilkd 147:244–253

von Hofacker N, Lehmkuhl U, Resch F et al. (2007) Regulationsstörungen im Säuglings- und Kleinkindalter. In: Deutsche Gesellschaft für Kinder- und Jugendpsychiatrie und -psychotherapie (Hrsg) Leitlinien zur Diagnostik und Therapie von psychischen Störungen im Säuglings-, Kindes- und Jugendalter. AWMF Online: http://www.awmf.org/leitlinien/detail/ll/028-041.html<https://mail.med.uni-heidelberg.de/leitlinien/detail/ll/,DanaInfo=www.awmf.org+028-041.html

von Kries R (2006) Exzessives Schreien bei jungen Säuglingen: Definitionen—Häufigkeiten—Risikofaktoren—natürlicher Verlauf—Prognose. Kinderarztl Prax 77:84–88

von Kries R, Kalies H, Papousek M (2006) Excessive crying beyond 3 months may herald other features of multiple regulatory problems. Arch Pediatr Adolesc Med 160:508–511

Wake M, Morton-Allen E, Poulakis Z et al (2006) Prevalence, stability, and outcomes of cry-fuss and sleep problems in the first 2 years of life: prospective community-based study. Pediatrics 117:836–842

Wessel MA, Cobb JC, Jackson EB et al (1954) Paroxysmal fussing in infancy, sometimes called "colic". Pediatrics 14:421–435

White BP, Gunnar MR, Larson MC et al (2000) Behavioral and physiological responsivity, sleep, and patterns of daily cortisol production in infants with and without colic. Child Dev 71(4):862–877

Winnicott DW (1990) Das Baby und seine Mutter. Klett-Cotta

Wollwerth de Chuquisengo R, Papoušek M (2004) Das Münchner Konzept einer kommunikationszentrierten Eltern-Säuglings-/Kleinkind-Beratung und –Psychotherapie. In: Papoušek M, Schieche M, Wurmser H (Hrsg) Regulationsstörungen der frühen Kindheit. Hans Huber, Bern, S281–309

Wurmser H (2007) Einfluss der pränatalen Stressbelastung der Mutter auf die kindliche Verhaltensregulation im ersten Lebensjahr. In: Brisch KH, Hellbrügge T (Hrsg) Die Anfänge der Eltern-Kind-Bindung. Klett-Cotta, Stuttgart, S129–156

Wurmser H (2009) Schrei, Schlaf- und Fütterstörung. Prävalenz, Persistenz, Prädiktoren und Langzeitprognose. Monatsschr Kinderheilkd 157:574–579

Wurmser H, Laubereau B, Hermann M et al (2001) Excessive infant crying: often not confined to the first 3 months of age. Early Hum Dev 64:1–6

Wurmser H, Papousek M, von Hofacker N et al (2004) Langzeitrisiken persistierenden exzessiven Säuglingsschreiens. In: Papoušek M, Schieche M, Wurmser H (Hrsg) Regulationsstörungen der frühen Kindheit. Hans Huber, Bern, S311–338

Zero To Three (2005) DC:0-3R. Diagnostic classification of mental health and development disorders of infancy and early childhood: revised edition. Zero To Three Press, Washington

Ziegler M, Wollwerth de Chuquisengo R, Papoušek M (2004) Exzessives Schreien im Säuglingsalter. In: Papoušek M, Schieche M, Wurmser H (Hrsg) Regulationsstörungen der frühen Kindheit. Hans Huber, Bern, S111–144

Zwart P, Vellema-Goud MAG, Brand PLP (2007) Characteristics of infants admitted to hospital for persistent colic, and comparison with healthy infants. Acta Paediatr 96:401–405

Sleep Disorders of Early Childhood

4

Kerstin Scholtes-Spang, Hortense Demant, and Marisa Benz

4.1 Definition of Early Childhood Sleep Initiation and Maintenance Disorders

Eight-month-old "S" had been waking up and crying as often as ten times per night. Her parents tried to help her settle back to sleep by carrying her around, pushing her in her stroller, and nursing her. "S" would fall asleep at the breast late in the evening and was usually put to bed when already asleep. At night, the mother took "S" into the parents' bed so that she would not have to get up so often to soothe her daughter. "S" was generally unhappy during the day and fussed frequently. She would have a 1-h nap in the late morning but, although she often appeared tired over the course of the day, would stubbornly resist opportunities to sleep. The parents were exhausted and under considerable strain. The father had moved out of the marital bedroom a few days previously due to the nightly disruptions and his lack of sleep, which impaired his concentration at work. The mother often felt overstrained and was also having difficulties concentrating. At night, the mother experienced strong feelings of resentment toward her daughter due to her own inability to soothe her child.

K. Scholtes-Spang, Dipl.Psych. (✉)
Institute for Psychosocial Prevention, University Hospital Heidelberg,
Bergheimer Str. 54, Heidelberg 69115, Germany
e-mail: kontakt@psychotherapie-scholtes.de

H. Demant, Dipl.Psych.
Psychotherapist for Adults, Poststraße 46, Heidelberg 69115, Germany
e-mail: Hortense.Demant@arcor.de

M. Benz, Dipl.Psych.
Florida State University, 4600 University Center, Tallahassee, FL 32306, USA
e-mail: mbenz@lsi.fsu.edu

M. Cierpka (ed.), *Regulatory Disorders in Infants*,
DOI 10.1007/978-3-319-43556-5_4

The case study of young "S" highlights a typical feature of early childhood sleep initiation and maintenance disorders: the infant's inability to fall asleep and/or settle back to sleep following nighttime awakenings, while the sleep per se is not disordered. Infants often demand support through increased crying behavior. They frequently appear exhausted, irritable, and constantly unhappy during the day. Due to their own lack of sleep, parents are likewise exhausted and irritable. Sleep situations are characterized by dysfunctional interaction patterns that perpetuate sleep initiation and maintenance disorders: offering extensive sleep aids (e.g., hour-long carrying around, playing, car rides) impedes the infant's development of self-regulatory skills in terms of self-soothing, which in turn results in increased demands for parental support (Papoušek 2007).

In addition to the above criteria, which emphasize the subjective experience of and psychological strain on those affected, the German Society for Child and Adolescent Psychiatry and Psychotherapy (*Deutsche Gesellschaft für Kinder- und Jugendpsychiatrie und Psychotherapie*) recommends the following criteria in their 2007 guidelines on "Regulatory disorders in infants and young children," which can be applied between the ages of 6 and 12 months:

Sleep Initiation Disorder

Sleep initiation only possible with parental support.

Average time to sleep initiation exceeds 30 min.

Sleep Maintenance Disorder

Waking on average more than three times per night for at least four nights per week, combined with the inability to settle back to sleep without parental support.

Nighttime awakening lasts on average longer than 30 min.

Phase shift in the circadian rhythm of sleep–wake phases.

Impaired waking state.

Sleeping in the parental bed (co-sleeping) should not necessarily be interpreted as a symptom of a sleeping disorder, since this practice is subject to broad cultural and interindividual variation and widespread in the first months of life. Of greater relevance is whether co-sleeping is perceived as problematic and as a strain on the parent–infant relationship.

4.2 Development of Sleep and Sleep Behavior

Parents often feel a sense of relief when provided with information on the development of sleep and sleep behavior in the context of prevention and intervention. The following section provides a short overview of the basics of the development of sleep and sleep behavior.

During the first months of life, sleep–wake phases adjust to the day–night rhythm and increase in regularity; sleep phases become longer and infants learn to fall asleep on their own as a part of their growing autonomy. As part of this process, sleep regulation is influenced by circadian and sleep homeostatic processes. The circadian process, which is already functional before birth, is a regular daily rhythm ("internal clock") synchronized by regularly recurring environmental factors, such as daylight (which acts as an external clock), social contact, and regular food intake (Jenni 2009). Together, a sleep-independent circadian process and a sleep-dependent homeostatic process govern sleep regulation (Borébly 1982): sleep deprivation builds up during the waking period and is diminished again by sleep. Pressure and propensity to sleep increase with growing sleep deprivation. Sleep homeostasis usually begins at the age of 2–3 months (Jenni et al. 2008) and, in contrast to circadian processes, is not present in neonates. As the two processes mature, the initial polyphasic cycle involving between six and eight sleep phases distributed over 24 h evolves in the long term into a biphasic cycle. Optimal attunement of the two processes described here forms the basis for stable and alert behavioral states during the day, as well as for peaceful and restorative sleep at night (Jenni 2009).

Neonatal sleep architecture is characterized by a high proportion of rapid eye movement (REM) sleep [50 % compared with 20 % in adults (Louis et al. 1997)], which explains infants' greater susceptibility to sleep disruption. Over the course of the first year of life, active REM phases and transitional phases become continuously shorter, being replaced by quiet, deep sleep (non-REM) and shifting to the second half of the night to the extent that, by the age of 1 year, sleep structure resembles adult sleep very closely. Reduced susceptibility to disruption and improved regulation of the transitions between waking and sleep, as well as between sleep phases, makes it possible for the infant to "sleep through the night"—the "Holy Grail" for many parents, bringing pride and relief.

Human sleep requirements at all ages are inherently subject to considerable variation. The Zurich longitudinal study showed that daily sleep duration in infancy is between 14 and 18 h, whereby a variation of between 10 and 20 h exists (Iglowstein et al. 2003). Therefore, in order to assess "restorative sleep," an infant's well-being during the day is taken into consideration, e.g., mood, ability to concentrate, daytime fatigue, age-appropriate play, and contact behavior.

The following overview offers information on infant sleep that may be helpful to parents:

- Initially, infant sleeping times are distributed virtually equally over the 24-h period. Sleep only starts to shift more to the nighttime over the course of the first year of life.
- The infant's organism adapts to a 24-h rhythm due to environmental factors such as daylight, noise, social contact, and regular food intake.

(continued)

(continued)

- The greater proportion of REM sleep phases in infants, combined with shorter and less frequent non-REM phases, explains the susceptibility of infant sleep to disruption.
- Particularly in the first 3 months of life, long waking periods do not generate sleep pressure, hence they do not improve an infant's ability to fall asleep or sleep longer.
- Between the ages of 3 and 6 months, the infant develops greater self-regulatory skills and is better able to fall asleep with the help of infant-controlled sleep aids.

4.3 Age-Typical Regulatory Development Tasks in the Context of Sleep

Up to the age of 3 months, the regulation and consolidation of behavioral states, from waking and active states back to quiet sleeping states, take the foreground. This includes structuring transitions between states and organizing them in a cyclical manner. Between the ages of 3 and 6 months, and as a result of the first biopsychosocial developmental spurt, active/alert waking phases, during which the infant's self-regulatory skills can be seen to develop further, become increasingly frequent. Approximately 70 % of 4-month-old infants are capable of falling asleep on their own and, upon awakening, of resuming sleep, assuming they are sufficiently tired and their basic needs are fulfilled. Dependence on external assistance to fall asleep decreases as the infant's own self-regulatory strategies, e.g., thumb- or pacifier-sucking, increase. The necessary readjustment and reorganizational processes appear to culminate at the age of 8 months, resulting in increased nighttime awakening, often accompanied by crying. From a developmental psychology perspective, the tasks at hand include closeness and distance regulation, coping with separation anxiety, and dealing with mother–infant separation processes (e.g., weaning). The central joint developmental tasks parents and infants face in the middle of the second year of life include establishing and regulating a good balance between the infant's need for autonomy and the associated resurgent need for closeness, both on the part of the infant and the parents, as well as the introduction and implementation of rules and boundaries, particularly with regard to bedtime rituals. At the ages of 3 and 4 years, a child's increasingly active fantasy can be responsible for a rise in sleep perturbation in the evenings or at night; children awake from nightmares full of anxiety, express their fear of, e.g., the dark, and seek the protective closeness of their parents (Largo 2001).

Due to the multitude and speed of changes that take place in the interplay between physical, psychological, and social processes in the developmental context of sleep, particular requirements, which differ according to the age of the child, are asked of the parents. In infancy, these include:

- Introducing regular sleep, wake, and quiet phases oriented to the infant's sleep requirements, as well as becoming accustomed to a regular bedtime ritual (Ziegler et al. 2004).
- Observing and responding to signals of receptiveness or the need for quiet, fatigue, overfatigue and overload, while at the same time avoiding overstimulation.
- Intuitively attuning regulatory support by means of body contact, nursing, rhythmic caressing and rocking, as well as conveying closeness, safety, and a sense of security.
- Promoting self-regulatory skills to fall asleep.
- Supporting the regulation of waking, sleeping, and wake–sleep transitions.

Toward the end of the first year of life, the number of tasks of emotional regulation starts to grow, such as coping with saying goodnight—a brief parting and temporary separation for the period of the night. From the age of 2 years onwards, negotiating bedtime can easily turn into a power struggle. An individually tailored solution to age-appropriate developmental tasks forms the basis on which to accomplish the next phase at hand. Insufficiently developed self-soothing skills in the infant, combined with the parents' lack of confidence in their infant's ability to accomplish tasks in the first year of life can, for instance, significantly hamper the parents in adopting appropriate attitudes toward their infant's growing need for autonomy in the second year of life.

4.4 Symptoms, Causes, and Parent–Child Communication in Early Childhood Sleep Initiation and Maintenance Disorders

Nighttime awakening and difficulties falling asleep in infancy are often transient, non-pathological manifestations that occur in the context of accomplishing developmental tasks or as a result of situations involving stress or change (e.g., starting kindergarten or school, moving to a new town, parent separation, or the birth of a sibling). The manifold adjustment and reorganization processes that take place over the course of the first year of life in terms of sleep–wake organization can also cause recurrent transient sleep disorders.

Infant overstimulation, overfatigue, and overload in the first 3 months of life may hamper the process by which a sleep–wake rhythm is consolidated. Difficulties accomplishing this developmental task often manifest in the form of increased fussing, crying, and general agitation over the course of the day, peaking in the late afternoon and early evening (between 5 p.m. and midnight), with comparatively quiet wake and sleep phases early and mid-morning. As a result, infants often fall asleep late in the evening, thereby starting their nighttime sleep late. Moreover, parents often report their impression that their infant appears to vigorously resist falling asleep. Extremely late bedtimes, combined with often excessively short and insufficiently restorative sleep phases during the day (<20 min), can lead to a cumulative sleep deficit in the infant, involving marked overstimulation often associated with excessive crying. Although initially helpful, the parents' deployment of considerable assistance in soothing and settling their infant to sleep in the early months can hamper the development of infant-controlled regulatory skills in the further course. In order to give the infant the opportunity to develop its own self-soothing skills, parents need to reduce their level of assistance and permit the infant to experience self-efficacy. Particularly parents of infants that are dysregulated in the early months find this adjustment challenging, since it requires them to have confidence in the growing self-regulatory skills of their infant. Thus, the infant's initial inability to independently master the transition between active or quiet wake phases into sleep can evolve into a persistent sleep initiation and maintenance disorder. Inadequate sleep hygiene (e.g., inconsistent sleeping times, lack of bedtime rituals), emotional stress (e.g., infant anxieties, acute stressors, chronic conflict situations), and disruptive environmental factors (e.g., noise, temperature, uncomfortable bed) all promote the development and persistence of sleep disorders (Papoušek et al. 2006).

Three-year-old "D" was in the habit of stalling his evening bedtime for hours: he would ask for another drink of water, ask his parents questions, call his mother or father into his room because it was too warm, too cold, too light, or too dark. He generally fell asleep at around 10 pm with a nightlight and the door open. He would wake up between three and four times a week and climb into his parents' bed, which he would then stubbornly refuse to leave. He was difficult to wake in the mornings and had problems concentrating in kindergarten, where he was forever yawning. Social contact made him sensitive and whiny. More recently, "D" had become increasingly prone to sudden emotional outbursts, during which he would shout at other children or throw things about.

The type and efficacy of parent–child communication at bedtime, as well as when soothing an infant after nighttime awakenings, play a central role in resolving the various stage-related developmental tasks. The example of "D" illustrates how misunderstandings and dysfunctional interaction can result in crisis-ridden developments (Papoušek 2007). Permanent overload on the parents, their own lack of sleep, their unsuccessful attempts to help their infant, and the associated feelings of failure or inadequacy all serve to increase the likelihood of impulsive actions on the part of the parents, thereby posing a risk for emotional or physical abuse in infancy and early childhood (Papoušek 2007). However, infant behavior may alter in other areas of development, such as social behavior, and, as with "D," lead to further problems.

4.5 Diagnostic Assessment

Studies show that, although children referred for sleep initiation and/or maintenance disorders according to the above definition do not wake up more frequently at night than do children without sleep disorders (Wolke et al. 1994), they do require more intensive support to settle (back) to sleep. Thus, in terms of clinical diagnosis, the actual number of disturbed nights, as well as the frequency and duration of waking episodes, is far less relevant compared with the subjective sense of strain on the mother or father, as well as on the parent–infant relationship.

Thus, considering a triad of symptoms in the initial diagnostic assessment is advised.

Symptom Triad of Early Childhood Sleep Disorders
The infant is unable to initiate sleep or resume sleep after nighttime awakening without considerable parental support. The parents experience overload syndrome involving a cumulative sleep deficit due to disrupted and insufficient sleep at night. Dysfunctional interaction patterns in the context of settling the infant to sleep perpetuate the sleep disorder. Parents, often stressed and irate after extensive and often elaborate strategies to help their infant fall asleep, e.g., carrying around for hours, playing, driving about in the car, yield to their infant's demands.

4.5.1 Diagnostic Questions

The following aspects can be considered when taking a disorder-specific patient history (Papoušek et al. 2006):

Sleep-Related Patient History

- Onset, conditions under which the disorder began, causes, triggers, course to date, type and success of previous interventions.
- The infant's current state of well-being when awake, behavior at bedtime, and nighttime awakening.
- Type and extent of current parental support to initiate sleep, bedtime ritual, sleep setting, and family sleeping habits.
- Subjective and objective stressors and resources of the mother, father, and their relationship.
- Behavioral problems in other everyday contexts (feeding, diaper changing, separation situations, boundary setting, play).

▶ The diagnostic workup of sleep initiation and maintenance disorders in early infancy should include an assessment of infant behavior that also takes the infant's self-regulatory skills outside the sleep context into consideration.

Physical Examination

- Investigation and co-treatment of possible somatic disorders that negatively impact sleep, e.g., food intolerance, allergy, atopic eczema, gastroesophageal reflux, airway obstruction, sleep apnea (Undine syndrome), organic brain damage involving absent/disrupted sleep–wake rhythm, seizures, chronic pain.
- Observation of self-regulatory skills and temperament factors (irritability, hypersensitivity to stimuli, distractibility, capacity to adjust, self-soothing, social openness) during direct contact with the infant.

Sleep Diaries (Papoušek et al. 2006)

- These are kept by the parents over several days and provide an overview of: sleep times and sleep requirements; frequency and duration of nighttime awakenings; type and extent of parental support to settle the infant to sleep; distribution of mealtimes over the day; phases of fussing and crying. Nighttime awakenings sometimes resolve, e.g., when sleeping times are adjusted to the infant's requirements in terms of timing and duration (Fig. 4.1).

Relational Questions

- Observation of the emotional relatedness between infant and parents.
- How do the parents see the settling-to-sleep ritual and bedtime interaction? What emotions does the crying evoke? To what do they attribute the nighttime crying bouts? How do they feel after being woken up for the third or fourth time?
- How are roles distributed between mother and father? Do the parents disagree on settling-to-sleep strategies?

Home video of typical bedtime interaction, taken by the parents where possible.

4.5.2 Differential Diagnosis

Classifying sleep disorders of early infancy as non-organic sleep disorders according to ICD-10 (F51.0) is inappropriate due to the definition and criteria that apply here; the ICD-10 classification remains reserved for adults. A diagnosis of "adjustment disorder (F 43.2) in the form of a regulatory disorder of infancy involving sleep initiation and/or maintenance disorders" is recommended from the age of 3 months. In the case of marked sleep problems and difficulties in sleep–wake organization before the age of 3 months, the diagnosis "adjustment disorder (F 43.2) in the form of a regulatory disorder of infancy involving excessive crying," with no explicit mention of sleeping problems, is recommended (Dilling et al. 2008). These are often precursors of subsequent sleep initiation and maintenance disorders.

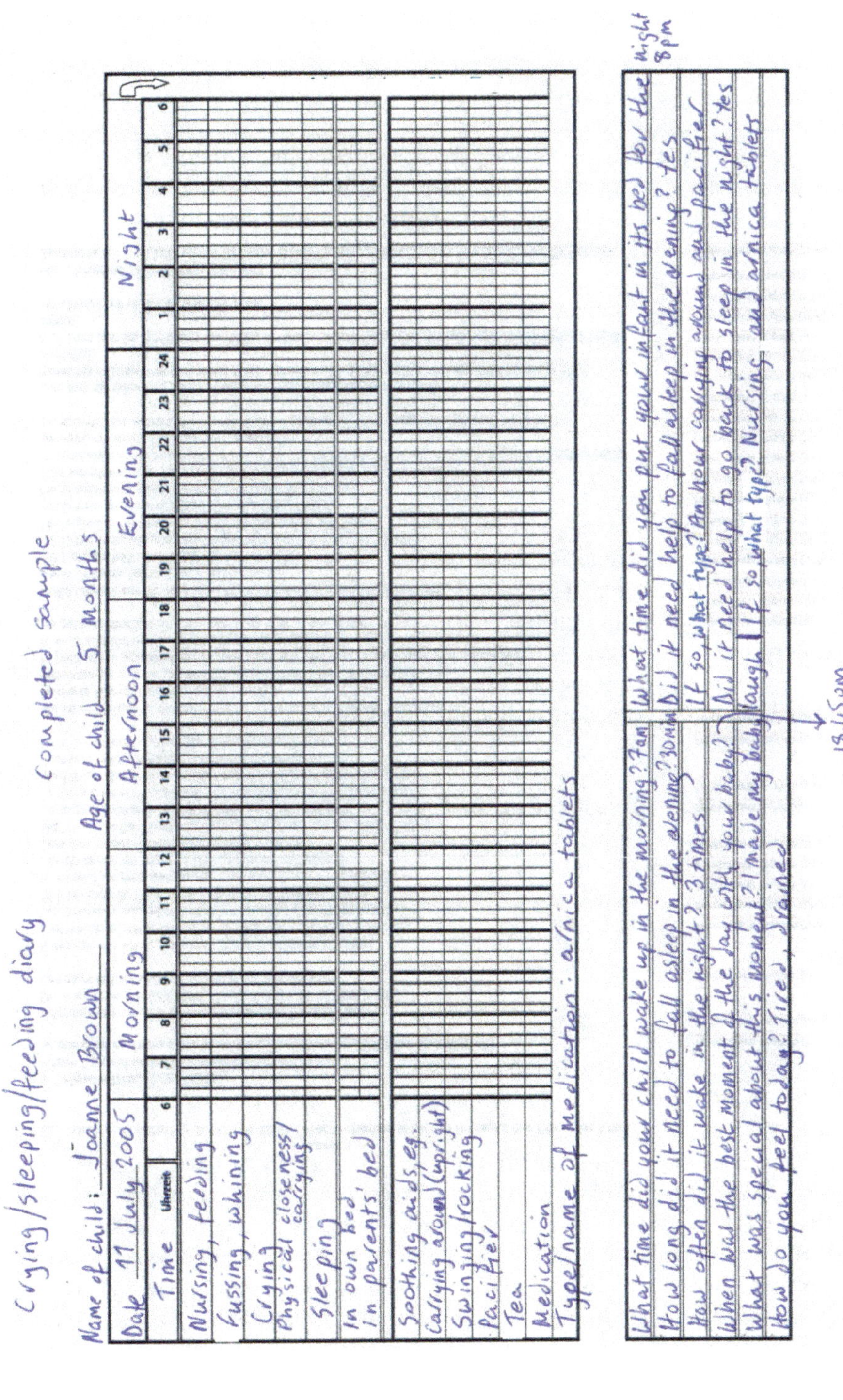

Fig 4.1 An example of a completed sleep diary. A template of the sleep diary can be found in the Appendix

4.6 Interventional Approaches

It is generally accepted that overstimulating and overloading the infant hampers both "switching off" during the daytime and sleep initiation at night. Thus, infants rely heavily on their parents for support during the first months of life (see Chaps. 2 and 3.) The process of adjusting parental support, or withdrawing it in a staged manner, requires the parents to be aware of their infant's skills in the domain of self-regulation and to support these skills. Ultimately, the parents must learn to trust that their infant is capable of taking the step of initiating sleep alone without coming to harm.

▶ Allowing the buildup of sleep pressure, e.g., by keeping the infant awake, as indicated for the treatment of adult sleep initiation disorders, is contraindicated in infants and young children on the basis that their circadian and sleep homeostatic processes are still developing and their self-soothing skills remain limited.

During parent interviews, both in the counseling and psychotherapeutic setting, it is essential to identify not only parental resources and skills, but also to ask questions about and assess parents' emotions, such as fears, hopes, expectations, and convictions. Only in this way it is possible to ensure that interventions appropriate for the family, and thus promising greater chances of success, are formulated. Interventions that can be successfully implemented reinforce the parents' sense of self-efficacy, thereby promoting access to their intuitive skills. Thus, a process of positive reciprocity between parents and infant can be set in motion early on.

4.6.1 Prevention-Focused Parent Counseling in Practice

Prevention-focused parent counseling to practice positive sleep habits and promote a regular sleep–wake rhythm in early infancy, particularly in dysregulated infants with excessive crying, can contribute to the effective prevention of sleep disorders later on.

- **Promoting regular sleep–wake cycles** comprising: waking up–nursing/feeding–wake period with dialogue/quiet observation–settling to sleep when tired
- Many infants still rely on their parents for regulatory support (physical contact, familiar odor/voice, gentle rocking, nursing) up to the age of 3–4 months, and hence: **parents should not worry about spoiling their infant!**
- **Recognize and learn to interpret infant signals** of receptiveness, the need for rest, fatigue, overstimulation, as well as hunger and physical discomfort, in order **to be better guided in terms of what to offer the infant.**
- **Avoid overfatigue.** Resting times or the opportunity to sleep should be offered promptly.

(continued)

- **Avoid overstimulation.** Overstimulation can occur, e.g., as a result of hours-long carrying about or vigorous rocking, or if attempts at continuous distraction are made when an infant expresses discontent. Therefore, shutting out or reducing stimulation prior to bedtime is recommended.
- Nighttime waking phases should remain as stimulation-free as possible (no light, no playing).
- ©Papousek, Rothenburg, Cierpka, and von Hofacker (2006) (Papoušek et al. 2006).

If an infant is still only able to fall asleep in close physical contact with its parents or while nursing even after the developmental spurt at 3 months, introducing a short interval between the soothing bedtime ritual and when the infant finally falls asleep in its own bed is recommended; the interval should then be extended stepwise. The infant is placed in its cot while relaxed but still awake and, initially while a parent is still present, is able to experience how it can fall asleep through self-regulation. If this succeeds, the parents can gradually say goodnight ever earlier so that the infant experiences that it can also fall asleep when its parents are not present.

4.6.2 Sleep Counseling in Practice

The parents of the now 11-month-old "S" attended parent–infant/toddler counseling. The introduction of an evening ritual including a bath, singing, and cuddling, which was recommended to her by friends, had not worked. Instead, the infant's crying had increased and bedtime in the evening had grown ever later. Since the mother was at the end of her tether, she continued to let "S" sleep in the parental bed, while the father still slept in the living room. Neither parent was happy with the situation and started by consulting their pediatrician, who recommended attending a counseling center. After this initial consultation, the parents were asked to observe their daughter over a few days: When did she show signs of fatigue? When did she need a rest? Could she already shield herself from external stimulation? By using these observations as a guide, the parents had the impression that "S" could be settled to sleep much earlier in the evening. Feeling that their daughter was extremely tired and having the impression that she needed help to switch off, the parents tolerated the crying that broke out upon renewed introduction of a soothing, low-stimulation bedtime ritual. Prompted by the counseling, the parents also asked themselves how they felt about their child sleeping in their bed: the mother still enjoyed the close physical contact with her infant, but also felt it disturbed her sleep. The father clearly stated that he felt his sexual needs were not being fulfilled as a result of his child's presence in the parental bed.

A combination of techniques implemented at the behavioral level while taking the individual situation, as well as parent and infant resources, into consideration have proven helpful in counseling for marked sleep initiation and maintenance disorders. The self-help approach referred to as "checking" (also known as the Ferber method) is a widely used and demonstrably effective behavioral intervention (see Ferber 1985). The "checking" procedure for infants aged from 6 months was elaborated for German-speaking countries by Kast-Zahn and Morgenroth (1995) in their book, "*Jedes Kind kann schlafen lernen*" ("Any child can learn to sleep") as follows:

- The infant should be able to recognize the beginning of the bedtime routine by its soothing going-to-bed/falling-asleep rituals, which take place outside the bed and with undivided attention. These rituals should take place at the same time every evening. The parents can let themselves be guided by their infant's signals of fatigue in order to identify the right moment to begin the bedtime ritual.
- The infant should be placed in its cot while awake so that it experiences the process of falling asleep. After initially staying with the infant for a short period, a move intended to ease the child's arrival in its bed, the parents say goodnight and leave the room. Some infants and parents find it helpful to leave the door ajar, so that the separation is not overly abrupt.
- It is to be expected that the infant cries during the intervention. Parents should be prepared for this. The crying can be an expression of:
- Protest at the breach of previous habits.
- A tenacious attempt to regain familiar ground.
- Testing boundaries.
- Separation anxiety and a sense of abandonment.
- The infant's use of sleep aids, such as a security blanket, a teddy, or a pacifier, helps it to cope with both the separation from its parents and the transition to sleep. These can be introduced in parent–infant interaction during the day, e.g., while diaper changing, thereby enabling the infant to internalize these objects as symbolic representations of its parents.
- If the infant begins to cry, the parents return at regular preset intervals—not determined by the crying—to give their child brief attention and reassurance, without taking it out of its cot or offering a bottle or the breast. It is essential during this process that the parents convey a sense of warmth and dependability to their infant and make it clear that it is not alone. Placing a hand briefly on the infant and talking in a soothing, monotone voice, for example, have proven to be effective. Interactions consisting of a clear, repetitive procedure instill the infant with a sense of security. The parents are reassured by their trust in the fact that their infant is essentially capable of soothing itself and falling asleep alone.

Once sleep initiation in the evening succeeds, the parents can implement the same procedure for nighttime awakening and crying (from Ferber 1985).

The checking intervention makes high demands on the infant's self-regulatory skills and attachment security, as well as on the parents' emotional resources. Due mainly to the parents' ambivalent feelings, their sense of reliving their own childhood experiences, and their fear of overstraining or even traumatizing their infant, these interventions are often unsuccessful, despite the positive scientific evidence. The likelihood of failure or early discontinuation is increased in the case of: highly ambivalent parents with scant resources, extremely dysregulated infants, and generalized regulatory disorders. For this reason, embedding a stepwise variant of this method in a broad counseling concept that focuses on the current difficulties in parent–child communication, the psychological status of the parents, and the infant's current developmental stage has proven its worth. The Ferber method promises success if the following requirements are met (Papoušek et al. 2006):

> Both parents should feel sure and agree that their infant is capable of learning to fall asleep alone. Both parents should agree that they are able to withstand the strain associated with carrying out the intervention (increased protest and crying). The infant should be in good physical and mental health. The intervention should begin at a point when both parents have sufficient time at their disposal and when no other significant changes are pending.

During the counseling session, it is important to establish the parents' individual needs for support in this process. As a precaution, their expectations, anxieties, and feelings of ambivalence should be discussed in advance in order to weigh the strain anticipated from the intervention against the strain created to date by the sleep disorder and its negative effects on the entire family (Schieche et al. 2004). Successful implementation of the intervention results in satisfying the needs of all involved in terms of peace and sleep, as well as an improvement in the well-being of the infant and the parents during the day, which in turn has a positive impact on wake-phase interaction. Experiencing their own self-efficacy has a positive effect on the emotional state of the parents and contributes to greater satisfaction in their relationship.

However, some parents prefer an even more stepwise approach which, while causing less acute strain, takes considerably longer. Here, the initial emphasis lies on adjusting the infant's bedtime to its sleep requirements and the regularity of its daily routine. Parent-controlled sleep aids are reduced very gradually in order to achieve a stepwise improvement in the infant's self-regulatory skills. In concrete implementation, individual adjustments to the procedure aimed at achieving greater autonomy for the infant in the sleep context can include the following:

- Carrying the infant around until it is soothed and calm.
- Placing the infant while awake in its cot.
- Conveying closeness by sitting next to the bed, firstly with physical contact (e.g., placing a hand on the infant's tummy), then without physical contact.
- Leaving the room after saying goodnight.
- Leaving the door open or ajar so that the infant can become accustomed to being alone in the room.

In order to help the infant acquire the self-soothing strategies it needs to go (back) to sleep at night, it is helpful to start introducing this procedure during the day. Introducing small boundary-setting and separation situations can underpin success here: by setting up specific times of divided and undivided attention, the infant learns that there are phases when it receives its parents' full attention, others when it needs to keep itself occupied for short periods of time. Since parents and infants find brief separation situations such as these easiest at the most rested time of day, they should be introduced early in the morning. Thus, the prospects of experiencing a sense of achievement is increased for all involved and trust in the infant's self-regulatory skills reinforced. At around the age of 1 year, a familiar transitional object (Winnicott 1951), e.g., a worn T-shirt belonging to the mother, a soft toy, or a security blanket, by serving as a proxy for closeness to the primary caregiver, can convey the sense of security the infant needs to fall asleep in that it reminds the infant of the physical presence of the caregiver even in that person's absence. Toys, in contrast, should be removed from the bed.

Any counseling concept should include acute and long-term relief for the parents and their relationship, for instance: through short breaks during the day together with the infant; involving both parents in, and making clear agreements on, the nighttime care of the infant; the possibilities of getting support from the social environment; as well as suggestions on how to tend the relationship.

4.6.3 Psychotherapy

At the initial interview, the mother of 23-month-old "P" reported that her daughter was waking up as often as ten times per night and only rarely managed to fall back asleep alone. She was only able to fall asleep in her cot if she could hold her mother's hand. According to the mother, pacifiers, soft toys, music, or a nightlight were insufficient to make "falling asleep palatable." "P" would wake up again after 2 h and switch to her parents' bed. The mother, who attended the parent–infant/toddler clinic on her own with her daughter since the father had work commitments, was ambivalent in her feelings: on the one hand she enjoyed the physical closeness to "P" who, in her eyes, "was growing up far too quickly," while on the other hand she questioned whether sleeping in the parents' bed might be harmful to her infant's development. When asked about her partner's point of view, the mother reported that he "wanted to let P sleep in their bed because she was still so little." During the day, "P" was quick to start fussing, nothing was right for her, and she would show extremely clingy behavior toward her mother. Attempts to tire "P" out by offering her more opportunities for motor stimulation had failed. Having read "Any child can learn to sleep," the mother considered the approach "brutal" and "could never do that."

With regard to her personal life, the mother reported how her significantly older husband had a child from an earlier relationship. Since she was the one who spent the most time with "P," she insisted on having the last word on all decisions. It was apparent that the mother had a clear need to be autonomous and take a controlling role, while at the same time she was overstretched by the current situation and felt she had little support from her husband. Mother and child frequently stayed with the mother's parents, often for several days. The family was considering moving closer to the grandparents. The mother expressed her desire to also have some free time, but insisted that this was only possible if her own mother looked after "P." On these occasions, the mother would slip away secretly, since she could not bear the protests her daughter made when she left. Upon her return, she would usually find "P" playing happily, which triggered feelings of ambivalence in her. On the one hand she was happy that "P" was happy and well, while on the other hand she found it difficult to accept that her daughter "no longer thought about her" after such a short time.

At the initial interview, the mother gave the impression of being tired, unconcentrated, and somewhat unkempt. She complained of her persistent lack of sleep, excessive ruminating in the evenings, difficulties falling asleep, and permanent physical tension. The little girl sat on her mother's lap during the entire interview and showed no interest in exploring the room. She fussed occasionally, requested something to eat or drink, and wanted to go home. Although the mother appeared attentive in her interaction with the child, she found it increasingly difficult to remain calm in the face of her daughter's demands and came across as tense, irate, and tearful. Eventually, she said despairingly: "If only I could understand her! When will she finally be able to talk?"

The parents encountered in specialist clinics, counseling centers, and psychotherapy practices are those for whom behavioral instruction and self-help strategies alone offer an inadequate solution. The questions "why is a child unable to fall asleep and maintain sleep alone" and "why are the parents unable to let their child sleep alone" can be considered on an individual basis. Conscious and unconscious factors that hamper the parents in their ability to either provide their infant with the skills it needs in the transition to initiating and maintaining asleep, or to withstand the associated perturbation in the infant, are considered from a diagnostic and therapeutic perspective. Unpleasant emotions that emerge, for example, in conjunction with falling asleep at night are often associated with the parents' own early childhood experiences, rekindled by pregnancy, birth, and the early phase with their infant according to the "ghosts in the nursery" concept (Fraiberg et al. 1975). Containment (Cierpka 2012, p. 88), the process by which the mother receives and preserves her infant's expressions of negative affect, is impossible against this background. The infant's crying in the sleep context can then for example trigger excessive responses in the parents, since they are unable to cope with the internal stress they experience. Feelings of guilt at expecting too much from their infant need to be compensated immediately with for example increased physical closeness, but are at the same time accompanied by feelings of ambivalence. Containment is closely linked with the capacity for mentalization (Fonagy et al. 2004) (see Cierpka 2012, p. 408), i.e., reflecting on and differentiating between one's own and others' emotional states, in turn making it possible to understand one's own and others' behavior. A capacity for mentalization enables parents to empathize with their infant's needs and, based on this empathy, understand signals such as crying as their child's way of expressing itself; they then use these signals to shape interaction with their infant in the sleep context as part of the attunement and support processes. This forms the basis for parents to perceive and correctly interpret their infant's signals in order to be able to provide developmentally appropriate support to initiate and maintain sleep. Attempts can be made together with parents in a psychotherapeutic process to empathize, guided by the infant's signals, with how the infant is feeling, respond to these signals, and assess the infant's possible responses. Interaction of this kind gives the infant a sense of being understood and supported. The parents are able to experience a sense of competence and self-efficacy, a sense lost by many mothers and fathers through repeated failure to soothe and help their infant fall asleep, thereby contributing to deep insecurity. The case of "P" represents a persistent sleep initiation and maintenance disorder beyond the age of 6 months and becomes more understandable in the context of the separation issues between parents and child associated with autonomous falling asleep and remaining asleep. According to attachment theory, falling asleep represents a separation experience, nighttime awakening a reunion. Investigations by Nolte et al. (2006) on the association between attachment patterns in 18-month-old toddlers and sleep disorders at the age of 30 months revealed that securely attached infants more frequently exhibited combined sleep initiation and maintenance disorders. One assumes that, while sensitive attunement and response to an infant's needs promote early attachment development, they hamper the steps toward developing the autonomy needed for an infant to fall asleep and maintain sleep alone. Insecurely attached children exhibited marked self-stimulatory behaviors (e.g., finger sucking), presumably to suppress negative affect and attachment behavior in the sleep context (Nolte et al. 2006).

Moreover, children can only cope independently with the demands made on them by autonomy development, and detach from their parents in order to sleep, when the parents condone and support their child's development of autonomy. The parents' own conflicts in dealing with their needs for closeness and autonomy may be rekindled or aggravated through experiencing their infant's developmental stages, and responded to according to their coping strategies. P's mother appeared to still be very close to her own mother and was recreating the same relationship structure with her daughter. Although perpetuating intense parental support to fall asleep may have been satisfying a need for closeness in P's parents, it was at the same time keeping the child in a position of dependency and hampering the development of her self-regulatory skills. Understanding the significance of infant sleep disorders through the prism of the parental biography permits issues to be processed in the psychotherapeutic setting; as a result, the parents are capable of supporting their infant's development and adjusting to its various developmental phases (Barth 1999). The same applies to sleep disorders in the context of generalized regulatory disorders, as well as impaired attachment security (Papoušek 2007), in which sleep training can elicit or exacerbate separation anxiety or feelings of abandonment.

4.7 Parasomnias

Parasomnias in childhood are generally transient maturational phenomena that disrupt sleep, but do not otherwise represent a primary disorder of sleep–wake regulation (Fonagy et al. 2004, Papoušek 2007).

Although they do not belong to early childhood regulatory disorders, parasomnias occur as early on as toward the end of the infant stage. They are subdivided into waking disorders, REM sleep-related parasomnias (e.g., nightmares), and other parasomnias (e.g., sleep-related enuresis) (Schramm and Riemann 1995).

Since parents of young children are often extremely unsettled by pavor nocturnus (sleep terror) due to its alarming symptoms, it will be discussed here as an example of the class of waking disorders that occur during the deep-sleep phase. Nightmares are the commonest form of REM sleep-related parasomnias in childhood.

Pavor nocturnus manifests as partial arousal from non-REM sleep and generally occurs in the first third of sleep at the end of the first deep-sleep phase. Sleep terror is accompanied by poor responsiveness to external stimuli and difficulty waking the child, followed by disorientation. Its occurrence is associated with stress, emotional strain, febrile disease, noise, or sleep deficit as triggering factors.

A sudden panicked cry from 18-month-old D's bedroom startled the parents 2 h after putting their son to bed. They found "D" with his eyes wide open and an alarming look of fear on his face. He was crying, tugging at his bedcovers, thrashing about wildly, and was in danger of hurting himself by banging his head. He was perspiring heavily and in a state of high tension. After a few minutes, he pulled himself up on the bars of his cot, shook the bars wildly, and continued his rant. He seemed to be out of his senses and, although he appeared to be awake, he was unresponsive. Alarmed, the parents tried to pick "D" up out of his cot. He refused to be touched and continued crying in an apparent state of panic. The parents had some difficulty waking "D." Once they had finally managed to shake him awake, he looked about, confused and barely responsive to his mother's soothing words. He let his parents place him back in his cot and very quickly resumed peaceful sleep. Although "D" was somewhat crotchety the next morning, the sleep terror had left no visible traces.

Many parents are shocked and startled by this kind of short episode (generally lasting not longer than 10 min) of pavor nocturnus. It is associated with strong vegetative arousal in children, while parents observe extreme fear. No forms of long-term physical or mental damage are known. The risk of injury during an attack of this kind is extremely remote if a child is in a safe environment.

In the case of nightmaress, children start up from a dream phase, are awake or easily awoken, and are oriented within moments. As a rule, children recall the dream vividly and in detail, both immediately after waking and the next morning (Fricke-Oekermann and Lehmkuhl 2008). Falling back to sleep is hampered by the recollection of frightening impressions from the dream. The frequent occurrence of nightmares puts considerable strain on parents and children, as well as causing secondary sleep initiation disorders.

The 3-year-old "M" was tossing about in his bed moaning; finally, he woke up with a start and cried out for his parents. He was sitting in his bed shaking and crying. He kept repeating the same fragments of sentences describing his fall from a climbing frame the day before. His mother took him in her arms and soothed him. His agitation, however, was slow to abate. After his mother had placed him back in his bed, "M" refused to shut his eyes and resisted sleep. Exhausted, the mother finally took "M" to the parents' bed, where he fell asleep within a few minutes.

4.7.1 Diagnostic Assessment

In addition to a detailed interview with the child and primary caregivers, as well as keeping a sleep diary, parents may find videoing nocturnal episodes helpful (Vella 2003). From a differential diagnostic perspective, frequent episodes of pavor nocturnus should prompt the exclusion of an epileptic event, as well as other neurological disorders (Deutsche Gesellschaft für Kinder- und Jugendpsychiatrie und Psychotherapie 2007). Interaction and attachment disorders between child and caregiver or other emotional stressors may underlie frequently recurring nightmares in infancy.

The child's well-being during the day and self-regulatory skills also need to be considered in the diagnostic workup of parasomnias. This provides, for instance, an indication of the extent to which the infant's sleep needs are being met and how well it is coping with age-appropriate developmental tasks in the sleep context. Pavor nocturnus in particular is frequently associated with underestimations of an infant's need for sleep.

As a sleep arousal disorder, pavor nocturnus is distinct from nightmaress in a number of respects:

- Sleep terror occurs during deep sleep, nightmares, in contrast, during REM sleep.
- In sleep arousal disorders such as sleep terror, those affected are difficult to wake and are subsequently disoriented. With nightmares, however, the child is readily awoken and exhibits little or no disorientation.
- Whereas a child falls back to sleep quickly and without difficulty following a sleep terror episode, nightmares frequently cause a delay in resuming sleep, often associated with anxiety.
- Concomitant physiological arousal, such as perspiring, tachypnea, and tachycardia, is marked in pavor nocturnus and seen only in milder form in nightmares.
- Those affected by pavor nocturnus have no recollection of the episode upon awakening. Nightmares, on the other hand, are often recalled in detail.

4.7.2 Treatment

The following interventions are helpful in sleep arousal disorders such as pavor nocturnus:

- Ensuring the sleeping environment is safe in order to avoid injury.
- Psychoeducation of parents on sleep arousal disorders as developmental phenomena.
- Advising parents not to unsettle their child with insistent questions the next day or to wake it during the night.
- Providing adequate sleep hygiene, e.g., maintaining a regular sleep–wake rhythm with sleep phases of sufficiently long duration.

There are also other possible stressors that could represent co-triggers, which need to be addressed (see Chap. 6, Sect. 6.3). Drug treatment or other psychotherapeutic measures are only rarely necessary in childhood (Fricke-Oekermann and Lehmkuhl 2008).

Parental fears and anxieties should be dealt with sensitively in dialogue with the parents. Parents often equate the alarming symptoms of sleep terror with "a serious disease"; hence they are sometimes only able to accept reassurance about the harmlessness of the disorder after a thorough diagnostic workup for somatic disorders accompanied by negative organic findings.

Nightmaress are as normal in childhood as dreaming about pleasant things. Thus, dreaming anxiety-provoking dreams does not per se represent a psychological disorder (Largo 2001). Intervention only becomes necessary when nightmares occur frequently (several times a week) over an extended period of time, and the child also seems to be anxious during the daytime as a result of what it experiences at night. Parent counseling on the significance of nightmares from a developmental psychology perspective and an infant's individual need to process experiences in their sleep can promote parental insight and relief. Dealing with developmental experiences of separation and creating a balance between aspirations for autonomy and the desire for dependence can trigger anxiety in an infant, anxiety that finds expression in nightmares, for instance. This important developmental task at the infant stage requires the parents to ensure that their infant experiences a sufficient sense of closeness and security on the one hand, while granting ample room for its need for autonomy on the other (Largo 2001). It may be necessary within the psychotherapy setting to address parents' autonomy-related issues, issues that interfere with their support of their infant's development (see Chap. 6, Sect. 6.3).

4.8 Pitfalls in Practice

Providing information on the symptoms, diagnosis, and treatment of sleep disorders in adults is contraindicated on the basis of particular development-related features. If developmental parameters are not taken into consideration in the diagnosis of and intervention for early childhood sleep initiation and maintenance disorders and parasomnias, intervention may not only fail but in fact aggravate symptoms. By way of example, the reader is referred to the attempts to "build-up sleep pressure in a young infant." Parents that receive this erroneous advice often report an escalating vicious circle. Moreover, children do not necessarily exhibit the "preoccupation with their sleep deficit" that is diagnostically relevant in adults, or their actual suffering from sleep deprivation in a clearly identifiable manner (Fricke-Oekermann and Lehmkuhl 2007). They appear, for instance, vaguely ill-tempered, cranky, sensitive, discontent, fussy, lethargic, or prone to particular motor restlessness. The task of interpreting these behaviors as signs of sleep deficit lies initially with the parents, who use them to "flag" their child's state.

In counseling and psychotherapeutic practice, the competencies and resources available to parents need to be included in intervention planning. A modification in infant sleep behavior can only be achieved by modifying the approach and attitude of the parents. Thus, strong and justifiable emphasis is placed at times on parental emotions, attitudes, and experiences. Paying too little attention to the strain and stress on parents jeopardizes interventions that need to be implemented and supported by parents at home and may destabilize the family system further.

Specific features in the infant also influence the success of treatment. Children's responses to interventions vary greatly depending on temperament, actual developmental age, and physical health. For this reason, a tailored approach is crucial. Not all children can learn the art of sleep in the same way and at the same time, but rather each does so at its own pace and by deploying its own skills.

4.9 Conclusion

The early identification of sleep initiation and maintenance disorders and parasomnias in infancy can help prevent a chronically unfavorable course of development. Informing parents on infant sleep behavior and their infant's specific sleep disorder, while taking age and developmental stage into account, can provide initial relief to the overall situation and promote an understanding of the issues at hand. The inclusion of developmental parameters is highly relevant in both diagnostic workup and intervention.

References

Barth R (1999) Schlafstörungen im Kontext der Autonomieentwicklung. Monatsschr Kinderheilkunde 147:488–492

Borébly AA (1982) A two process model of sleep regulation. Hum Neurobiol 1:195–204

Cierpka M (ed) (2012) Frühe Kindheit 0–3 Jahre. Springer, Heidelberg

Deutsche Gesellschaft für Kinder- und Jugendpsychiatrie und Psychotherapie u. a. (Hrsg) (2007) Leitlinien zur Diagnostik und Therapie von psychischen Störungen im Säuglings-, Kindes- und Jugendalter. Deutscher Ärzte Verlag. 3. überarbeitete Auflage. Online unter http://www.awmf.org/uploads/tx_szleitlinien/028-028_S1_Regulationsstoerungen_im_Saeuglingsalter__u.a._F98.2__11-2006_11-2011.pdf

Dilling H, Mombour W, Schmidt MH (2008) Internationale Klassifikation psychischer Störungen. ICD-10 Kapitel V (F). Huber, Bern

Ferber R (1985) Solve your child's sleep problems. Simon and Schuster, New York

Fonagy P, Gergely G, Jurist EL, Target M (2004) Affektregulierung, Mentalisierung und die Entwicklung des Selbst. Klett-Cotta, Stuttgart

Fraiberg S, Adelson E, Shapiro V (1975) Ghosts in the nursery. A psychoanalytical approach to the problems of impaired infant-mother relationships. J Am Acad Child Psychiatr 14:387–421

Fricke-Oekermann L, Lehmkuhl G (2007) Nichtorganische Schlafstörungen im Kindesalter. Monatsschr Kinderheilkd 7:616–623

Fricke-Oekermann L, Lehmkuhl G (2008) Schlafstörungen. Interior coil Petermann F (Hrsg) Lehrbuch der klinischen Kinderpsychologie. Hogrefe Verlag, Göttingen, pp S603–S620

Iglowstein I, Jenni OG, Molinari L, Largo RL (2003) Sleep duration from Infancy to adolescence: reference values and generational trends. Pediatrics 111:302–307

Jenni OG (2009) Säuglingsschreien und Schlaf-Wach-regulation. Monatsschr Kinderheilkd 157:551–557

Jenni OG, Benz C, Largo RH (2008) Schlafstörungen in den ersten beiden Lebensjahren. Interior coil Borke J, Eickhorst A (Hrsg) Systemische Entwicklungsberatung in der frühen Kindheit. Facultas, Wien, pp S164–S188

Kast-Zahn A, Morgenroth H (1995) Jedes Kind kann schlafen lernen: Vom Baby bis zum Schulkind: Wie sie Schlafprobleme ihres Kindes vermeiden und lösen können. ObersteBrink-Verlag, Ratingen

Largo RH (2001) Babyjahre. Piper, München

Louis J, Cannard C, Bastuji H, Challamel J (1997) Sleep ontogenesis revisited: a longitudinal 24-hour home polygraphic study on 15 normal infants during the first two years of life. Sleep 20:323–333

Nolte N, Pott W, Pauli-Pott U (2006) Schlafstörungen und Bindungsqualität im Kleinkindalter. Psychother Psychosom Med Psychol 56:154–161

Papoušek M (2007) Frühkindliche Regulationsstörungen. In: Mattejat F (Hrsg), Lehrbuch der Psychotherapie vol. 4: Verhaltenstherapie mit Kindern, Jugendlichen und ihren Familien. CIP-Medien, München, pp S407–S420

Papoušek M, Rothenburg S, Cierpka M, von Hofacker N (2006) Regulationsstörungen in der frühen Kindheit. CD-basierte Fortbildung. Stiftung Kindergesundheit

Schieche M, Rupprecht C, Papoušek M (2004) Schlafstörungen: aktuelle Ergebnisse und klinische Erfahrungen. Interior coil Papoušek M, Schieche M, Wurmser H (Hrsg) Regulationsstörungen der frühen Kindheit. Huber, Bern, pp S145–S170

Schramm E, Riemann D (1995) ICSD—Internationale Klassifikation der Schlafstörungen. PVU-Beltz, Weinheim

Vella S (2003) Abklärungen von Schlafstörungen im Kindes- und Jugendalter und der Stellenwert der Polysomnographie. Paediatrica 3:49–54

Winnicott D (1951) Übergangsobjekte und Übergangsphänomene. In: Winnicott D (Hrsg) (1974) Von der Kinderheilkunde zur Psychoanalyse. München, Kindler

Wolke D, Meyer R, Orth B, Riegel K (1994) Häufigkeit und Persistenz von Ein- und Durchschlafproblemen im Vorschulalter: Ergebnisse einer prospektiven Untersuchung an einer repräsentativen Stichprobe in Bayern. Prax Kinderpsychol Kinderpsychiatr 43:331–339

Ziegler M, Wollwerth de Chuquisengo R, Papoušek M (2004) Exzessives Schreien im frühen Säuglingsalter. Interior coil Papoušek M, Schieche M, Wurmser H (Hrsg) Regulationsstörungen der frühen Kindheit. Huber, Bern, pp S111–S144

Feeding Disorders in Infants and Young Children

5

Consolata Thiel-Bonney and Nikolaus von Hofacker

5.1 Drinking, Eating, and Feeding: Developing Eating Skills in a Social Context

Eating and drinking represent basic human biological needs and are essential for survival. In addition to this, however, children and parents require fulfilling emotional and social experiences in dialogue with one another, in mutual play, as well as in feeding and being fed in order to get to know one other, experience a sense of satisfaction and competence, consolidate their relationship, and enjoy physical/mental well-being in a context of positive reciprocity.

A healthy neonate is capable of signaling hunger and satiation and of independently regulating the quantities of food and drink it consumes (Papoušek 2002). In its further development, the infant is able to adjust to new tastes, different consistencies and textures, and to master the transition from drinking to spoon-feeding. Exploiting particularly sensitive time windows, e.g., between the ages of 4 and 8 months, for the introduction of new tastes and textures, makes this developmental task easier to accomplish. In addition to hunger, thirst, and appetite, which all play an important role in intrinsically motivating the infant to eat, the infant also has a need to actively participate in feeding interaction and, ultimately, to eat independently. The parents support their infant here on a regulatory level, offering food in a manner intuitively attuned to its hunger and satiation signals, as well as its motor, cognitive, and socioemotional skills (Papoušek 2002).

C. Thiel-Bonney, M.D. (✉)
Center for Children, Adolescents and Families, Hospital Hochried,
Hochried 1-12, Murnau 82418, Germany
e-mail: cthiel-bonney@gmx.de

N. von Hofacker, M.D.
Private Practice for Infant, Child and Adolescent Psychiatry,
August-Exter-Straße 4, München 81245, Germany
e-mail: hofacker@ae-4.de

M. Cierpka (ed.), *Regulatory Disorders in Infants*,
DOI 10.1007/978-3-319-43556-5_5

Table 5.1 Early childhood developmental tasks in the feeding and eating context

Age	Food	Developmental and adjustment task
1–3 Months	Breastfeeding/bottle-feeding	Sucking (breast/bottle), hunger and satiation rhythm
3–6 Months	Bottle-feeding, initiation of pureed food	Transition to bottle-feeding, more intense sucking, adjustment to spoon-feeding
6 Months–1 year	Spoon-feeding, pieces increase in size, coarse and easy to handle	New tastes, consistencies, and textures, increasingly in a sitting position
2 Years	Food coarsely chopped and cut small, raw fruit and vegetables, followed by regular mealtimes at table; drinking from a cup	Independent eating and drinking
3 Years	Solid food diet	Increasing adoption of family and cultural conventions

Infant developmental tasks in the feeding context are summarized in Table 5.1 (for a differentiated overview, see Papoušek et al. 2004; Wolke 2005; van den Engel-Hoek 2008). A complex and coordinated interplay between a variety of somatopsychological and interactional processes underlies unencumbered food intake. Recently published recommendations aim to support parents and physicians in this process (Koletzko et al. 2013), and provide a compass for parents to navigate their way through the jungle of contradictory messages transmitted by a wide variety of media. Adjustment problems are often encountered when tackling the developmental tasks list below. If the parents and infant fail to accomplish these tasks together, deep-seated parental insecurity and anxieties may ensue, often prompting the parents to seek medical advice.

5.2 Definition and Symptom Triad of a Feeding Disorder

Definition of a Feeding Disorder

According to the Guidelines, a Feeding Disorder Exists When:

- The disorder has persisted for at least 1 month and feeding interaction is perceived as problematic and stressful by the parents
- Individual mealtimes last on average longer than 45 min and/or
- The interval between mealtimes is less than 2 h

A feeding disorder may be associated with a failure to thrive, which is characterized by the following criteria according to the specialist guidelines (von Hofacker et al., 2004; GPGE 2007):

Definition of Failure to Thrive

- For infants with a birth weight ≥3rd percentile:
  - Weight loss < 3rd percentile and/or
  - A change of more than two percentile curves due to weight loss or stagnation over a period of at least 2 respectively 3 months (child aged ≤6 months or >6 months)
- For infants with a birth weight <3rd percentile:
  - Any failure to gain weight over at least 1 month
  - Low weight for length

Failure to gain weight or weight loss generally lead to a growth disorder.

The high rate of "comorbidity" between organic risk factors and problems in feeding interaction indicate from the outset a complex interplay between somatic, psychosocial, and interactional aspects in the development of feeding disorders. Therefore, the distinction between organic and non-organic feeding disorders and failure to thrive is no longer valid (Benoit 2000; Papoušek 2002; von Hofacker et al., 2004; Wolke 2005; Bryant-Waugh et al. 2010). Feeding disorders cannot be viewed in isolation from the relational context in which they develop. Like other early childhood regulatory disorders (see also ► Chaps. 1, 3, 4, and 8, this volume), they are characterized by a *triad of symptoms* (Papoušek et al. 2004; von Hofacker et al. 2007):

Triad of Symptoms in Feeding Disorders

- Impaired development of infant regulatory skills in the feeding context and in eating/drinking behavior.
- Dysfunctional interactional and communication patterns between parents and infant in the feeding context; impaired parental co-regulatory support.
- Parental overload syndrome with strained or impaired parent–infant relationship.

The multifactorial genesis of feeding problems makes an interdisciplinary collaboration in their diagnostic workup and treatment essential.

5.2.1 Disorder of Infant Behavioral Regulation in the Feeding Context

Many infants and toddlers with feeding problems transmit unclear signals of hunger and satiation, thereby hampering communication in the feeding context (Lindberg et al. 1996). The infants appear not to be hungry, turn their heads away, spit their food out, or passively refuse to eat. Some children resist sitting at the table, are very easily distracted, and stop eating upon any form of interesting external stimulation; others will allow themselves to be fed only when distraction is offered. Some children exhibit extremely fussy eating behavior (Jacobi et al. 2003; Papoušek et al. 2004; Zero To Three 2005), while others put up fierce and anxious resistance to stimulation in the orofacial or pharyngeal area, or indeed upon catching sight of their bottle or plate even before mealtimes.

In addition to feeding problems, particularly young infants often exhibit other regulatory problems (► Chap. 3, this volume), which hamper eating and the introduction of an appropriate sleep/mealtime/play rhythm. In desperation, parents resort to breastfeeding at night or feeding their infant while it dozes.

5.2.2 Dysfunctional Interaction

Parents of children that eat poorly quickly find themselves under immense emotional pressure—after all, they are the "guarantors" for their infant's nutrition and thriving. If an infant does not eat adequately at mealtimes, the parents often feed it again after a short interval for fear it could lose weight. Mealtimes become longer, are filled with tension, and it is not uncommon for infants to be fed by force or by using pressure in order to achieve sufficient caloric intake. Soon, "eating" becomes the overriding theme in the family—happy, playful interaction becomes a rarity. One father described how he perceived his child as "nothing more than a stomach." It becomes increasingly difficult for parents to create a pleasant atmosphere during mealtimes and to give their infant positive feedback when, e.g., it signals hunger, interest in its food, or a desire to eat. Motivating an infant to eat by, e.g., distracting it with opportunities to play, can have the effect of making refusal to eat particularly "interesting" for the infant (Lindberg et al. 2006; Papoušek et al. 2004). In a strained context of this kind, the infant increasingly resists its parents' control of and restrictions on its need for self-regulation in eating. Social togetherness descends into a cycle of negative reciprocity (see also Ammaniti et al. 2004).

5.2.3 Parental Overload Syndrome

Particularly mothers of children with feeding problems soon see themselves questioned in their primordial role as their infant's "nurturer" and the person responsible for its survival (see also *"The Motherhood Constellation,"* Stern 1998). Moreover, in cases where the infant's survival was or is threatened by premature birth, disease, or disability, parents may experience greater anxiety in the context of feeding interaction from the very outset. They feel exhausted and held—helpless and powerless—at the mercy of their infant's refusal to eat. Wounded self-esteem, depression, and/or fierce conflicts of ambivalence involving feelings of guilt and angry/aggressive impulses may ensue.

5.3 Prevalence, Course, and Prognosis

Transient feeding problems are common in the development of healthy infants, being reported by approximately a third of parents in the first year of life (Forsyth and Canny 1991). Mild to moderate feeding disorders, on the other hand, are seen in 20–25 % of children in the first years of life (Fergusson et al. 1985; Wright et al. 2007), while severe feeding disorders affect significantly fewer children (3–12 %). The prevalence of failure to thrive is around 3–4 %; it was 7 % in a population covered by the Munich Program for Fussy Babies (von Hofacker et al., 2004). Between 35 and 80 % of infants with developmental disorders are affected by feeding disorders (Burklow et al. 1998).

Feeding disorders and failure to thrive exhibit a significant rate of persistence into school age (Dahl et al. 1994; Wolke et al. 1990; McDermott et al. 2008). At the same time, failure to thrive in particular is associated with risks to a child's health development and longitudinal growth (Dahl 1987; Benoit 2000; Lindberg et al. 2006; Wright et al. 2007). Findings on cognitive development in feeding disorders without failure to thrive are less homogeneous (Wolke et al. 1990; Drewett et al. 1999; Benoit 2000; Chatoor et al. 2004); a recent investigation by Wolke et al. (2009) found crying and feeding problems to have a slight yet significant effect on cognitive development in at-risk preschool infants. Children's socioemotional development appears to be strained in all forms of feeding disorders, with an increased rate of infant behavioral problems, including most notably hyperactive and anxious/depressive symptoms (Dahl 1987; Dahl and Sundelin 1992; Burklow et al. 1998; Wolke 2005; McDermott et al. 2008).

5.4 Risk Factors for the Development of Feeding Disorders

Systemic and multifactorial perspectives on the development of feeding problems are gaining acceptance in research efforts and in the literature. Feeding disorders and failure to thrive occur in a complex interplay between multiple organic, psychosocial, parental, and infant factors (Papoušek et al. 2004) and can be understood in terms of a biopsychosocial cycle of negative reciprocity .

5.4.1 Organic Risk Factors

In population samples, organic disease is found to be the sole cause of feeding disorders in less than 10 % of cases (Sect. 5.2; Drewett et al. 2002; Wolke 2005). The rate of medical risk factors in clinical samples is 25–80 %, depending on the population investigated (Benoit 2000; Rommel et al. 2003). All diseases associated with chronic loss of appetite, vomiting, as well as impaired food intake and digestion can be directly related to feeding problems (Papoušek 2002; von Hofacker 2014). Even in primarily healthy feeding-disordered infants and young children, mild, transient neurological abnormalities that possibly hamper a child's food intake are seen at a rate of 43 % (von Hofacker et al., 2004). Children with feeding problems are more likely to have a low birth weight (Unlü et al. 2008). Given the high survival rate among extremely premature infants, it is important to remain vigilant of oral-motor and sensory problems, as well as impaired coordination of sucking/swallowing/breathing (Mathisen et al. 1989; von Hofacker et al., 2004; Papoušek et al. 2004; Arvedson 2008).

At over a third, preterm infants and underweight or immature infants are already overrepresented in the group of feeding-disordered infants (Hawdon et al. 2000; Rommel et al. 2003; Thiel-Bonney 2006). Preterm infants attended the Heidelberg parent–infant/toddler outpatient clinic (Cierpka 2012, Chap. 30) due to feeding problems significantly more often compared with their full-term counterparts. Thus, the relative risk of requiring recourse to counseling rises with decreasing birth weight. Preterm infants with low to extremely low birth weight are at particular risk of developing a feeding disorder (Erb et al. 2014).

Sensory problems can influence food acceptance and hamper infants in their transition to new tastes and textures. Studies have shown that some adults (the so-called "supertasters") experience taste far more intensely than others—the density of their lingual papillae is significantly greater (von Hofacker et al., 2004; Chatoor 2012).

In cases where physical examination yields no indication of an organic cause, the likelihood of more invasive investigations doing so is extremely remote (von Hofacker et al., 2004). Therefore, invasive investigations should be approached with caution, not least to protect the infant from experiencing further aversive oral stimulation.

5.4.2 Problems of Behavioral Regulation and Temperament Factors

Additionally, associated regulatory problems are often more relevant than organic causal factors (Miller-Loncar et al. 2004; von Hofacker et al., 2004; Wolke 2005; von Kries et al. 2006). In a sample from the Munich Program for Fussy Babies, feeding disorders were very often related to other regulatory problems (e.g., sleep problems, excessive crying and defiance, dysphoric fussiness, aggressive behaviors) (von Hofacker et al., 2004).

Moreover, the infant's temperament has a crucial effect on its behavior in the feeding context. "Difficult" temperament traits, such as fussiness/being difficult, unpredictability, poor ability to adjust, irritability, stubbornness, poor consolability (von Hofacker et al., 2004), and negative affectivity ("mealtime negativity"; Farrow and Blissett 2006b) hamper the infant in its adjustment to new tastes and textures and make it difficult for parents to give their infant appropriate support in the feeding situation. At the same time, infant temperament traits and parental interactive behavior often interact with each other (Wolke et al. 1990; Hagekull et al. 1997).

5.4.3 Traumatic Early Childhood Experiences

The previous history of feedings disorders and failure to thrive often includes traumatic experiences in infancy in the face, mouth, throat, and gastrointestinal tract, e.g., in the context of intensive care, medical interventions, surgical procedures, and examinations, as well as diseases associated with pain (e.g., gastroesophageal reflux). A traumatic experience related to swallowing and a resultant fear of choking (Chatoor et al. 1988) or, unfortunately all too often, the use of force during feeding (restraining the infant, opening its mouth with force, feeding despite crying) can have the effect that all food intake is associated with the fear of repeated aversive stimulation. As a result, the infant exhibits anxious to phobic resistance to all contact and stimulation in the orofacial and pharyngeal region and refuses to eat or swallow food (Chatoor et al. 2001). A "posttraumatic feeding disorder" develops.

5.4.4 Parental and Familial Risk Factors

Contrary to earlier research, there appears to be virtually no relationship between sociodemographic factors, such as social class, socioeconomic status, gender, education, parent age, and number of siblings, and feeding disorders (Wolke 2005; Wright et al. 2007). Having said that, a subgroup of families with multiple psychosocial risk factors and dysfunctional family relational patterns has been identified in clinical samples of children with severe failure to thrive (Benoit 2000; Papoušek et al. 2004). However, failure to thrive as a direct manifestation of emotional deprivation and neglect is seen in only 9 % of cases (Wolke 2005).

Parental, biological, and psychosocial risk factors are closely interlinked with infant risk factors. Data from the Munich Program for Fussy Babies reveal a high rate of prenatal, perinatal, and postnatal risk factors that can negatively impact intuitive parenting skills in the feeding context and infant self-regulation (von Hofacker et al., 2004; Papoušek et al. 2004).

Psychosocial maternal and parental risk factors before and after birth, such as depression, anxiety, and marital conflicts, were observed significantly more frequently in the setting of childhood feeding disorders in the first 3 years of life (von Hofacker et al., 2004; Wright et al. 2006), whereby parental psychological risk factors evidently influence the perception of feeding problems (McDermott et al. 2008).

Furthermore, recent studies have emphasized the relationship between maternal eating disorders and early childhood feeding problems, and even low body weight already at birth (Sollid et al. 2004; Blissett et al. 2005; Blissett and Meyer 2006; Micali et al. 2009): feeding interaction is often characterized by more conflict at mealtimes if mothers are themselves eating-disordered. Mothers exhibit difficulties recognizing their infant's signals at mealtimes and responding to these appropriately, making them less able to support their infant's need for autonomy during mealtimes. Controlling and intrusive behaviors, as well as negative emotionality are more frequently observed in the feeding context (Stein et al. 1994; Stein et al. 1999), which interferes negatively with the infant's need to self-regulate its feeding behavior (Farrow and Blissett 2006a, 2008; Scaglioni et al. 2008; Haycraft and Blissett 2008; Reba-Harrelson et al. 2010). Overall, early childhood conflicts at mealtimes appear to represent risk factors more for the development of nonspecific eating disorders in adolescence and early adulthood, while indicators pointing to the development of specific eating disorders (anorexia, bulimia) are currently lacking (Kotler et al. 2001; see also Cooper et al. 2004).

5.4.5 Feeding Disorders and Attachment

Feeding disorders, particularly when associated with failure to thrive, may strain the relationship between infant and parents to a considerably greater extent than excessive crying or severe sleeping problems. Conversely, parental problems in developing and structuring a positive relationship (also in the sense of "bonding") with their infant can negatively affect infant eating behavior. A strained parent–infant relationship in the context of a feeding disorder can compromise infant bonding (Brinich et al. 1989; Chatoor et al. 1998; Ward et al. 2000; Papoušek et al. 2004).

5.5 Diagnostic Workup

The somatic and psychosocial diagnostic workup should be embedded in an integrative and interdisciplinary process from the outset. Only in this way is it possible to adequately assess the complex interplay between somatic, psychosocial, interactional, and relational factors at play in a feeding disorder.

5.5.1 Diagnostic Classification According to the ICD-10, DSM-V, and DC: 0-3R

Professional and standardized criteria for the diagnosis of feeding disorders are still lacking (Papoušek et al. 2004). Although the diagnostic classification system developed for the first 3 years of life, DC: 0-3R, classifies feeding disorders into subgroups on the basis of preset criteria, it has not yet received full international acceptance. "Feeding disorder" is the only regulatory disorder of early childhood to be included in the ICD-10 (Dilling et al. 2010) and DSM-V diagnostic systems (see box for overview). The complexity of the disorder is only poorly reflected in the ICD-10 classification, whereas the DSM-V, although attempting a more specific formulation and suggesting classification into subgroups, fails to go further than the DC: 0-3R in terms of criteria-based differentiation.

5.5.2 Feeding Disorder in the DC: 0–3R (Zero To Three 2005)

In light of their long-standing research activities and extensive therapeutic experience, the working group directed by Irene Chatoor (2012) incorporated their differentiated classification system of early childhood "feeding behavior disorder" in the diagnostic classification 0–3R of the working group "Zero To Three" as early as 2005 (Zero To Three 2005). The subgroups shown in the box come under Axis I, "clinical disorders." The introduction of Axis II for the classification of parent–infant relationships meant that the classification scheme was able to take the developmental factors of the first years of life into particular account (von Hofacker et al., 2004). Axes III–V are concerned exclusively with medical conditions/specific developmental disorders, psychosocial risk factors, and emotional and social functioning (see Chap. 1).

Feeding Disorder According to the Diagnostic Classification DC:0–3R (Zero To Three 2005)

- Axis I Feeding disorders, 600 et seq.

601. Feeding Disorder of Homeostatic Regulation
- Onset in neonatal age.
- Difficulties in the infant to achieve or maintain a quiet, well-balanced waking state during feeding (regulatory disorder).
- The infant gains too little, or loses, weight.

602. Feeding Disorder of Caregiver–Infant Reciprocity
- Onset generally between the ages of 2–8 months.
- Lack of social reciprocity with the caregiver (e.g., eye contact, smiling, vocalization); often a sign of neglect.
- Failure to thrive.
- Poor relatedness and failure to thrive cannot be attributed to a physical disease or deep-seated developmental disorder alone.
- Often seen in conjunction with maternal/parental mental illness, poverty, alcohol or drug abuse, neglect, and abuse.

603. Infantile Anorexia
- Onset before the age of 3 years, usually between 8 and 18 months during the transition from bottle-feeding to spoon-feeding and when learning to eat independently.
- Duration of at least 1 month.
- The infant displays virtually no signs of hunger or interest in food, yet shows great interest in exploration and/or interaction with the caregiver.

(continued)

- A marked deficit in thriving/growth is present.
- There is no temporal relationship between food refusal and a traumatic event, nor is refusal the result of a medical disease.

This feeding disorder corresponds to the "restrictive" subgroup in the DSM-V category "avoidant/restrictive food intake disorder."

604. Sensory Food Aversion

- The infant consistently refuses certain foods on the basis of consistency, taste, texture, and/or smell.
- Refusal begins during the introduction of a new food.
- When offered its preferred food, the infant eats without protest.
- Nutritional deficits or delayed oral-motor and speech development may occur.
- Failure to thrive is not usually seen.

This feeding disorder corresponds to the "avoidant" subgroup in the DSM-V category "avoidant/restrictive food intake disorder."

605. Feeding Disorder Associated with Somatic Disease

- Although the infant begins mealtimes willingly, it shows ever greater signs of stress in the further course of eating, ultimately refusing further food intake.
- A concurrent medical disease to which the feeding problems can be attributed is present.
- Medical treatment improves the feeding difficulties, yet is not able to fully resolve the problem.
- The infant's weight gain is insufficient or it loses weight.

606. Posttraumatic Feeding Disorder (PTFD)

- Food refusal follows a significant aversive experience or repeated interventions in the oropharyngeal region or gastrointestinal tract responsible for causing the infant to experience intense stress.
- Onset can be at any age.
- Recalling the traumatic event is stressful for the infant and triggers anticipatory anxiety reactions, for instance when the child is placed in a feeding position. Resistive behavior increases at the sight of food and the infant shows considerable opposition to swallowing the food placed in its mouth. It avoids, e.g., all oral or solid food, will only be bottle-fed while asleep, or does not bottle-feed at all but does accept spoon-feeding.
- Food refusal represents an acute or long-term threat to the infant's health, nutritional status, and growth, as well as impairment to its (oral-motor) feeding development.

Although the classification of eating behavior disorders in the DC:0–3R is the subject of controversy in German-speaking countries (Kroll 2011), it is enjoying increasing popularity and application in the wake of a number of training workshops held by Chatoor, as well as the translation of her book (Chatoor 2012), due to its good clinical practicability. Chatoor's observations, however, are confined to a particular clinical setting and the proposed subgroups, treatment programs, and results have not undergone sufficient empirical validation (Bryant-Waugh and Lask; von Hofacker et al., 2004; von Gontard 2010).

Feeding Disorder in Early Childhood According to ICD-10 (F98.2) (Dilling et al. 2010)

According to the ICD-10, this is a specific early-childhood feeding disorder with a variety of manifestations. The disorder includes food refusal and extremely selective eating behavior in the setting of:

- Adequate food supply.
- A reasonably competent caregiver.
- Absence of organic disease.

The feeding disorder may be accompanied by rumination. Since minor feeding difficulties in early childhood are extremely widespread, a disorder should only be diagnosed if:

- **Its extent clearly lies outside the normal range.**
- **The feeding problem is qualitatively abnormal.**
- **The infant fails to gain weight or loses weight over a period of at least 1 month.**

Factors Requiring Exclusion Include

- Situations in which the infant accepts food without protest from adults that are not its usual caregivers.
- Organic disease that can plausibly explain food refusal.
- Broader psychiatric disorders.
- Feeding difficulties in the context of errors in care.
- Feeding problems in neonates.

The ICD-10 exhibits manifold flaws and inaccuracies, e.g., the question of how one should define a "reasonably competent caregiver." A number of the problems in this definition were avoided in the DSM-V, e.g., the categorical exclusion of organic or psychiatric disease; moreover, the presence of failure to thrive is not mandatory—"marked interference with psychosocial functioning" is adequate. It is hoped that the ICD-11 will further develop and differentiate the criteria established in DSM-V.

Feeding Disorder in Infants and Toddlers According to DSM-V (APA 2013)

According to the DSM-V, feeding and eating disorders in infants and toddlers fall under category 307.59, "avoidant restrictive food intake disorder." However, a prerequisite here is that the feeding and eating disorder is not part of a medical or psychiatric disease classifiable elsewhere. Where this is the case, the primary diagnosis should be classified, unless the feeding disorder is so severe that it requires treatment as a discrete and specific disorder alongside the primary diagnosis (see below). Avoidant restrictive food intake disorder is defined as followed:

(a) Failure to meet appropriate nutritional and/or energy needs associated with one (or more) of the following:
  - Significant weight loss (or failure to achieve expected weight or longitudinal growth).
  - Significant nutritional deficiency.
  - Tube feeding.
  - Marked impairment to psychosocial functioning.

(b) The disturbance is not better explained by a lack of available food or by an associated culturally sanctioned practice.

(c) The eating disturbance does not occur exclusively in conjunction with anorexia nervosa or bulimia nervosa, and there is no evidence of a body image disturbance.

(d) When associated with concomitant medical or psychiatric disease, the severity of the disorder must be sufficiently severe to warrant treatment as a separate entity.

Criterion A explicitly states that only one of the four diagnostic sub-criteria listed, hence also a "marked interference with psychosocial functioning" alone, i.e., in the absence of concomitant failure to thrive, is sufficient to meet this criterion. This represents a definite improvement on ICD-10. The term "avoidant restrictive feeding and eating disorder" is aimed at three essential subgroups of feeding and eating disorders that have been similarly described, albeit using different terms, both in the DC: 0-3R for infants and toddlers and by the English working group under Rachel Bryant-Waugh et al. (2010) for children. One subgroup includes children that eat too little ("infantile anorexia/DC: 0-3R," "restrictive eating disorder"/Bryant-Waugh et al. 2010); a second subgroup relates to children that, while they eat enough, eat highly selectively ("sensory food aversion"/DC: 0-3R, "selective feeding disorder"/Bryant-Waugh et al. 2010); while a third subgroup develops a conditioned, anxious aversion on the basis of aversive experiences ("posttraumatic feeding disorder/DC: 0-3R," "conditioned dysphagia"/Bryant-Waugh et al. 2010). All three subgroups fall under the category "avoidant restrictive food intake disorder" in DSM-V. Although, unlike DC: 0-3R (Zero To Three 2005), the DSM-V makes no detailed differentiation into subgroups, it does explicitly include, under the sections "diagnostic criteria" and "development and course," infants that correspond to the "feeding disorder of state regulation" and the "feeding disorder of caregiver–infant reciprocity" in DC: 0-3R. Thus, with the exception of feeding disorders in the context of an underlying medical disease, which, according to the DSM-V criteria should be classified elsewhere, all five feeding disorders in the DC: 0-3 R have been included in the 307.59 category of the DSM-V.

Since "the feeding of young children is fundamentally a relational and multisystemic process," Davies and colleagues (2006) propose criteria for a "feeding disorder between parent and child" that encompasses the entire complexity of the feeding disorder from the outset. Thus, a multiaxial diagnostic workup should consider the following in equal measure: infant factors (medical, developmental, and behavioral characteristics), parental factors, the parent–child relationship, as well as the social and nutritional context of feeding.

5.5.3 Diagnostic Steps in the Feeding Context

The guideline-based diagnostic workup (von Hofacker et al., 2004; see also von Hofacker 2009) includes:

- Taking a disease-specific patient history of symptoms relating to each of the following:
  - Infant and parents.
  - Interaction and relationship.
  - Family/infant environment.
- (Video-supported) behavioral observation and analysis of feeding interaction, as well as other interactive contexts.
- Behavior protocols and diaries (e.g., crying, feeding, sleeping diary (see ► Chap. 1).
- Symptom-specific questionnaires, e.g.,
  - Questionnaire on crying, feeding, and sleeping (Groß et al. 2007).
  - Questionnaire on previous eating and feeding history (von Hofacker 2002).
  - Patient history questionnaire on early childhood feeding disorder and weaning from tube feeding (Wilken and Jotzo 2009).
- Parent questionnaire on:
  - Infant behavior (e.g., Child Behavior Checklist 1½–5; Achenbach and Rescorla 2000).
  - Infant temperament (e.g., ICQ, Bates, Freeland and Lounsbury 1979).
  - Parental stress (e.g., Parenting Stress Index, Abidin 1983).
- Structured assessment of the parent–infant relationship (e.g., Parent-Infant Relationship Global Assessment Scale (PIR-GAS) in the DC:0–3R (Zero To Three 2005).

In order to identify functional and dysfunctional patterns and to provide parents with as concrete advice as possible, it is particularly important to observe a feeding and

Table 5.2 Assessment of feeding interaction and assessment of infant behavior, parental behavior, and interactional and relational characteristics

Infant behavior	Parental behavior	Interactional and relational characteristics
– Mood – Eating/feeding skills (sucking activity, chewing, swallowing) – Signs of interest in active, independent participation – Clarity of infant signals of appetite, hunger, thirst, satiation – Indication of particular sensory features, selective food aversion – Distractibility, anxious aversion, provocative, defiant behaviors	– Positioning of infant and caregiver – Prevailing mood of the caregiver(s) – Mealtime structure and clarity of beginning, end, and boundaries – Responsivity to functional vs. dysfunctional infant behaviors – Positive/negative verbal and nonverbal support and feedback given to the infant; consistency of the messages conveyed – Type and appropriateness of motivational support, distraction vs. control, pressure, force – Support for infant autonomy and self-regulation during food intake – Extent to which parent(s) serve as a model	– Successful sequences of positive reciprocity, successful feeding behavior adapted to infant signals and needs – Dysfunctional, inappropriate interaction patterns – Extent of tension, conflicts, and power play during the meal – Indications of inconsistent behavior patterns on the couple level; couple conflicts

eating disorder and, where possible, make a video recording of the feeding situation; this can subsequently be discussed with the parents in a resource-oriented manner (see also ► Chap. 10). The simplest approach here is to ask the parents to film—using either a camera or smartphone—the feeding and eating situation at home (home video), preferably during a family mealtime, and bring this with them to their appointment. The feeding and eating situation is then analyzed on the level of the triad comprising infant, parent, and interaction (Papoušek et al. 2004; von Hofacker et al., 2004; Table 5.2).

The severity of a feeding disorder (von Hofacker et al., 2004; Papoušek et al. 2004) is measured according to the following:

- The duration of the feeding problem.
- The extent to which regulatory problems are generalized and pervasive (e.g., in conjunction with excessive crying, defiant behavior, and sleeping problems).
- The level of impairment to the infant's somatic (failure to thrive), mental, psychosocial, and speech development, as well as to its ability to accomplish developmental tasks.
- The extent of strain on the parent–infant relationship.

5.6 Counseling and Therapy

Therapy for early childhood eating disorders can only succeed in the context of a viable relationship between the parents and the therapist(s). Prior to the initial therapeutic contact, the family has often followed a tortuous path through a variety of institutions, which has served to deepen their sense of insecurity and guilt.

The mother of a feeding-disordered infant reported: "We've already been everywhere, but the doctors couldn't find an organic problem. Now they've sent us to you, saying that our 18-month-old son's eating problem is definitely psychological. Since I'm the one who's generally responsible for meals, I suppose I've been doing everything wrong. I feel as if it's my fault that he doesn't eat. We are at out wits' end!"

Any counseling and therapeutic concept should include somatic, developmental, and behavioral interventions, as well as a consideration of psychodynamic and family-centered aspects. Bolstered by an understanding and respectful attitude from the therapist(s), the parents feel that not only their fears, but also the skills they deploy in their efforts for their infant, are acknowledged and appreciated. This is the only way to afford parents the freedom to articulate the feelings they sometimes have toward their infant, ranging from ambivalence to aggressive impulses, and to develop confidence in their own strengths—strengths they will need to harness in the therapeutic process.

It is common for several therapists to be involved in an infant's treatment, e.g., pediatricians, speech therapists, occupational therapists, physiotherapists, psychotherapists, and pediatric psychosomatic medicine specialists. Although it is easier to make a constellation of this kind available in the partial or full inpatient setting rather than in an outpatient setting, we also recommend establishing individual treatment "networks" in the outpatient sector to support affected families. The success of treatment crucially depends on cooperation between all parties involved in the process. Only seamless collaboration between therapists can guarantee the greatest possible level of security for the infant and its parents, who are otherwise quick to feel at the mercy of differing opinions and approaches.

The "therapeutic decision tree" (Papoušek et al. 2004) summarizes the procedures used in the counseling and therapy of feeding disorders. The therapeutic spectrum explained below covers four levels, ranging from a transient crisis in the feeding context despite sufficient infant and parental resources, to severe impairments to the parent–infant relationship.

5.6.1 Somatic Level

Underlying and concomitant somatic diseases (Sect. 5.4.1) need to be adequately taken into consideration and, where necessary, co-treated. The parents can only commit themselves emotionally to the often stressful and protracted therapeutic process when they do not have to carry the full burden of their infant's well-being alone. In this connection, we advise caution when dealing with outpatient- and in particular internet-based tube weaning programs. If infants grow/thrive adequately and develop normally, parents should receive reassurance from the treating physicians that more extensive physical examinations are not indicated (Bernard-Bonnin 2006). Nutritional counseling is helpful, particularly in the case of stagnant weight gain, to at least temporarily increase caloric intake at mealtimes (e.g., with calorie-fortified foods or high-calorie food supplements). Physiotherapy, speech therapy, and ergotherapy are indispensable in many cases, most notably in the treatment of infants with problems of (oral) sensory and motor development. However, good medical management is not always a guarantee that the feeding problem will subsequently be resolved (Bernard-Bonnin 2006; Nelson et al. 1998; Mathisen et al. 1999).

5.6.2 Developmental Level

Developmental psychological counseling aims to inform and advise parents on: the maturation and development of infant eating behavior (Sect. 5.1); the willingness to adjust to new eating habits; the significance of hunger and satiation in the regulation of food intake; qualitatively and quantitatively age-appropriate nutrition; and recognizing and responding in a developmentally appropriate manner to infant signals in the feeding context. Counseling includes discussing the developmental psychological issues faced by the infant and its parents (e.g., the infant's increased need for autonomy), how these issues are embedded in the subject of feeding, and how the parents can appropriately take them into account in the mealtime context.

Finally, a set of "eating rules" (see overview in the box below), oriented to the infant's developmental stage and individually coordinated with the parents, are introduced. These rules are aimed at permitting the infant to develop hunger- and satiation-guided self-regulation of food intake (von Hofacker et al., 2004).

Eating Rules (According to Papousek et al. 2004; von Hofacker et al., 2004; Bernand-Bonnin 2006)

- Fixed mealtimes embedded in a regular daily routine, ideally together with other family members (learning from role models, social reinforcement).
- No snacks between meals; water ad libitum—not, however, immediately before meals.
- The parents determine when, how often, and what the infant eats.
- The infant determines whether and how much it eats.
- A pleasant and relaxed atmosphere should be created during mealtimes.
- Infant hunger and satiation signals should be observed: no food without a signal from the infant!
- Small portions should be offered.

- No playing or distraction during mealtimes.
- Pressure or force should be avoided; no force-feeding.
- Interest in eating and active participation should receive positive feedback; age-appropriate increases in independent eating behavior should be supported and reinforced.
- Signs of infant avoidance, aversion, and distraction should be ignored; a break from the meal can potentially be taken until the infant shows renewed interest.
- Duration of mealtime: maximum 30 min.
- Set boundaries according to preset rules in the case of inappropriate eating behavior, e.g., by clearing away food after 10–15 min if the infant is only playing with food, or ending the mealtime if the infant throws food about in anger.
- The infant's mouth should only be wiped when the mealtime is over. Food should not be used as a reward or gift.

If the feeding disorder is associated with other regulatory problems (e.g., sleeping problems), these should be treated first or concomitantly; this often leads to an improvement in the regulation of food intake (von Hofacker et al., 2004). In the case of early regulatory disorders (e.g., in conjunction with excessive crying, increased irritability, and chronic fussiness; see also Sect. 5.4.2), parents receive support and instruction on how to soothe their infant and encourage its self-regulation (von Hofacker et al., 2004). Ideally, parents should respond to their infant's first hunger signals by feeding it in a waking and rested state in an age-appropriate position.

A 4-month-old infant was referred to an outpatient clinic for fussy babies due to a marked regulatory disorder involving excessive crying, distinctly disordered sleep–wake regulation, and feeding problems. The infant was awakening up to 10 times per night, could be soothed only with a bottle, and needed to be carried around day and night to remain pacified. The infant had virtually no calm wake phases and cried particularly loudly when hungry. He then drank so fast that he choked himself, as a result of which he subsequently refused the bottle. Both parents, the mother in particular, were suffering from chronic exhaustion and were at the end of their strength.

The intervention initially comprised elaborating a hierarchical approach together with the parents as to how the infant's sleep–wake regulation could be improved. With the help of an ergotherapist, ways were found (e.g., baby hammock) for the infant to soothe itself during crying and fussing phases without being carried about. The parents learned in particular to look out for

(continued)

signs of overstimulation and fatigue. Nighttime feeding was reduced to two bottle-feeding sessions. Over the course of 1 week, the infant managed to sleep for up to 4 h at a time; moreover, the sleep initiation situation improved noticeably and no longer followed its usual protracted course lasting over 1 h. Due to the improved and restive night's sleep, wake regulation during the day improved considerably: the infant had ever longer, more alert, and calmer wake phases, during which the feeding situation was generally relaxed. Thereafter, food was only offered when the infant was in a quiet behavioral state, at regular intervals, and no longer for soothing purposes.

In general, it is important to ensure that mealtimes take place in calm and undisturbed conditions—this applies in particular to mealtimes with older, easily distractable children. The latter, moreover, should be required to remain at the table until the joint meal is finished, since this group of children often only eat adequately if the mealtime lasts a sufficiently long period; the incentive to start a new game is generally stronger than the incentive to spend long enough on the subject of "eating" to the point where adequate satiation is achieved [see also "Infantile Anorexia" and in the overview in Sect. 5.5.2 and Chatoor (2012)].

5.6.3 Interactional and Communicational Level

Interaction- and communication-centered counseling aims to heighten parents' sensitization to their infant's needs (see ► Chap. 3). Generally with the help of video feedback (Thiel-Bonney 2002; see ► Chap. 10), parents are instructed and encouraged to respond in a developmentally appropriate manner and contingent on their infant's signals. Video recordings are made not only in strained contexts (e.g., feeding, putting to bed, boundary setting), but also in moments of unencumbered interaction (e.g., playing), in order to identify resources and reinforce parental skills. As part of this process, the therapist becomes a mouthpiece for the infant, "translating" its signals in such a way that the parents gain greater insight into their infant and are better able to respond to it sensitively (see also Wilken et al. 2008). This is achieved by, e.g., asking parents how they interpret a particular signal from their infant (e.g., aversion to drinking or eating); which other possible interpretation this signal could have (e.g., "rejection of the mother" vs. "desire to do something on its own"); and which response from the parents is able to support their infant's self-regulation and autonomy, thereby helping to ease tension at mealtimes. When working with video sequences, parents are initially shown a successful feeding episode in an approach that serves to reinforce their skills and identify their resources; then, together with the therapist, they consider what it was that made that particular episode relaxed for parents and infant. Dysfunctional sequences are then examined and discussed in a subsequent step. A joint discussion then ensues on how successful aspects can be carried over to other feeding episodes. The father should always be included in these discussions and in the observation of instances of dyadic and triadic communication.

Concern about the nutrition of an infant with a feeding disorder generally dominates everyday family life; dialogue, play, and relaxation are virtually nonexistent. Therefore, therapeutic support to achieve moments together in interactional and relational harmony is of particular importance.

5.6.3.1 Particular Features of Sensory Food Aversion and Posttraumatic Feeding Disorders

Due to sensory hypersensitivity in some infants, combined with parental behaviors, the spectrum of food is often significantly limited. Hunger alone is insufficient to simply resolve an infant's resistance to food in the setting of sensory food aversion or a posttraumatic feeding disorder. In the course of "systematic and gradual desensitization," the infant with sensory food aversion becomes accustomed to previously refused foods according to a stepwise and preset plan; the behavior of parents as role models, and possibly also of siblings, plays an essential role here.

Lucas, an 18-month-old infant, had developed ever fussier eating behavior since the introduction of coarser food at the age of 10 months. He had continued to tolerate soft foods such as banana or soft cooked vegetables for a time, but meanwhile accepted only finely pureed food, reacting to even the smallest bits in his food by pulling faces, expressing his disgust, and sometimes also retching. Clinical patient history and examination yielded no indication of oral-motor problems. The temperament questionnaire showed increased aversion to new stimuli and changes in routine, accompanied by prolonged adjustment phases and increased anxiety.

Much like with an anxiety disorder, a hierarchy of the refused foods was formulated together with the parents, and the food that elicited the least aversive reactions (banana) and which Lucas had already accepted once started to be introduced regularly in the weekly menu. The parents ate banana together with Lucas and encouraged him to eat small amounts, giving him correspondingly positive feedback when he put pieces of banana in his mouth. At first Lucas refused banana as a snack between meals; he was offered banana again after an interval between food intake, and his preferred food was only offered once he had tried a small piece of banana. Once Lucas had become accustomed to banana over a period of 2 weeks, he was offered the next food on the food hierarchy list. Within 8 weeks, it was possible to significantly improve his acceptance of coarse food and broaden his food spectrum using this approach.

Desensitization in posttraumatic feeding disorders follows a somewhat different approach. Here, the infant is offered small amounts of food at short intervals (e.g., every 2 h) until the threshold of the first anxious reaction is reached; this should be done without force-feeding (von Hofacker et al., 2004). Aversive stimuli or unpleasant experiences should be avoided at all costs. Infants are initially allowed to experiment freely in play with their food ("play-eating," Dunitz-Scheer et al. 2001; "baby picnic," Wilken et al. 2008). Exposing infants to foods of different tastes and consistencies outside the feeding situation, i.e., by leaving food lying about near the infant, encourages their autonomous and anxiety-free familiarization with the food while playing and promotes a gradual reduction in their refusal of these foods.

Additional desensitization in the orofacial region is often necessary in cases where any form of stimulation in the mouth area elicits aversion. In a first step, the infant should experience orofacial stimulation outside the feeding context, firstly through playful stroking and light massaging of the body, followed by touching of the head, upper half of the face, and finally the mouth area (cheeks, chin, and lips), using hands as well as toys (Wolke 2005). Concomitant oral-motor/orofacial therapy, starter toothbrush sets, reaching for a spoon, and playing with eating utensils promote infant exploration and desensitization. In this way, infants and toddlers learn to perceive a wide variety of sensory stimuli as pleasant and unthreatening forms of stimulation independent of hunger (see also van den Engel-Hoek 2008).

Alternative approaches, such as repeatedly exceeding the infant's threshold of resistance ("flooding"), e.g., by repeatedly touching the infant's lips quickly with food despite their aversion to it, requires a particularly experienced and confident therapist; however, there is as yet scant empirical evidence to support this approach and, in the author's view, it is ethically unacceptable given the previous traumatic experiences of most of these children (Benoit and Coolbear 1998; see overview of behavioral therapy methods in Wolke 2005).

Temporary *feeding while asleep* over a period of 2–3 months can be helpful in infants with posttraumatic food refusal of acute onset, combined with a stepwise "deactivation" of anxious aversion in the waking state. Ideally, the infant receives so much nutrition through feedings while asleep that it only needs to be fed up to the first sign of an anxious aversive reaction during wake phases. Eventually, the quantity of food intake during the day can slowly be increased.

Whereas infants with sensory food aversion generally eat sufficiently yet highly selectively, children with posttraumatic feeding disorders often initially require tube feeding. Although *tube weaning* can be carried out on an outpatient basis when certain requirements are met, it is usually performed in an inpatient setting and will not be discussed in more detail here. Dunitz-Scheer et al. (2001) described a novel group of young patients they referred to as "tube-dependent." These are children that are generally primarily fed via nasogastric tube due to premature birth or surgical intervention and subsequently, since the transition to self-directed learning to eat has not taken place, become dependent on tube feeding. For this reason, the anticipated duration of feeding via gastric tube should always be discussed and secondary preventive measures taken in order to prevent tube dependency.

5.6.4 Psychodynamic Relational Level: Parent–Infant/Toddler Psychotherapy

Given the vital significance of nutrition and the concern surrounding an infant's thriving and survival, parents faced with a feeding problem are often under considerable strain. The parents' own deep-seated anxieties, often rooted in experiences of loss, may be triggered during the several family meals that take place over the course of a day (see Sect. 5.4.4). The parents feel deeply challenged and adrift (Wilken et al. 2008) and require a supportive therapeutic relationship to help them face their own insecurities, anxieties, and ambivalences, as well as to discover their own and their infant's resources and strengths. For this reason, concomitant psychodynamic psychotherapy sessions are indispensable.

Experiences, memories, and fantasies from the parental biographies (see also ► Chap. 3) may resurface during feeding interaction in the form of "ghosts" from the parents' past and start to "direct" the scenes played out on the stage of family mealtimes (Jacubeit 2004). The parents no longer see their "real" child before them, with its strengths and weaknesses, but repeat instead relational patterns from their pasts in interaction with their baby. This can result in a distorted/negative perception and misinterpretation of their infant's signals and hamper them in providing it developmentally appropriate support. In such cases, early childhood neglect, experiences of separation, loss, and trauma (violence, sexual abuse) in the parental biography should be taken into consideration. In the case of organic disease or sensory motor problems in the infant, parents require a high level of flexibility and willingness to adjust in order to provide their infant with appropriate support at mealtimes. If primary caregivers have their own stressors in the form of concern about the infant's health (e.g., following premature birth), latent marital conflicts, transgenerational conflicts (e.g., conflicts relating to independence/autonomy), or their own psychiatric illness, these will impair their intuitive skills and become superimposed on interaction in the feeding context (Jacubeit 2004). The examples of parent statements listed in the box below were made in the counseling context and reveal a number of psychodynamic aspects that can (co-)shape dysfunctional parent–infant interaction.

Psychodynamic Aspects of Feeding Interaction

- Anxiety relating to survival, thriving, and growth.
  - "My baby almost starved in my tummy, then he was born too early—and now I still can't manage to feed him enough."
- Separation anxiety.
  - "My first baby had a heart defect and couldn't drink—she died shortly after birth. I'm not going to let that happen again!"
- Control/force vs. autonomy.
  - "She always wants to feed herself—but she's not even able to do that yet!"
  - "Better a bit of pressure than the tube."

(continued)

- Symbiosis, self-esteem, own neediness/narcissistic disorder.
  - "Although once again I made a lot of effort cooking, she still wouldn't eat for me."
  - "If my daughter eats badly, I'm going to have a bad day."
- Marital conflicts.
  - "My husband trusts her to eat enough on her own and regulate her eating herself—she'd starve if things were left to him!"
  - "As with eating, my wife always wants to tell everyone what to do!"
- Parental feeding disorders
  - "I was always very thin and people used to force me to eat. Now I'm overweight and have lost all feel for quantities—but my child shouldn't ever put on as much weight as I have!" (paternal obcsity).
  - "If she doesn't finish her food, I eat the leftovers then make myself sick." (maternal bulimia).

Observing social togetherness during mealtimes reveals important interactional patterns and conflicts in an unusually emotional density—they are literally "on the table" (von Hofacker et al., 2004). In order to identify how the feeding problem is embedded in the relational constellation and what type of (psycho-)therapeutic support the infant and its family need, it is crucially important to broaden the therapeutic perspective from the dyad and the triad to complex family relational structures; at the same time, observing a joint meal in the therapeutic setting or by means of a home video is indispensable.

A mother presented with her 15-month-old daughter, Clara, due to an eating problem. The patient history revealed a normal feeding history up until the infant had started eating independently at the age of 11 months. Feeding and eating situations had become increasingly conflict-laden as Clara's need for autonomy grew. In particular her need to play with her food, take it in her hands, and experiment with it was virtually intolerable to her mother, who was obsessively concerned with cleanliness. Conflict-laden mealtimes during which the mother attempted to contain Clara's need for exploration while she fed the infant in a controlled manner—attempts vehemently refused by Clara—were lasting for up to 1 h.

The feeding problem was accompanied by a sleeping problem, which was putting a strain on the mother: Clara and her mother slept in a bed together, while the father slept in the living room. The mother reported that she herself had slept in the same bed as her mother until the age of 16, then quickly

(continued)

moved out of home at the age of 17 with her boyfriend to start her professional training. At the time of the consultation, she still had a very close relationship with her mother and spoke to her on the phone daily. Although she would have liked Clara to learn to sleep in her own bed and wanted to share a bed with her husband again, her mother had urgently advised her against this, warning her that she would impair the child's attachment development.

The first aim of intervention was to address the transgenerational autonomy–dependency conflict. The mother's own need for autonomy was reinforced. In the course of a sleep intervention and with the father's support, Clara quickly learned to fall asleep and remain asleep in her own bed. This success bolstered the mother's self-confidence and self-esteem, and she was increasingly able to better distance herself from her own mother. Parallel to this, she began to positively support and enjoy Clara's need for autonomy and her active participation in the eating situation. She started to address her compulsive symptoms during psychotherapy on her own.

However, the eating situation represents not only the "stage" for daily struggles and conflicts, but also provides the backdrop for: caring and closeness; regulatory processes and positive social interaction between parents and infant; the pleasant exchange of communication; and the infant's development of hand and oral-motor activity, exploratory behavior, attention control, and need for autonomy. This sphere of positive experiences needs to be (re-)gained together with the parents and their infant.

5.6.5 Indications for In- and Out-Patient Treatment

Outpatient counseling based on sound developmental psychology and focused on interaction is indicated when:

- The infant's physical well-being (e.g., thriving) is not—or not hazardously—impaired and there are no indications of previous traumatic experiences.
- The primary caregiver (still) has sufficient psychosocial resources at their disposal and access to their intuitive skills.
- The parent–infant relationship has not suffered any relevant impairment and there is no danger of child neglect or abuse.
- The infant disorder has not extended to other contexts and has not been present for more than 3 months.

Parent–infant/toddler psychotherapy is indicated (von Hofacker et al., 2004) when:

- The feeding disorder is of more than 3 months' standing and developmental counseling has achieved no substantial improvement in symptoms.
- Other interactional contexts are also affected and/or there have been no prolonged phases of undisturbed infant development.
- The feeding disorder is associated with dysfunctional, maladaptive interaction patterns and a risk of neglect and abuse.
- Parent–infant relationships are clearly strained/disordered, e.g., as observed in a hostile, aggressive attitude, distorted perception of the infant's needs, attribution of guilt, impaired intuitive parenting skills, and limited emotional access to the infant.

In the presence of organic and/or mental/psychiatric illness [e.g., severe overload syndrome, (postpartum) depression, anxiety disorders, psychosis] in the parents or major partnership conflicts, the mother/father should be referred for individual, e.g., psychotherapeutic/psychiatric treatment or couples counseling/therapy.

Partial or full inpatient treatment, including admission of the primary caregiver, becomes necessary in cases in which: outpatient treatment yields inadequate results, the implementation of interactional and relational interventions in everyday domestic life fails, the infant has marked organic/constitutional risk factors (e.g., due to premature birth, organic disease, severe failure to thrive), and/or the parents suffer from severe psychopathology. In the case of an immediate risk to the physical or mental well-being of the infant, serious risk factors in the psychosocial environment/social isolation, severe interactional and relational perturbation, and/or parental exhaustion, partial inpatient admission enables close monitoring of the situation and multimodal treatment by an interdisciplinary team. As in specialty clinics, (day) clinics should also offer the following: pediatrics (in particular neuropediatrics and gastroenterology), developmental psychology, and, where required, speech therapy, ergotherapy, physiotherapy, and parent–infant/toddler psychotherapy. The mother/parents are able to delegate the monitoring of caloric intake to the pediatrician, which often comes as a significant relief to them. The treatment team should be specially trained to calmly advise and support the mother and father at this time of high emotional tension and provide them and their infant with the space needed to develop and experience self-efficacy, autonomy, and competence. Severe failure to thrive, marked posttraumatic feeding disorders, and tube weaning are generally treated in an inpatient setting.

5.6.5.1 Case Report

"If things carry on like this, we're all going to fall apart! His eating behavior is going to drive us to distraction!" Full of tension, anxiety, and resentment, the parents of the 2.5-year-old Simon reported the persistent eating difficulties their son had had since birth (at normal body weight).

Simon would eat only a few selected foods, and these he would keep in his mouth—where he would "sort" them—for long times. Whatever he didn't like, he spat out again. He "angrily and aggressively" resisted his parents' attempts to feed him.

Mealtimes took up hours of the mother's time and generally involved either distraction or force. In her desperate attempt to "get something down him," the mother would follow Simon from room to room trying to feed him something "on the side."

Prior to the first appointment in our clinic, the family pediatrician had referred the infant to the pediatric hospital for an evaluation of his failure to thrive, and informed the parents that their son was in a dangerous physical condition and required "immediate tube feeding." His body weight was just under the 3rd percentile. However, the hospital physician first contacted us, since he had reservations about tube feeding and feared that this measure "could rob Simon of every last bit of interest in eating."

As part of the *patient history*, the parents reported that the mother had become pregnant with Simon following ICSI treatment. Simon had already fed poorly in the first 2 weeks of life. Fearing for his survival, the mother had started feeding her infant pureed food at the age of 3 months, which he "also refused." Only with considerable effort was she able to maintain his weight above the 3rd percentile. Relationship formation following Simon's birth had been severely strained, since the mother was unable to see her son for 2 days due to complications, after which time she regarded him as a "stranger." Moreover, he had experienced "crying bouts" from the age of 3 days onwards, as a result of which the parents had enjoyed only very few relaxed and pleasant moments in everyday life with their baby. The infant's crying and fussing had not abated until after the age of 6 months.

In the *examination setting*, Simon presented as an alert, happy, sensitive toddler that listened very attentively to his parents and made short comments in return while he played, in an unfocused manner, a game from which he was easily distracted by external stimuli. He found a yogurt and began to try this on his own initiative. Both parents immediately focused their full attention on Simon and, under their controlling and dysfunctional attempts to "support" him in eating, he immediately lost all interest in the food.

The parents brought a *home video* to their second appointment; in this, Simon could initially be seen to happily eat his lunch in a normal manner. As soon as the infant was satiated and demonstrated less interest in eating, his mother began to make controlling attempts to feed him. Simon finally pushed his plate away angrily and wanted to leave the table—an escalating power struggle ensued.

In a second scene, the mother, father, and maternal grandmother were sitting at the table, their full attention focused on Simon. The tense silence at the table was only interrupted by short, sharp requests from the mother for Simon to finally start eating. At the same time, the mother and grandmother kept taking Simon's plate away, since his food had gone cold and needed to be warmed up. Intrusive feeding attempts finally led to the toddler putting up massive resistance and completely refusing any food.

The feeding situation had become a power struggle between parents and toddler, during which strong affects of disappointment, powerlessness, and anger became manifest. The grandmother, who lived in her own yet not self-contained apartment within the family house, was often present at mealtimes.

During the therapy session, the mother was quick to raise her voice and become prohibitory, while the father took a more reserved and lenient stance. Parental communication was concerned almost exclusively with the toddler's eating behavior; the father would phone home from work almost hourly to find out how much Simon had eaten.

From a psychodynamically relevant perspective, Simon's mother described early depressive symptoms and a marked problem with self-esteem. After a phase of being overweight during adolescence, she had developed anorexia, which she had since overcome. To date, she had "always taken care of everyone in the family, but it was never enough." She now saw herself as an inadequate mother and, particularly in the eating context, felt rejected by her son. Her self-confidence was closely aligned to her son's behavior, leading to a pronounced controlling relational mode and a parentification of the child: in response to her frequent promptings—and thereby assuming responsibility for her emotional well-being—Simon would keep having to reassure her: "Mummy is the best!"

The father tried as much as possible to keep out of conflicts and his involvement in the "nitty-gritty" of everyday life appeared to be limited; bearing in mind his previous biographical experiences, this was understandable.

The *couple dynamics* appeared to be covertly conflictual: the parents tended to deny conflicts outside the feeding context. Conflicts were clearly waged primarily through interaction with Simon, who, in the case of tension, would assume responsibility and reunite the parents through ritualized actions.

From a *family dynamics* perspective, it was apparent that there was a very serious problem in terms of autonomy and distance from the grandmother and within the couple. Simon would evade parental boundary setting by "simply going up to granny." The mother harbored considerable feelings of ambivalence: on the one hand she wanted Simon to "listen" to her and enjoy his food, while on the other she admired his ability to get his own way with his willpower and his "No!"—something she had never been able to do herself.

5.7 Course of Therapy

Six sessions in an alternating counseling constellation (parents/child; grandmother/mother/child; mother alone) were held. It was important to firstly convey *information* on Simon's upcoming steps toward autonomy, his strengths, and the pleasant moments with him in everyday life in order to make these tangible to the parents and agree with them that they should avoid intrusive feeding interaction. Simon was to be allowed to experiment independently with food between mealtimes and to help prepare meals. Meanwhile, he began to try different foods. Efforts to involve the father more intensively in everyday life and to organize family mealtimes (with the introduction of the "eating rules," Sect. 5.6.2), during which Simon's parents granted him greater freedom, were successful. The child was increasingly able to take the initiative in the context of *play*; with guidance, the parents slowly withdrew their control and supported Simon with encouraging words. During the period that followed, the father appeared to be less emotionally rigid and came across as happier and "more alive" in the context of contact. Father and son enjoyed exhilarating, physically oriented "father–son" games.

Since the whole family was involved in the therapy, agreements were reached on when Simon could spend time with his grandmother and how the adults should behave in boundary-setting situations. The mother assumed more responsibility.

To the mother's surprise, the grandmother showed herself to be understanding of the situation and willing to lend her support to the family. Against the backdrop of these positive developments, the mother was able to take steps toward autonomy from her own mother. Bolstered by this, she was able to adequately support her son's developmentally appropriate steps toward autonomy and respond suitably to him in conflict situations. Observing that their son, a lively, happy boy, was able to signal when he was hungry and when he was satiated, the parents slowly began to lose their fears about his survival, and the parent–child relationship was strengthened. Simon showed interest in mealtimes and had made a satisfactory gain in weight.

Six months later, the parents returned to discuss seemingly compulsive behavior in their toddler, as well as new boundary-setting conflicts. Simon's weight had remained stable and the eating situation had eased further in the intervening months. The parents reported how they continued to communicate well with each other as a couple and were able to come to successful arrangements with the grandmother. The problems they referred to were all but resolved following an additional therapy session, by which time the parents felt sufficiently confident about their handling of Simon.

Conclusion Feeding disorders tend to become persistent, thereby jeopardizing the further physical, mental, and socioemotional development of the infant, as well as relational development within the family. They need to be taken seriously, recognized, and treated promptly. While taking the symptom triad consisting of infant/parental risk factors and interactional anomalies into consideration, interdisciplinary therapy on a number of different and complementary levels forms the basis for prevention aimed at minimizing subsequent developmental and relational disorders and enabling parents and child to enjoy pleasant social togetherness.

References

Abidin R (1983) Parenting stress index: manual, administration booklet and research update. Pediatric Psychology Press, Charlottesville, VA

Achenbach TM, Rescorla LA (2000) CBCL/1,5–5 & C-TRF/1,5–5 Profiles. Research Center for Children, Youth, and Families, Burlington

Ammaniti M, Ambruzzi AM, Lucarelli L (2004) Malnutrition and dysfunctional mother-child feeding interactions: clinical assessment and research implications. J Am Coll Nutr 23(3):259–271

Arvedson JC (2008) Assessment of pediatric dysphagia and feeding disorders: clinical and instrumental approaches. Dev Disabil Res Rev 14:118–127

Bates JE, Freeland CA, Lounsbury ML (1979) Measurement of infant difficultness. Child Dev 50:794–803

Benoit D (2000) Feeding disorders, failure to thrive, and obesity. In: Zeanah CH (Hrsg) Handbook of infant mental health, 2. Aufl. Guilford Press, New York, pp S377–S391

Benoit D, Coolbear J (1998) Post-traumatic feeding disorders in infancy: behaviour predicting treatment outcome. Infant Ment Health J 19(41):409–421

Bernard-Bonnin AC (2006) Feeding problems of infants and toddlers. Can Fam Physician 52:1247–1251

Blissett J, Meyer C (2006) The mediating role of psychopathology in the relationship between unhealthy core beliefs and feeding difficulties in an nonclinical group. Int J Eat Disord 39:763–771

Blissett J, Meyer C, Farrow C et al (2005) Maternal core beliefs and children's feeding problems. Int J Eat Disord 37:127–134

Brinich EB, Drotar DD, Brinich PM (1989) Die Bedeutung der Bindungssicherheit vom Kind zur Mutter für die psychische und physische Entwicklung von gedeihschwachen Kindern. Prax Kinderpsychol Kinderpsychiatr 38:70–77

Bryant-Waugh R, Markham L, Kreipe RE, Walsh BT (2010) Feeding and eating disorders in childhood. Int J Eat Disord 43(2):98–111

Burklow KA, Phelps AN, Schultz JR et al (1998) Classifying complex pediatric feeding disorders. J Pediatr Gastroenterol Nutr 27:143–147

Chatoor I, Conley C, Dickson L (1988) Food refusal after an incident of cocking: a posttraumatic eating disorder. J Am Acad Child Adolesc Psychiatry 27(1):105–110

Chatoor I, Ganiban J, Colin VN, Harmon RJ (1998) Attachment and feeding problems: a reexamination of nonorganic failure to thrive and attachment insecurity. J Am Acad Child Adolesc Psychiatry 37(11):1217–1224

Chatoor I, Ganiban J, Harrison J, Hirsch R (2001) Observation of feeding in the diagnosis of posttraumatic feeding disorder of infancy. J Am Acad Child Adolesc Psychiatry 40(5):59S–602S

Chatoor I, Surles J, Ganiban J et al (2004) Failure to thrive and cognitive development in toddlers with infantile anorexia. Pediatrics 113(5):440–447

Chatoor I (2012) Fütterstörungen bei Säuglingen und Kleinkindern. Klassifikation: Diagnostik und Behandlung. Klett Cotta, Stuttgart

Cooper PJ, Whelan E, Woolgar M et al (2004) Association between childhood feeding problems and maternal eating disorder: role of the family environment. Br J Psychiatry 184:210–215

Dahl M (1987) Early feeding problems in an affluent society. III. Follow-up at two years—natural course, health, behaviour and development. Acta Paediatr Scand 76(6):872–880

Dahl M, Rydell AM, Sundelin C (1994) Children with early refusal to eat: follow-up during primary school. Acta Paediatr 83:54–58

Dahl M, Sundelin C (1992) Feeding problems in an affluent society. Follow-up at four years of age in children with early refusal to eat. Acta Paediatr 81(8):575–579

Davies WH, Satter E, Berlin KS et al (2006) Reconceptualizing feeding and feeding disorders in interpersonal context: the case for a relational disorder. J Fam Psychol 20(3):409–417

Dilling H, Mombour W, Schmidt MH (Hrsg) (2010) Internationale Klassifikation psychischer Störungen, ICD-10, Kapitel V (F). Hans Huber, Bern

Drewett RF, Corbett SS, Wright CM (1999) Cognitive and educational attainments at school age of children who failed to thrive in infancy: a population-based study. J Child Psychol Psychiatry 40(4):551–561

Drewett RF, Kasese-Hare M, Wright C (2002) Feeding behaviour in young children who fail to thrive. Appetite 40:55–60

Dunitz-Scheer M, Wilken M, Scheitenberger S et al (2001) Sondenentwöhnung in der frühen Kindheit. Monatsschr Kinderheilkd 149:1348–1359

Erb L, Thiel-Bonney C, Cierpka M (2014) Zum Zusammenhang von Frühgeburtlichkeit und frühkindlichen Fütterstörungen. Ärztliche Psychotherapie und Psychosomatische Medizin 9:19–25

Farrow C, Blissett J (2006a) Breast-feeding, maternal feeding practices and mealtime negativity at one year. Appetite 46(1):49–56

Farrow C, Blissett J (2006b) Maternal cognitions, psychopathologic symptoms, and infant temperament as predictors of early infant feeding problems: a longitudinal study. Int J Eat Disord 39:128–134

Farrow C, Blissett J (2008) Controlling feeding practices. Cause or consequence of early child weight. Pediatrics 121:164–169

Fergusson DM, Horwood LJ, Shannon FT (1985) Relationship between family life events, maternal depression and child rearing problems. Pediatrics 73:773–788

Forsyth BWC, Canny PF (1991) Perceptions of vulnerability 3 1/2 years after problems of feeding and crying behavior in early infancy. Pediatrics 88:757–763

Groß S, Reck C, Thiel-Bonney C, Cierpka M (2007) Fragebogen zum Schreien, Füttern und Schlafen. Unveröffentlichtes Manuskript, Universitätsklinikum Heidelberg

Hagekull B, Bohlin G, Rydell AM (1997) Maternal sensitivity, infant temperament, and the development of earl feeding problems. Infant Ment Health J 18(1):92–106

Hawdon JM, Beauregard N, Kennedy G, Slattery J (2000) Identification of neonates at risk of developing feeding problems in infancy. Dev Med Child Neurol 42:235–239

Haycraft E, Blissett J (2008) Controlling feeding practices and psychopathology in an non-clinical sample of mothers and fathers. Eat Behav 9:484–492

Jacobi C, Agras WS, Bryson S, Hammer LD (2003) Bahavioral validation, precursors, and concomitants of picky eating in childhood. J Am Acad Child Adolesc Psychiatry 42(1):76–84

Jacubeit T (2004) Gespenster am Esstisch. Psychodynamische Aspekte in der Behandlung von Fütterstörungen. In: Papoušek M, Schieche M, Wurmser H (Hrsg) Regulationsstörungen der frühen Kindheit. Frühe Risiken und Hilfen im Entwicklungskontext der Eltem-Kind-Beziehungen. Hans Huber, Bern, pp S263–S280

Koletzko B, Armbruster M, Bauer CP, Bös K, Cierpka M, Crème RM, Dieminger B, Flothkötter M, Graf C, Heindl I, Hellmers C, Kersting M, Krawinkel M, Plöger A, Przyembel H, Reichert-Garschhammer E, Schäfer T, Wahn U, Vetter K, Wabitsch M, Weißenborn A, Wiegand S (2013) Ernährung und Bewegung im Kleinkindalter. Handlungsempfehlungen des Netzwerks “Gesund ins Leben—Netzwerk Junge Familie”, ein Projekt von IN FORM. Monatsschr Kinderheilkd 161:1187–1200

Kotler LA, Cohen P, Davies M et al (2001) Longitudinal relationship between childhood, adolescent, and adult eating disorders. J Am Acad Child Adolesc Psychiatry 40(12):1434–1440

Kroll M (2011) Interdisziplinäre Eltern-Kind Behandlung von schweren komplexen Fütterstörungen. Prax Kinderpsychol Kinderpsychiatr 60(6):452–465

Lindberg L, Bohlin G, Hagekull B, Palmerus K (1996) Interactions between mothers and infants showing food refusal. Infant Ment Health J 17(4):334–347

Lindberg L, Ostberg M, Isacson IM, Dannaeus M (2006) Feeding disorders related to nutrition. Acta Paediatr 95(4):425–429

Mathisen B, Skuse D, Wolke D, Reilly S (1989) Oral-motor dysfunction and failure to thrive among inner-city infants. Dev Med Child Neurol 31:293–302

Mathisen B, Worrall L, Masel J et al (1999) Feeding problems in infants with gastro-oesophageal reflux disease: a controlled study. J Paediatr Child Health 35:163–169

McDermott BM, Mamun A, Najman J et al (2008) Preschool children perceived by mothers as irregular eaters: physical and psychosocial predictors from a birth cohort study. J Dev Behav Pediatr 29:197–205

Micali N, Simonoff E, Treasure J (2009) Infant feeding and weight in the first year of life in babies of women with eating disorders. J Pediatr 154:55–60

Miller-Loncar C, Bigsby R, High P et al (2004) Infant colic and feeding difficulties. Arch Dis Child 89:908–912

Nelson SP, Chen EH, Syniar GM et al (1998) One-year followup of symptoms of gastroesophageal refl ux during infancy. Pediatrics 102(6):e67

Papoušek M (2002) Störungen des Säuglingsalters. In: Esser G (Hrsg) Lehrbuch der Klinischen Psychologie und Psychotherapie des Kindes- und Jugendalters. Thieme, Stuttgart, pp S80–S100

Papoušek M, Rothenburg S, Cierpka M, von Hofacker N (2004) Regulationsstörungen der frühen Kindheit. CD-basierte Fortbildung. Stiftung Kindergesundheit, München

Reba-Harrelson L, VonHolle A, Hamer RM et al (2010) Patterns of maternal feeding and child eating associated with eating disorders in the Norwegian mother child cohort study (Moba). Eat Behav 11(1):54–61

Rommel N, De Meyer AM, Feenstra L, Veereman-Wauters G (2003) The complexity of feeding problems in 700 infants and young children presenting to a tertiary care institution. J Pediatr Gastroenterol Nutr 37(1):75–84

Scaglioni S, Salvioni M, Galimberti C (2008) Influence of parental attitudes in the development of children eating behaviour. Br J Nutr 99(Suppl 1):22–25

Sollid CP, Wisborg K, Hjort J, Secher NJ (2004) Eating disorder that was diagnosed before pregnancy and pregnancy outcome. Am J Obstet Gynecol 190(1):206–210

Stein A, Woolley H, Cooper SD, Fairburn CG (1994) An observational study of mothers with eating disorders and their infants. J Child Psychol Psychiatry 35(4):733–748

Stein A, Woolley H, McPherson K (1999) Conflict between mothers with eating disorders and their infants during mealtimes. Br J Psychiatry 175:455–461

Stern D (1998) Die Mutterschaftskonstellation. Eine vergleichende Darstellung verschiedener Formen der Mutter-Kind-Psychotherapie. Klett-Cotta, Stuttgart

Thiel-Bonney C (2002) Beratung von Eltern mit Säuglingen und Kleinkindern. Videogestützte Verhaltensbeobachtung und Videomikroanalyse als Interventionsmöglichkeit. Psychotherapeut 47:381–384

Thiel-Bonney C (2006, unveröffentlicht). Deskriptive Daten aus dem Elternfragebogen der Interdisziplinären Spezialambulanz für Eltern mit Säuglingen und Kleinkindern. Institut für Psychosomatische Kooperationsforschung und Familientherapie, Heidelberg

Unlü G, Aras S, Eminağaoğlu N et al (2008) Developmental characteristics of children aged 1–6 years with food refusal. Public Health Nurs 25(1):2–9

van den Engel-Hoek L (2008) Fütterstörungen. Ein Ratgeber für Ess- und Trinkprobleme bei Kleinkindern. SchulzKirchner Verlag, Idstein

von Gontard A (2010) Säuglings- und Kleinkindpsychiatrie. Ein Lehrbuch. Kohlhammer, Stuttgart

von Hofacker N (2009) Frühkindliche Fütterstörungen. Neuere Entwicklungen und ihre Relevanz für die Praxis. Monatsschr Kinderheilkd 157:567–573

von Hofacker N (2014) Fütter- und Essstörungen im Säuglings- und Kleinkindalter. Interior coil. In: Rosenecker J (ed) Pädiatrische Differenzialdiagnostik. Springer, Heidelberg, Berlin

von Hofacker N, Tortorelia S, Sobanski P (2002) Fragebogen zur Ess- und Fütteranamnese. Unveröffentlichtes Manuskript, Klinikum München Harlaching

von Hofacker N, Papoušek M, Wurmser H (2004) Fütter- und Gedeihstörungen im Säuglings- und Kleinkindalter. In: Papoušek M, Schieche M, Wurmser H (Hrsg) Regulationsstörungen der frühen Kindheit. Frühe Risiken una Hilfen im Entwicklungskontext der Eltern-Kind-Beziehungen. Hans Huber, Bern, pp S171–S199

von Hofacker N, Lehmkuhl U, Resch F et al (2007) Regulationsstörungen Im Säuglings- und Kleinkindalter. In: Deutsche Gesellschaft für Kinder- und Jugend psychiatrie und -psychothérapie (Hrsg) Leitlinien zur Diagnostik und Therapie von psychischen Störungen im Säuglings-, Kindes- und Jugendalter. AWMF Online. http://mrw.il ni-duesseldorf.de/AWMF/ll/028-028.htm

von Kries R, Kalies H, Papoušek M (2006) Excessive crying beyond 3 months may herald other features of multiple regulatory problems. Arch Pediatr Adolesc Med 160:508–511

Wilken M, Jotzo M (2009, unveröffentlicht) Anamnesebogen frühkindliche Fütterstörung und Sondenentwöhnung (AFS). Pädiatrisches Dysphagiezentrum, Darmstadt

Wilken M, Jotzo M, Dunitz-Scheer M (2008) Therapie frühkindlicher Fütterstörungen. In: Borke J, Eickhorst A (Hrsg) Systemische Entwicklungsberatung in der frühen Kindheit. Facultas, Wien, pp S189–S208

Wolke D (2005) Fütter- und Essstörungen im Säuglings- und Kleinkindalter. In: Schlottke P, Silbereisen RK, Schneider S, Lauth GW (Hrsg) Störungen im Kindes- und Jugendalter - Grundlagen und Störungen im Entwicklungsverlauf, Bd 5. Hogrefe, Göttingen, pp S381–S417

Wolke D, Skuse D, Mathisen B (1990) Behavioural style in failure-to-thrive infants: a preliminary communication. J Pediatr Psychol 15(2):237–254

Ward MJ, Lee SS, Lipper EG (2000) Failure-to-thrive is associated with disorganized infant-mother attachment and unresolved maternal attachment. Infant Ment Health J 21(61):428–442

Wolke D, Schmid G, Schreier A, Meyer R (2009) Crying and feeding problems in infancy and cognitive outcome in preschool children born at risk: a prospective population study. J Dev Behav Pediatr 30(3):226–238

Wright CM, Parkinson KN, Drewett RF (2006) The influence of maternal socioeconomic and emotional factors on infant weight gain and weight faltering (failure to thrive): data from a prospective birth cohort. Arch Dis Child 91:312–317

Wright CM, Parkinson KN, Shipton D, Drewett RF (2007) How do toddler eating problems relate to their eating behaviour, food preferences, and growth. Pediatrics 120(4):1069–1075

Zero To Three (2005) Diagnostic classifi cation of mental health and developmental disorders of infancy and early childhood: Revised edition (DC:0–3R). Zero To Three Press, Washington, DC

Developmentally Appropriate and Excessive Clinginess

6

Kerstin Scholtes-Spang and Marisa Benz

6.1 Clinginess: An Overview

Clinginess represents an early means at the infant's disposal to react to anxiety and find protection and reassurance by seeking or maintaining physical proximity to a trusted person. As such, clinginess does not represent a pathological reaction per se, but rather an initially age-appropriate means of reacting to an anxiety-inducing situation by activating attachment behavior. Maintaining physical proximity to the primary caregiver is generally associated with anxious facial expressions, fear-filled vocalizations (e.g., crying, which may escalate to panicky screaming), and gaze aversion. Typical anxieties in the first 3 years of life include anxiety elicited by sudden and loud noises, as well as strangers and unknown situations (also known as "8-month anxiety"), which usually begin between the ages of 6 and 9 months and persist to the age of 30 months. Separation anxiety occurs somewhat later, peaking in the second and third years of life (Largo 2001).

Particularly in the first 3 years of life, infants rely on co-regulation from their trusted caregiver—the person to whom they can turn when they need security, protection, contact, and communication—to help them develop skills to regulate negative emotions, such as anxiety, frustration, and anger (Dornes 2001). The ability to mentalize, i.e., empathize with their infant's emotional distress, enables parents to support their infant on the path to independently overcoming its anxieties and, thus,

K. Scholtes-Spang, Dipl.Psych. (✉)
Institute for Psychosocial Prevention, University Hospital Heidelberg,
Bergheimer Str. 54, Heidelberg 69115, Germany
e-mail: kontakt@psychotherapie-scholtes.de

M. Benz, Dipl.Psych.
Florida State University, 4600 University Center, Tallahassee, FL 32306, USA
e-mail: mbenz@lsi.fsu.edu

M. Cierpka (ed.), *Regulatory Disorders in Infants*,
DOI 10.1007/978-3-319-43556-5_6

also to its longer-term development of anxiety tolerance. As part of this process, the parents must be able to withstand recurrent states of stress, detach themselves from their infant's anxieties, and also compose themselves. If parents are unable to detach themselves from their infant's anxieties and experience anxiety themselves, or project their own anxieties onto their infant, a cycle of reciprocal affect contagion in the absence of appropriate soothing strategies ensues. In her concept of developmental lines, Anna Freud described how "mastering the internal world and adjusting to the external world advances in stages" (1968, p. 2183). Accomplishing this developmental task "well enough" according to the concept of fit (Thomas and Chess 1977) fosters the development of an inner sense of security and a means to autonomously overcome anxiety.

Excessive, persistent clinginess that exceeds developmentally appropriate behavior is associated with a variety of risk factors (see Sect. 6.3.1) and may be a manifestation of a problem of emotional regulation, as well as a developmental, relational, or attachment disorder. The dysfunctional interaction patterns between parents and infant in this context, which are colored by considerable tension and ambivalence in closeness–distance regulation, represent an enormous strain on and hazard to the parent–infant relationship.

Principal Symptoms of Persistent and Excessive Shyness and Clinginess

- Excessive clinging to the primary caregiver despite the absence of a perceivable threat, e.g., in unchallenging situations.
- Demanding permanent attention.
- Difficulty or inability of the primary caregiver to clearly and sufficiently detach themselves in situations in which this would be appropriate.
- Age-inappropriate inhibition of willingness to play and explore despite the presence of the primary caregiver, accompanied by signs of anxious inhibition.

(Deutsche Gesellschaft für Kinder- und Jugendpsychiatrie und Psychotherapie Hrsg 2007)

▶ From a diagnostic perspective, excessive clinginess in infancy falls under the category of adjustment disorders in the form of early childhood regulatory disorders (ICD-10, F43.2). On the basis of the observation that early childhood regulatory disorders are often precursors of behavioral abnormalities in later childhood (e.g., Laucht et al. 2004), a persistent deficit in the domain of self-soothing can lead, for instance, to an emotional disorder with separation anxiety (ICD-10, F93.0) or social phobia (ICD-10, F40.1) being diagnosed in later childhood or adolescence.

6.2 Clinginess in the Course of Normal Development

In the course of their advancing physical, motor, cognitive, and social development, infants are increasingly confronted with new environmental stimuli, demands, and challenges between the age of 6 months and 1 year. Being confronted with the unfamiliar causes brief, but sometimes prolonged confusion and anxiety. In order to cope, recurrent processes of reorientation and adjustment are required.

The 8-month-old Antonia sat on her mother's lap with her back to her mother. A friend of the mother's was visiting and sat opposite mother and child. Attentive and interested, Antonia observed this person who she barely knew from her safe place at a distance. At the same time, she was fiddling with a spoon, which eventually fell to the floor. The mother's friend picked up the spoon and, with friendly words and facial expressions, drew closer to the infant to put the spoon back in Antonia's hand. Antonia became agitated and turned toward her mother. As soon as the friend touched the infant's hand, Antonia started to make more pronounced defensive movements, wriggled about on her mother's lap, whined and fussed, turned her face away, and clung tightly to her mother's sweater. The mother soothed Antonia by intensifying physical contact and talking softly to the infant, while the friend withdrew. The latter handed the spoon to the mother, who passed it to Antonia. Antonia continued playing quietly, while the "strange woman" continued talking to the mother from a distance. Antonia interrupted her game occasionally to observe the friend.

The two adults in the example above demonstrate good empathy for Antonia's experience and are able to understand her distress. Adequate interpretation of the infant's signal, "Don't come too close to me (yet)," results in Antonia being able to soothe and distance herself on the visible level of interaction. However, it is also important that she continues to have the opportunity to get close to the adult if she wishes; this enables the infant to familiarize herself with something or someone strange, unknown, or new and prevents the development of avoidance behavior.

Shyness with strangers, also referred to as 8-month anxiety, involving the typical reactions exhibited by Antonia, is often interpreted as a sign of a primarily cognitive developmental shift, i.e., the infant's new ability to distinguish between people (Largo 2001). The ability to differentiate between people based on their importance is associated with the more conscious perception of the possibility of losing the familiar (Cierpka and Windaus 2007). However, fear of the unknown—often accompanied by the infant's vehement rejection thereof and search for the proximity of trusted figures—can also be understood from an evolutionary perspective: "With the fear of strangers, nature ensures that the infant remains close to those people that care for its physical and psychological well-being in a dependable manner in the first years of life" (Largo 2001, p. 70). Anxiety and fear emerge as new emotional systems of interaction in conjunction with locomotor development between the ages of 6 and 12 months and person-specific attachment; this shift can also be interpreted as a mechanism to protect the infant (Papoušek and von Hofacker 2004). In line with this interpretation, shyness with strangers can be understood as a precursor to separation anxiety, which reaches its peak in the second and third years of life. Fussing and dissatisfaction are often observed on the behavioral level during this period of greater separation anxiety. Infants appear indecisive: they approach an interesting person or object, and then seek the proximity of their parents again, oscillating between these seemingly still irreconcilable poles. They are not as yet able to occupy themselves alone and appear to need abundant attention and affection. Margaret Mahler (1975/2003) describes this in her considerations on the separation–individuation process. She makes a distinction between the "track of individuation," characterized by the evolution of intrapsychic autonomy, perception, memory, cognition, and reality testing, and the "track of separation," characterized by differentiation, distancing, boundary formation, and disengagement from the primary caregiver. Optimal situations appear to be those in which the perception of separation from the mother or father runs parallel to the infant's autonomous, independent functioning. In the course of development, the infant's ambivalence between closeness and the need for autonomy can manifest as what Mahler et al. (1978) refer to as a rapprochement crisis.

Jonathon (20 months) started crying every time he was picked up from the child care provider by his mother or father. In the mornings, he needed an intense settling-in phase to cope with the separation. During the day, he was highly active in the exploration of his environment and needed intensive support from the child care provider to settle or fall asleep. The parents always offered Jonathon immediate physical closeness, told him that they had missed him during the day, and stayed and played with him for a few minutes before leaving for home. After 3 weeks, Jonathon greeted his mother with a beaming smile, led her by the hand to a large toy truck and enthusiastically showed her how it tipped and emptied.

In addition to infant factors, the relational desires and psychological needs of the parents also influence the shape this phase takes. In their treatment model, Cierpka and Cierpka (2000) illustrate this with the image of scales: autonomy and closeness need to be balanced in all aspects thrown on the scales by parents and child (see Chap. 7, "Age-Appropriate vs. Persistent Defiance and Aggressive Behavior"). New opportunities arising in the course of motor development for the infant to actively discover its environment and create distance between itself and its mother or father often result in short but extremely intense phases of increased clinginess (Mahler 1975/2003). If motor skills lag behind the infant's drive to explore, frustration and boredom often ensue. Many infants press to be carried about more in order to reach the objects of their interest. This need automatically results in increased closeness between infant and parent; infants are often seen as demanding, while parents feel used as a means of transport. From the age of around 6 months, infants exhibit the need for reassurance in unknown or generally unsettling situations: they use their parents' emotional expressions as a guide to their own emotional assessment of a situation ("Should I touch that other child?"). This phenomenon, referred to as social referencing, guides the infant's actions during this phase (Campos and Stenberg 1981). In the course of intersubjective affective attunement, emotionally attuned parents intuitively pick up on their infant's affects and mirror them, without exerting too much influence on the action level. They transmit information on their affective appraisal of a situation to their infant via facial expressions, gestures, or verbally, thereby fostering the infant's ability to self-soothe ("Is this situation one I need to be scared in?"), as well as accomplish its affective action goals.

Emboldened by his father's nods and smiles and filled with curiosity, Robin (9 months) crawled toward an infant of his own age. When the infant, apparently also interested, moved toward him somewhat boisterously, Robin cried out anxiously, looked for his father, and was rooted to the spot with terror. The father registered Robin's anxiety, knelt down beside him, took him reassuringly in his arms, and verbalized his infant's state using empathic intonation: "Oh dear, you weren't expecting that little boy to come toward you so quickly! That gave you a fright, didn't it!" Robin calmed down and, feeling safe in his father's proximity, was able to turn his attention once again to the object of his interest.

This example of a father picking up on his infant's affective dynamics signalizes parental referencing and makes it easier for the infant to become aware of its subjective emotional state. The father expresses his infant's affect in a different modality using his voice, gestures, and facial expressions, thereby contributing to the modulation of his infant's arousal.

In addition to the modulating function described in the example, which serves affective attunement (Stern 1985), parents also act as a "container" in the Bion sense (Bion 1962/1984). This means the maternal and paternal willingness to empathize understandingly with the infant's state, endure the unpleasant state with the infant, and, e.g., enable the experience to be processed by putting it into words. This allows the infant to increase its scope for internal processing. If the infant learns that it will receive regulatory support, e.g., when it cries, the attachment figure becomes a safe base to which the infant can turn. If the infant primarily experiences rejection by the attachment figure when it cries, it will attempt to minimize or hide negative feelings in order to avoid rejection. If the attachment figure's behavior toward the infant's crying is unpredictable, some infants will try to ensure the protective proximity they crave through exaggerated attachment behavior involving excessive clinginess, demandingness, crying, and defiance, despite running the risk of rejection (Papoušek and von Hofacker 2004). However, some infants respond to inconsistent parental behavior with withdrawal and relationship avoidance behavior, signalizing that they need attention, e.g., by means other than crying. Toward the age of 12 months, transitional objects take on greater significance as aids to coping with the negative feelings elicited by separation situations in the course of early detachment from the parents (Winnicott 1951).

6.3 Excessive Clinginess

Excessive clinginess is a sign that the steps toward parent–infant detachment have not yet been adequately mastered. Unprocessed, often unconscious separation anxieties on the part of the parents generally form the backdrop to this phenomenon. As a result, insufficient security and confidence in its own coping skills are conveyed to the infant, even in non-threatening separation contexts. The parent–infant relationship generally appears strained and at risk. The infant's functional level is impaired and it becomes difficult, if not impossible, for it to accomplish the developmental steps at hand.

A mother who appeared tense, complained of her 11-month-old daughter, Louisa: "I don't have a minute to myself; she's always crawling behind me! And when I put her in her playpen so that I can unpack the dishwasher in peace, she goes completely crazy. And she won't be pacified by anyone but me. Even at night, my husband doesn't have a chance." Louisa, who was playing on the floor with a piece of paper, kept looking at her mother. Once the mother had calmed down somewhat, she responded to some of the infant's attempts at contact; she spoke to Louisa, e.g., when she cried after hitting her head: "What's the matter? I'm here, aren't I!" The mother neither offered the infant physical contact, nor did she speak to her; there were no moments of shared pleasure. The mother saw her relationship to her daughter as "one-sided and tiring." During the further course of the interview, the mother suddenly jumped up and quickly said to the therapist: "I need to go to the restroom," and left the room. Louisa remained frozen to the spot on the floor, staring at the door through which her mother had just disappeared. She glanced only briefly at the therapist, then started to cry loudly.

Symptom Triad of Excessive Clinginess

Excessive clinginess from the perspective of the symptom triad of early childhood regulatory disorders (Papoušek 2004; see also Chap. 1, "Developmental Crises") is described as follows:

(continued)

- *The infant* is not yet sufficiently capable of deploying self-directed soothing strategies to cope with states of inner tension, e.g., anxiety, confusion, frustration, or boredom. It relies primarily on attachment figures, generally its parents, for soothing. For this reason, the infant attempts to create or maintain physical proximity to its parents.
- *The parents* have the sense that their attempts at soothing and encouragement are inadequate and, as a result of their infant's persistent need for closeness, suffer from overload syndrome.
- *Dysfunctional interaction patterns* in the context of soothing and encouragement serve to perpetuate excessive clinginess. The parents, under strain, maintain closeness and fail to create clear detachment contexts.

▶ Prevalence

Whereas there is extensive information in the literature on emotional and behavioral disorders at preschool age, disorders of this kind in infancy and young childhood, although discussed in terms of their developmental psychological aspects, have not yet been investigated in direct relation to clinical disorders (see, e.g., Belsky et al. 1996; Calkins 2002; Crockenberg and Leerkes 2000; Laucht 2002).

Of the parents that attended the parent–infant/toddler clinic at the Heidelberg University Hospital with their infants between 1999 and 2009, 21 % gave separation anxiety as the reason for their visit (Thiel-Bonney 2009). This is often associated on a behavioral level with excessive clinginess, as well as impaired exploratory behavior (disinterest in play) or sleep disorders.

6.3.1 Aspects Requiring Particular Attention in Practice: Typical Trigger Situations and Risk Factors

Anxiety and fear emerge in a developmentally appropriate manner in the course of locomotor development as important affects in interaction and person-specific attachment at around the age of 9 months (Bowlby 1969). Weaning is an external step toward detachment often occurring at around the same time. The infant is no longer exclusively dependent on its mother for care and a spatial separation becomes possible. The fact that the infant sleeps in its own bed can also be seen as a step toward growing separateness. At the same time, the infant increasingly turns its attention to the outside world and starts to explore its environment. Either on all fours or on its feet, the child can move away from its parents of its own accord and lay claim to a wider radius of activity. Infants often feel alone when confronted with the experiences their conquests bring, and which may initially be perceived as threatening, thereby triggering anxiety or fear. The ability to consciously differentiate between primary attachment figures and strangers can, for instance, cause infants distress, even though they appeared unaffected by the proximity of strangers in the preceding months.

Other age-typical triggers of anxiety in the first 3 years of life include experiences of social separation, e.g., frequent or abrupt change of caregiver, premature or forced entry to a child care center, a strange environment due to moving home or going on vacation, changes in the family constellation (e.g., birth of a sibling or parental divorce), as well as a real or perceived interruption to a relationship (e.g., hospitalization of the mother).

On a physiological level, anxiety or fear manifest themselves as heightened arousal accompanied by behavioral inhibition (Papoušek and von Hofacker 2004), resulting in impaired exploratory behavior. From a psychophysiological perspective, the "acute stress response" (or hyperarousal) first described by Cannon (1929), with its alternatives of fight or flight, is triggered. Depending on the infant's motor skills, its clinginess in the sense of the stress response, "flight from the fear-inducing moment," may be the only appropriate reaction at that moment. Interpersonal regulation of the infant's anxiety by the caregiver is essential to coping with such situations (Papoušek and von Hofacker 2004). Kagan and Snidman (1999) see a relationship between the temperament factors of behavioral inhibition ("novelty inhibited"), greater irritability, and lower capacity for emotional regulation and an increased susceptibility to developing emotional disorders. Möhler et al. (2008) showed that generally negative hyperreactivity to unknown stimuli in very early childhood, e.g., increased crying in response to unknown events, objects, or people is associated with the onset of behavioral inhibition in the second year of life. It is possible that early social anxiety inhibits social learning, which would explain the effects this has on the further developmental course.

Interactional and relational experiences the infant has with its parents represent further risk factors. According to Fonagy et al. (2004), affect regulation and personality develop via the process of mentalization. Affective states are marked by a mechanism of affect mirroring, e.g., facial expressions or parents' vocal responses, in the context of parent–infant interaction. Affective states are then experienced by the infant as its own states and, ultimately, become concepts when the parents make it clear that it is the infant's and not their own affective state that is being expressed (Resch 2004). A prerequisite here is that the parents have the intrinsic ability to reflect mental experiences and translate these into language, affective responses, or actions. Parents that are limited in their ability to do this due to their own (early) childhood experiences and/or own anxiety symptoms are potentially incapable of making these translations. As a result, the reciprocal contagion of anxiety pervades interaction between parents and infant. Since there is no clear differentiation between who is scared of what now, these parents serve no soothing function for their infant. Parents may unconsciously expect their infant to soothe them as part of an interpersonal defense mechanism via parentification. This can contribute to an entanglement (Minuchin 1977/1997) between parents and infant, which undermines the development of detachment on both sides. A "good enough mother," according to Winnicott (1973), "starts off with an almost complete adaptation to her infant's needs, and as time proceeds she adapts less and less completely, gradually, according to the infant's growing ability to deal with her failure" (Winnicott 1973, p. 20). The mutual clinginess of mother/father and infant in the spiral of anxiety described above, however, maintains infant and parents in a state of dependence. The infant is prevented from developing self-directed strategies of anxiety regulation. Pathological parental resistance via projective identification can also contribute to the persistence of excessive clinginess. Parents are able to become active in the soothing of their infant, while they no longer perceive in themselves the anxieties that they have shifted to the infant. Parental separation anxiety is staved off in the context of these interpersonal dynamics. The parents "read" their own characteristics or perceptions into their infant—characteristics or perceptions that do not suit its developmental stage or character (Fraiberg et al. 1975). This can become harmful for the infant's well-being when it is attributed with a high level of intentionality, as in the following statement of a mother about her 5-month-old son: "He doesn't give me a moment's peace—he wants to torment me!" Resolving a distorted perception such as this can generally only be achieved in a psychotherapeutic setting.

On the relational level, parents and infant need to adapt to the "developmental paradox" (Trad 1993). The acquisition of new skills in the domain of self-regulation can result in a stronger sense of connectedness and intimacy in the family system. On the other hand, it also results in greater autonomy and detachment from one another from a developmental psychological perspective on the part of the infant, and from a lifecycle perspective on the part of the parents. The likelihood of clinginess manifesting increases if the family system fails to adapt to this paradox, primarily in the transition from dyad to triad (Cierpka and Cierpka 2000).

6.3.2 Infant Aspects Requiring Particular Attention

- A striking feature of the infant's behavior is its frequent, situation-unspecific demand for physical contact. Parents describe how their infant is literally tied to their apron strings. Breastfed infants frequently appear to demand the breast. The apparent demands for physical contact are accompanied by anxious, sometimes panicky crying.
- The infant expends a disproportionate amount of energy in soliciting parental attention and establishing contact. The infant fails to withdraw its attention from its parents to the extent needed for exploration and play. Infants are unable to engage in a play activity, switch activities regularly, or appear consistently unhappy due to the fact that they feel torn between play and proximity to their parents.
- When closeness or physical contact between parent and infant do occur, one observes that this often fails to result in soothing of the infant, but instead perpetuates a mood of tension.

(continued)

- Clinginess may be associated with social inhibition. This is characterized by an age-inappropriate, persistent inhibition of openness in strange environments or to unknown people. Infants often cling, motionless and in a state of high physical tension, to the arms or on the lap of the primary caregiver. They exhibit increased anxiety reactions, such as turning away or crying, upon attempts to approach them.
- Excessive separation anxiety that persists beyond the expected phase of increased anxiety to separation between the ages of 6 and 12 months is also associated with clinginess. Where separation between the primary caregiver and infant does occur, this results in marked, age-inappropriate reactions to separation, such as clinginess, crying, and panicky sobbing. Attempts at consolation, often colored by the primary caregiver's massive feelings of guilt, insecurity, and anxiety, generally fail to soothe the infant, since it is impossible to convey a sense of security to the child against this backdrop (Papoušek and von Hofacker 2004).

6.3.3 Aspects Requiring Attention in the Parent Interview

The parents' behavior toward their infant's attempts at contact generally appears insecure and ambivalent. The infant's signals are often misunderstood, or not recognized as such, while the parents frequently ask themselves what their infant wants from them. Parents often defer their own needs in daily life in favor of their infant's demands in the belief that this will satisfy their infant. Failure on the infant's part to react positively to this deferment puts strain on the relationship. Communication between parents and infant fails when clinginess is interpreted by the parents exclusively as attachment behavior and not as a soothing strategy. The infant's needs in terms of co-regulation, e.g., of anxiety, fatigue, boredom, or for entertainment, can no longer be clearly recognized and, as such, cannot be clearly addressed. The parents' sense of helplessness can result in them also experiencing greater resentment. This suppressed resentment gives rise in turn to a pattern of higher, yet dysfunctional responsivity. One gets the impression that parents do not allow themselves to take their attention off their infant for even a moment. Parents occasionally express a desire for detachment and time for themselves; however, they have no concept whatsoever of how this time window could be filled. Here again, their ambivalence becomes tangible and often gives rise to the notion that the infant's clinginess also fulfills an important parental function.

The parents find it difficult to let the infant out of the focus of their attention and thereby afford it greater freedom. For instance, they can barely follow a conversation with another adult, alternating their attention between the infant and the adult. Some parents also describe the impression that their infant becomes particularly demanding and clingy whenever they want to do something "for themselves" (e.g., make a telephone call, drink a cup of coffee), and ascribe intentionality to the infant in the form of aggression directed at them.

Parent–infant interactions are often characterized by an anxious and aggressive undertone. Parents frequently appear to be physically yet not emotionally available and struggle with detachment from their infant. Common observations include seemingly automated stroking or rocking of the infant as tension rises, or something between caring attention and rejection that does not appear to be guided by the infant's needs.

Asking the parents about their experiences of separation and how they currently deal with leave-taking and separation helps in the understanding of observed interactions and communication patterns. Demands arising in the context of infant development can reactivate suppressed conflicts in the parents. As a result, the parental coping mechanisms deployed to date may become destabilized and reinforce latent anxieties.

6.4 Treatment Approaches

Parents often seek help in a fog of helplessness, shame, and anger; in many cases, they suspect that their own unresolved issues will emerge from the difficulties their infant (sometimes in a dramatic way) exhibits (Fraiberg et al. 1975). The parents' view of their infant, among other aspects, is an essential factor in the selection of the appropriate approach: Are they able to see their infant's clinginess as an escalation in the context of a developmental task? Are they prepared to give their infant help when needed, and maintain a positive view of the infant despite all the difficulties? If yes, then they are likely to benefit from developmental psychological information. Do negative moments between parents and infant clearly predominate? Do the parents respond to their infant with only scant empathy and negative expectations? Have the difficulties persisted for more than 3 months and are other areas of development also affected (e.g., sleeping)? When this is the case, the optimal approach may be to elaborate individual options to provide developmental and relational support in the context of psychosocial counseling. Parent–infant/toddler psychotherapy is indicated in cases where a low-frequency counseling setting over a limited timescale is insufficient to implement changes and reduce psychological strain, e.g., in the case of structural limitations or neurotic conflicts in the parents, pronounced psychosocial risk factors, or a generalized early childhood regulatory disorder.

6.4.1 Developmental Psychological Information

Clinginess represents a means for the infant to respond to anxiety when it has insufficient self-directed, autonomous self-soothing strategies at its disposal. The parents' insight and understanding that their infant is still reliant on them for support are fundamental to conveying developmental psychological information.

Information on the infant's developmental stage and the developmental tasks it has already accomplished, as well as a consideration of the skills and deployable resources it has already gained (e.g., "can already play happily on her own," "explores his environment visually") can foster a positive and supportive approach on the part of the parents.

▶ Ways of Coping with Detachment Situations and Developing Anxiety Tolerance in Infants and Toddlers

- Conveying security and calmness in separation situations.
- Responding to and fulfilling the infant's need for closeness in stressful situations.
- Transmitting clear parental signals prior to a separation, even "small" separations (e.g., "I'm just going to sit on the chair there and read my book. You carry on playing here for a while with your building bricks. I'll come back to you in a minute.")
- Supporting the infant's self-directed play and exploration through encouragement and by conveying a sense of security (e.g., "You look very interested in the big doll over there on the shelf—shall we go over there together? I'll stay right next to you.")
- Introducing soothing aids that are person-independent and which the infant can reach on its own. Transitional objects of this kind, usually soft toys or security blankets, can fulfill a consoling and soothing function in lieu of the parents and represent an important companion for the infant at times of greater anxiety during the parents' absence.
- Verbal support aimed at modulating the infant's affects, but also at promoting insight into the infant's situation (e.g., "You don't quite know what to make of Uncle Billy, do you, so you're careful to start with. Take a look at him first—I'm right here with you. Maybe you'll want to play with him afterwards.")

6.4.2 Psychosocial Counseling

When brought to the child care provider, Mark (12 months) would cling to his parents, cry desperately and with growing intensity, and was barely consolable. This surprised and shocked his parents considerably, since they had only ever known their son as a happy and uncomplicated infant. Since visiting the child care provider, he had also started clinging to them more in other contexts. The parents were also concerned that Mark appeared highly irritable, reacted more strongly to separations and boundary setting than usual, and was unable to soothe himself, yet rejected help from his parents. Up until that point, Mark had spent a lot of time at home with one or both parents and his 5-year-old sister. His parents reported how he always observed new situations and people with interest, preferably from the proximity of his mother or father, only

(continued)

managing to detach himself and approach the things that interested him after a warm-up period. Since starting to settle in at the child care provider, it took him longer to be able to explore new things; often, he did not want to detach himself from his parents at all. At home, Mark occupied himself alone "when he wanted to." The mother would take advantage of the moments when Mark was engrossed in an activity to "slip away." She could not endure her son's crying when she tried to explain to him that she needed to leave. For this reason, she would wait next to Mark, impatient and irritated, until he was no longer paying attention to her. She sometimes had the feeling that Mark deliberately wanted to annoy her. Gratified, but also somewhat unsettled, the mother reported how Mark, who had never been a "cuddly baby," was now frequently seeking physical closeness. The parents also mentioned that Mark would only fall asleep in their presence and spent the second half of the night in their bed, which disturbed them. The mother in particular felt under pressure in relation to Mark settling-in at the child care, since she wanted to resume work and had scheduled a date for this with her employer: "Things need to have worked out with the child care by then." At the same time, the parents wondered whether they were expecting too much of their son.

Up until that time, Mark appeared to have had little opportunity to gather experience of separation situations. The parents had avoided establishing clear detachment contexts and separation situations recognizable as such to the infant. Closeness–distance regulation appeared as yet to be inadequately coordinated between parents and infant. Mark had until now determined when distance between him and his parents was permissible, while the parents adjusted themselves to him and subordinated their own needs to his. The parents and their infant had not yet succeeded in finding a good balance between closeness that offered comfort, security, and soothing, and autonomy that promised to satisfy the infant's curiosity and broaden his experience. When the parents were themselves in a state of emotional equilibrium, they noticed their infant's insecurity. They suspected that the separations they initiated presented Mark with difficulties that he was not yet able to cope with alone. On the other hand, the parents were less able to empathize in the same way when they themselves felt under strain or internal pressure. They felt anger, fueled in all likelihood by the fact that they regularly sacrificed their own wishes for the presumed needs of their infant. The parents saw Mark as the cause of their anger and ascribed to him intentionality directed at them. The sleep initiation and maintenance disorder they also reported is often associated with clinginess, since this domain likewise involves steps toward boundary-setting, detachment, and separation—tasks the parents and child needed to master.

Following an assessment of previous detachment processes, it was agreed during counseling that, together with the parents, individual approaches would be elaborated to offer Mark age-appropriate support in separation situations. In a first step, the question of what the parents felt they and their son were capable of needed to be answered. The parents suggested that they did not want to give Mark the feeling they were letting him down. They were aware that Mark relied on them heavily for support in terms of soothing and feeling secure. The introduction of a transitional object was proposed in order to facilitate the parents' gradual reduction of their still intensive support, while at the same time encouraging Mark to develop autonomous self-soothing strategies. The father suddenly remembered his "cuddly dolphin," which had helped him fall asleep every night up until school age. Opportunities for Mark and his parents to practice and gain experience with detachment and separation in everyday life were developed. This included, for instance, orchestrating small separation and reunion situations initiated by the parents in daily routine, and making separations identifiable as such by consciously taking leave of Mark in order that he could adjust to the situation. By anticipating Mark's potential protests, the parents were able to lower their expectations, thereby avoiding disappointment. Since it was particularly difficult for the mother to detach herself from Mark's proximity-seeking behavior, and she often resentfully and reluctantly gave in to his demands, the suggestion was made that the father provide her with back-up in such situations. The parents' growing insight in terms of detachment, as well as opportunities for closeness, combined with their understanding of the ongoing regulatory challenges facing Mark, conveyed a sense of security to the infant.

Experiencing when his parents left, but also learning that he could adjust to this separation when given clear prior signals and knowing that they would return, resulted in a marked reduction in Mark's protest crying and clinginess over a 2-week period. The soft toy that had been accompanying Mark everywhere for several weeks was embedded in the leave-taking ritual at the child care provider. The toy became less important as Mark became more accustomed to the procedure associated with being dropped off at child care; nevertheless, the toy continued to accompany Mark and would always be "waiting" for him on the coat rack after goodbyes. With great affection and delight, the parents reported on Mark's development and expressed their pride at having mastered this difficult time together as a family. They also felt ready to make near-term changes in the sleeping situation.

6.4.3 Parent–Infant Psychotherapy

Parent–infant psychotherapy may be indicated in those cases where developmental psychological information or psychosocial counseling is insufficient to achieve a significant change in symptoms. Impaired or distorted parental perception and interpretation of the infant's behavior, a generalized regulatory problem, or the emergence of maladaptive interaction patterns also constitute indications.

The "scales" model according to Cierpka and Cierpka (2000) enables one to consider the interplay between parental and infant autonomy and need for closeness as related to the onset of excessive clinginess. The central assumption is that, together, the parents and infant have an influence on the equilibrium of the scales, and hence also on the configuration and persistence of manifesting symptoms.

Both parents and infant throw not only negative aspects, but also resources on the scales (see also Figs. 7.1 and 7.2 in Chap. 7, "Age-Appropriate vs. Persistent Defiance and Aggressive Behavior").

Excessive clinginess can emerge as a result of various constellations in the parent–infant dynamics pertaining to autonomy and attachment:

1. The infant has a strong need for autonomy in the context of its pronounced curiosity behavior ("novelty seeking" according to Cloninger 1987). Due to the infant's resultant active exploratory behavior, it frequently finds itself in situations in which it is overchallenged; it then relies on the parents for soothing. Experiencing this repeatedly can potentially lead to the infant no longer daring to leave its parents' side, since it depends on the proximity of its parents for a sense of security, albeit that the parents do not actively offer this closeness. It may also arise that the parents restrict their infant's exploratory behavior on the basis that the infant's uneasiness elicits their own anxiety.
2. The infant responds anxiously to novelty ("novelty inhibited" according to Cloninger 1987) and prefers to remain closely attached to the parents. It reacts with anxious clinginess to the parents' encouragement to pay more interest in its environment. In adjusting to the infant's signals, the parents can offer little to foster autonomy and find themselves inextricably intertwined with the infant.
3. The parents' need for autonomy is high; therefore, they suppress, e.g., their own need for closeness. They want their infant to be independent and detached. The parents force detachment and separation to occur prematurely. If this causes the infant to experience overload and anxiety, it may respond in the form of increased clinginess toward its caregivers.
4. Due to their own considerable need for closeness, the parents enjoy the strong attachment to their infant. The infant's steps toward autonomy trigger anxiety in the parents and they wish to keep their infant close at hand. An interpersonal parental defense mechanism via projective identification results in the infant experiencing parental anxiety as its own and responding with increased clinginess.

A mother first attended the parent–infant/toddler clinic alone with her 23-month-old son, Max. She reported how Max continually wanted to play with her nipples with his hands for soothing purposes. In the mother's opinion, he demanded the breast in situations where he felt insecure or anxious; she reported that, in such situations, she felt able to understand his need for soothing. She continued: "Well you see, the breast is all he has: he never took a pacifier and I'm not about to start with something like that now." Although the mother was able to understand Max's behavior, she now found it inappropriate and embarrassing. She described how she would nevertheless put up with it, albeit in a state of heightening tension and irritation, sometimes even

(continued)

with revulsion, until Max stopped. The situations she found most challenging were those in which she would set boundaries for Max and he would subsequently express his anger toward her by crying, while at the same time repeatedly demanding the breast. She described an everyday situation: "We were in a toy shop. Max started unpacking boxes that were on display. I told him to stop doing that and picked him up. He started screaming defiantly—everyone was looking at me and I simply couldn't pacify this screaming child. I just wanted the ground to open up and swallow me. I tried reasoning with him—promised him something or other. But he just kept screaming 'Breast! Breast!' I suddenly got incredibly angry. I don't know anymore how we got out of the shop; all I can remember is that outside I grabbed him and shouted: 'What is it you want from me? Just leave me in peace; I'm there for you the whole time!' Once we got back home, I was terribly ashamed at having lost my self-control like that. Max was paralyzed with fear; I think I really scared him. I held him in my arms for a long time and when he reached into my blouse, I didn't stop him."

In terms of the conflict around autonomy and attachment, the above example equates to the constellation described in point (3).

Max was the second child in the family. After a long and unwelcomed period of childlessness, the parents had decided to undertake in vitro fertilization. After a number of failed attempts and one miscarriage, the mother had become pregnant and given birth to Max's older brother. She had spontaneously become pregnant with Max 4 months after the birth of her first child. The mother reported that this had been a considerable shock to her, that she had been in denial about the pregnancy, and felt she was losing control over her life. She had only ever wanted one child and still did not feel prepared for the task of raising two children adequately. It appeared that, even before Max was born, she had blamed him for "invading" her life and sabotaging her chances of self-determination and independence. Max was retrospectively described as an excessively crying infant. Again, the mother felt at the infant's mercy, since none of her efforts succeeded in soothing him (see Chap. 3, "Excessive Crying"). She noticed that physical closeness had a soothing effect on the infant, hence she offered him this, despite feeling "forced" to do so. She reported that she was unable to recall any pleasant "cuddle times" and, still today, felt predominantly negative emotions when she saw him or came into physical contact with him: "I feel as if I have to put down a protective shield that keeps me together and lets me live more or less anxiety-free." She described how she felt dominated by Max, since he did not allow her the space she needed.

At the therapist's invitation, the father also attended meetings over the course of therapy. He perceived Max as primarily anxious and helpless in the situations his wife described. In his opinion, the mother's and infant's arousal was mutually escalated in such situations. He suppressed his frequent urge to take his son in his arms and soothe him in his wife's presence, since this would send her into a fury. The mother accused her husband of reinforcing Max in the belief that he had a right to pester her physically. This scene clearly illustrated the degree of distortion in the mother's perception of Max in that she attributed a high level of intentionality to him. The father was able to empathize with Max, perceive his distress in detachment situations with the mother, and had an intuitive idea as to how to resolve the problem, i.e., offering a soothing aid. He agreed with his partner that, as yet, Max had no means of soothing other than playing with the breast. This, he believed, was responsible for Max's unhealthy attachment to his mother. It was established that the mother doubted on the one hand that her husband was capable of soothing Max, while on the other she was worried that he may indeed be able to do so and that she, as a result, would become less important to Max. The maternal gatekeeping behavior identified here was hampering the deployment of paternal resources and the formation of a relationship between father and son. It can be understood in the context of the mother's fear of losing control—in this case control of soothing the infant. The mother came to understand in the course of therapy that Max was overchallenged by detachment situations and sought physical closeness as a soothing mechanism. The resultant conscious perception of her own desire for closeness triggered considerable anxiety in the mother, leading to more controlling behaviors.

In the further course, the mother attended individual psychotherapy sessions. Recognizing her own anxiety, she was able to hand over child-care tasks to her husband. In a first step, the father was very well able to couple Max's need for closeness with appropriate positive encouragement to explore, particularly in the context of joint play situations. This enabled Max to develop autonomous soothing strategies in separation situations and helped him to cope better with irritation and frustration. Although the infant's growing autonomy also in other domains temporarily exacerbated the mother's anxieties, these could be identified as her own anxieties and worked through during psychotherapy independent of the infant.

6.5 Conclusion

Managing separation in the course of autonomy development and coping with the infant's resultant anxieties after the age of 6 months represent a double-pronged challenge for the parents and infant to master together. Since the infant's self-soothing skills are not yet fully developed, primary caregivers (generally the parents, but also child-care personnel) are called upon in this transitional phase to help the infant regulate its emotional states. The primary goals of counseling are to foster an understanding of clinginess as an initially appropriate response on the part of the infant to anxiety, and to find ways for the infant to acquire autonomous self-regulatory skills. Early childhood regulatory disorders, temperament factors, possible parental psychopathology, as well as early relational and interactional experiences may impact the course and need to be taken into consideration when establishing the indication.

References

Belsky J, Woodworth S, Crnic K (1996) Trouble in the second year: three questions about family interactions. Child Dev 67:556–578
Bion W (1962/1984) A theory of thinking. Second thoughts: selected papers on psychoanalysis. Karnac, London
Bowlby J (1969) Attachment and loss. Basic Books, New York
Calkins SD (2002) Does aversive behavior during toddlerhood matter? The effects of difficult temperament on maternal perceptions and behavior. Infant Mental Health J 23:381–402
Campos JJ, Stenberg CR (1981) Perception, appraisal, and emotions: the onset of social referencing. In: Lamb ME, Sherrod LR (Hrsg) Infant social cognition: empirical and social considerations. Erlbaum, Hillside, NJ, S 273–314
Cannon WB (1929) Bodily changes in pain, hunger, fear, and rage. Appleton Century Crofts, New York
Cierpka M, Cierpka A (2000) Beratung von Familien mit zwei- bis dreijährigen Kindern. Prax Kinderpsychol Kinderpsychiatr 49(8):563–579
Cierpka M, Windaus E (Hrsg) (2007) Psychoanalytische Säuglings-Kleinkind-Eltern-Psychotherapie. Konzepte, Leitlinien, Manual. Brandes & Apsel, Frankfurt a.M.
Cloninger CR (1987) A systematic method for clinical description and classification of personality variants. A proposal. Arch Gen Psychiatry 44:573–588
Crockenberg S, Leerkes E (2000) Infant social and emotional development in family context. In: Zeanah CH Jr. (Hrsg) Handbook of infant mental health, 2. Aufl. Guilford Press, New York, S 60–90
Dornes M (2001) Die frühe Kindheit. Entwicklungspsychologie der ersten Lebensjahre. Fischer, Frankfurt a.M.
Deutsche Gesellschaft für Kinder- und Jugendpsychiatrie und Psychotherapie (Hrsg) (2007) Leitlinien zur Diagnostik und Therapie von psychischen Störungen im Säuglings-, Kindes- und Jugendalter. Deutscher Ärzte Verlag, Köln
Fonagy P, Gergely G, Jurist EL, Target M (2004) Affektregulierung, Mentalisierung und die Entwicklung des Selbst. Klett-Cotta, Stuttgart
Fraiberg S, Adelson E, Shapiro V (1975) Ghosts in the nursery. A psychoanalytical approach to the problems of impaired infant-mother relationships. J Am Acad Child Adolesc Psychiatry 14:387–422
Freud A (1968) Wege und Irrwege in der Kinderentwicklung. Klett, Stuttgart
ICD-10. http://www.dimdi.de/static/de/klassi/diagnosen/icd10/index.htm. Accessed 15 Feb 2011
Kagan J, Snidman N (1999) Early childhood predictors of adult anxiety disorders. Biol Psychiatry 46:1536–1541
Largo RH (2001) Babyjahre. Die frühkindliche Entwicklung aus biologischer Sicht. Piper, München
Laucht M (2002) Störungen des Kleinkind- und Vorschulalters. In: Esser G (Hrsg) Lehrbuch der klinischen Psychologie und Psychotherapie des Kindes- und Jugendalters. Thieme, Stuttgart, S 102–118
Laucht M, Schmidt MH, Esser G (2004) Frühkindliche Regulationsprobleme: Vorläufer von Verhaltensauffälligkeiten des späteren Kindesalters? In: Papoušek M, Schieche M, Wurmser M (Hrsg) Regulationsstörungen der frühen Kindheit. Hans Huber, Bern, S 339–356
Mahler M (1975/2003) Die psychische Geburt des Menschen, Symbiose und Individuation, 18. Aufl. Fischer, Frankfurt a.M
Mahler MS, Pine F, Bergman A (1978) Die psychische Geburt des Menschen. Fischer, Frankfurt a.M
Minuchin S (1977/1997) Familie und Familientherapie, Theorie und Praxis struktureller Familientherapie. Lambertus, Freiburg
Möhler E, Kagan J, Oelkers-Ax R, Brunner R, Poustka L, Haffner J et al (2008) Infant predictors of behavioural inhibition. Br J Dev Psychol 26:145–150

Papoušek M (2004) Regulationsstörungen der frühen Kindheit: Klinische Evidenz für ein neues diagnostische Konzept. In: Papoušek M, Schieche M, Wurmser H (Hrsg) Regulationsstörungen der frühen Kindheit: Frühe Risiken und Hilfen im Entwicklungskontext der Eltern-Kind-Beziehungen. Hans Huber, Bern, S 77–110

Papoušek M, von Hofacker N (2004) Klammern, Trotzen, Toben—Störungen der emotionalen Verhaltensregulation des späten Säuglingsalters und Kleinkindalters. In: Papoušek M, Schieche M, Wurmser H (Hrsg) Regulationsstörungen der frühen Kindheit: Frühe Risiken und Hilfen im Entwicklungskontext der Eltern-Kind-Beziehungen. Hans Huber, Bern, S 201–232

Resch F (2004) Entwicklungspsychopathologie der frühen Kindheit im interdisziplinären Spannungsfeld. In: Papoušek M, Schieche M, Wurmser H (Hrsg) Regulationsstörungen der frühen Kindheit. Frühe Risiken und Hilfen im Entwicklungskontext der Eltern-Kind-Beziehung. Hans Huber, Bern, S 31–49

Stern D (1985) The interpersonal world of the infant. Basic Books, New York

Thiel-Bonney C (2009, unveröffentlicht). Deskriptive Daten aus dem Elternfragebogen der Interdisziplinären Spezialsprechstunde für Eltern und Säuglingen und Kleinkindern. Institut für Psychosomatische Kooperationsforschung und Familientherapie, Heidelberg

Thomas, A, & Chess, S (1977).Temperament and development. New York: Brunner/Mazel. The Temperament Trap: Recognizing and Accommodating Children's Personalities

Trad PV (1993) Short-term parent-infant psychotherapy. Basic Books, New York

Winnicott D (1951) Übergangsobjekte und Übergangsphänomene. In: Winnicott D (Hrsg) Von der Kinderheilkunde zur Psychoanalyse. Kindler, München, S 293–312

Winnicott DW (1973) Vom Spiel zur Kreativität. Klett, Stuttgart

7 Developmentally Appropriate vs. Persistent Defiant and Aggressive Behavior

Manfred Cierpka and Astrid Cierpka

Case Report

Max (24 months) had become increasingly defiant in the preceding 6 months. He sometimes threw tantrums of such intensity that he would injure himself. His mother, exhausted and perplexed, was just managing to hide her anger under the surface. Her voice sounded husky as if she had a lump in her throat. It was necessary for her to attend the initial session alone in order to unburden herself. It was not until the second session that she brought her son with her. When the therapist went to greet mother and son in the waiting room, Max was engrossed in playing with the cars he had brought with him. The mother seized him relatively abruptly and took him into the therapy room. Max started to cry as soon as he was in his mother's arms. He made it clear with his gestures that he wanted to go back into the waiting room. "No! No! No!" he screamed repeatedly. He did not want to play in the therapy room, but rather in the other room. When his mother failed to give in to his demands, remaining instead in the therapy room and sitting down, Max flew into a tantrum. He threw himself on the floor, then wanted to go back on his mother's lap, then back on the floor again—up and down. He stiffened his body and rolled about on the floor. With patches of perspiration appearing at her armpits, the mother tried to calm her toddler. He, however, hit her, while she on the other hand stroked his head. "I have to put up with this madness for several hours a day," she interposed, almost shouting to be heard over her son. "I'm scared that I'll do something to him one day."

M. Cierpka, M.D. (✉)
Institute for Psychosocial Prevention, University Hospital Heidelberg,
Bergheimer Str. 54, Heidelberg 69115, Germany
e-mail: manfred.cierpka@med.uni-heidelberg.de

A. Cierpka, Dipl.Soz.Arb.
Private Practice, Keplerstr. 1, Heidelberg 69120, Germany

M. Cierpka (ed.), *Regulatory Disorders in Infants*,
DOI 10.1007/978-3-319-43556-5_7

Definition of Defiance and Temper Tantrums

Defiance in toddlerhood is always a response to self-initiated frustration or frustration caused by a third party. Defiance in a toddler is not driven by intention, but is instead an expression of the child's failure to emotionally regulate its frustration. Momentary and temporary loss of contact with the environment is characteristic. The toddler is "beside itself" (Metzger 1972), "thrown off track." Temper tantrums generally last between 30 s and 5 min—sometimes longer in the case of excessive defiance. A temper tantrum goes through the following phases (Potegal and Davidson; Potegal et al. 2003):

1. The triggering situation.
2. The "knee-jerk reaction": the toddler is "beside itself." The oppositional behavior ranges from verbal "No!" and "Don't want to!" to shouting and screaming, and ultimately to crying and whimpering. Finally, the child is completely exhausted.
3. The drama ends, the child experiences relief, and seeks the closeness of its mother or father.
4. Once the "fit" is over, infants frequently fail to remember what it was they wanted in the first place.

Max likewise appeared transformed after his temper tantrum. His mother had taken him back into the waiting room, where he played alone for a few minutes while his crying abated. He then decided of his own accord to cross the hallway back into the therapy room and continue playing there. It was as if the temper tantrum had never taken place.

Defiance should not be confused with other forms of noncompliance. Disobedience belongs to oppositional behavior and will be discussed later. A child sometimes acts more reasonably than an adult in its apparent disobedience and intentional noncompliance. One can by all means assume that a child may be right about something even at such a young age. In the case of defiant behavior, one should always bear in mind that a toddler might be responding with noncompliance due to shyness or inhibition.

7.1 Developmentally Appropriate Defiance

7.1.1 Prevalence

Based on the US classification of childhood into different ages, "toddler" refers in the following to children aged between 13 and 36 months.

Defiance is a transient developmental phenomenon in virtually all children. Seen in 80 % of 17-month-old infants, it peaks in 2-year-olds and slowly abates thereafter up to the age of 5 years (Shaw et al. 2000, 2001). There are no apparent boy–girl differences in the prevalence of normal defiance (Potegal and Davidson 2003; Österman and Björkquist 2010). Normal defiance also encompasses the first instances of developmentally appropriate physical and verbal aggression. Up to 80 % of infants and toddlers aged between 12 and 17 months exhibit aggressive behaviors. Data show that 70 % of all toddlers take toys away from other children, 46 % push and shove others, and 21–27 % bite, scratch, kick, hit, and pull hair (Tremblay et al. 1999). This behavior peaks in frequency at 2 years. Aggression of this kind is part of the normal development of boys and girls. Temper tantrums also belong to the spectrum of normal behavior at this age. Indeed, Belsky et al. (1996) found defiance problems in 62 % of 15- to 21-month-old first-born boys included in a random sample, while Österman and Björkquist (2010) found a rate of 87 % in children aged up to 9 years. Defiant behavior typically diminishes in frequency and intensity in the fourth year of life (Potegal et al. 2003; MacFarlane et al. 1954), a decline associated with increased language attainment (Dionne et al. 2003). There is evidence that temper tantrums in children are a universal problem (Bhatia et al. 1990; Johnson 2003; Tomm and Suzuki 1990; Fouts et al. 2005). However, there are significant cultural differences in terms of how this problem is addressed.

7.1.2 Defiance as a Regulatory Phenomenon

Defiance and, indeed, temper tantrums are associated with strong emotions that need to be regulated by the child. With its defiance, the toddler gains more time to cope with its intense feelings. When this fails, a temper tantrum may ensue. From a phenomenological perspective, the toddler's temper tantrum is not dissimilar to the angry and often irrational protests of the adolescent or to the adult's "blind fury." Strong emotions spiral out of control.

In the second year of life, the toddler is better able to express positive as well as negative emotions. This results in toddlers being able to strongly express emotions such as happiness and anger without immediately losing control. However, since the toddler has become more aware of itself, new emotions such as shame and pride emerge. The emergence of shame only becomes possible when the still fragile "self" sees itself as unable to fulfill its own (or others') demands and is disappointed in itself. Pride at an achievement or a new experience is also a particular novelty at this age. These new developmental steps are associated with the need to control emotions and modulate them according to context. The development of emotions follows distinct stages spanning from infancy and toddlerhood to preschool age. Whereas the infant can rely on its caregivers for interactional and mostly dyadic regulation of its emotionality (co-regulation) in the first year of life, it outgrows the dyadic relationship after infancy by virtue of its growing autonomy. Dyadic emotional regulation is gradually replaced by self-regulation of emotions. A reliable and supportive caregiver remains essential in order for self-regulation in toddlerhood to develop successfully. Although the toddler is already capable of coping with its emotional arousal in many instances, this continuity is regularly interrupted and the toddler once again requires short-term support from its stable caregiver, particularly when it experiences frustration or is unable to cope with the emotional transformation from great pride to bitter disappointment.

In the second year of life, further cognitive maturation takes places, bringing with it growing skills of self- and object perception. The toddler learns to distinguish better between itself and others. This is associated with the development of its own will and desires. Greater autonomy results in the toddler developing a new need for efficacy. It enjoys new challenges and is proud of its achievements. As its skills grow, so does its struggle for independence: it wants to do more itself or have more for itself. This increase in conscious volition (Bischof-Köhler 1998) leads in interaction with parents as well as peers to a greater tendency toward self-assertion, which can be dogged by conflict.

The child's new developmental steps mean new insecurities for the parents. Any trend toward independence triggers separation anxieties. Since the toddler is not equal to many of the challenges it faces and its safety is at times compromised, it continues to rely on its parents for support and boundary-setting. In summary: in the second year of life, the focus is no longer on autonomy *or* closeness and attachment, but rather on a balance *between* autonomy and attachment.

This is a period of transformation that can also be associated with crises for the parents. During this phase of increasing autonomy, the parents need to have a particular understanding of the "paradox of development" (Trad 1993, p. 23): while the acquisition of new skills in the parent–toddler system leads to a stronger sense of attachment and intimacy on the one hand, it results on the other in greater autonomy and hence detachment from one another—from a developmental psychological perspective on the part of the infant and from a life cycle perspective on the part of the parents. If the system is able to adjust to this relational paradox, the toddler is capable of taking a further developmental psychological step toward object constancy and the parents are afforded new relational qualities in their partnership.

During this affectively challenging phase, infants require stable caregivers and parents that are capable of attunement and agreement. In this sensitive phase of ever more frequent aggressive behavior, infants need parents that are able to empathize with these phase-typical difficulties and view them from the infant's perspective. The experiences of those involved in parent–infant interaction result in an intersubjective system that is created out of the experiential world of dealing with power and powerlessness, as well as control and submission. The internalization of this intersubjective system expands on the "relational patterns" described by Stern (1992) by adding the themes "power and powerlessness" and "control and submission."

7.1.3 Trigger Situations

Frustrations arise constantly in daily life. They are triggered when the infant is restricted from carrying out its intended action, its needs are not fulfilled, or when the intended action surpasses its abilities and it experiences disappointment in itself. Frustration is anchored in the conflict between infant wishes and parental intentions. Hunger or fatigue can additionally contribute to reducing the stress tolerance required to cope with frustration. Examples:

- A child is engrossed in play and flies into a tantrum when the parents say "Come on, we've got to go."
- Getting dressed, washing, and brushing teeth are seen as acts of parental exercise of power.
- The toddler dawdles while getting dressed—the parents show their impatience.
- The toddler refuses to have its safety belt fastened in the car, even though this measure is required for its own safety.
- The parents want to collect their toddler from kindergarten—the infant, however, would like to stay longer.
- The toddler is tired and wants to go to bed—but it doesn't really want to go to bed.

Although defiance usually occurs in familiar surroundings, it sometimes also occurs in public settings. This can prove particularly stressful for the parents due to the embarrassment factor. Interestingly, excessive defiance occurs in the presence of adults, not however peers.

7.1.4 Information and Developmental Psychological Counseling for Parents

Parents should be made aware of the fact that excessive defiance is a transient phenomenon. They require patience and equanimity during the excessive-defiance phase. They also need a certain degree of ingenuity and imagination to divert their child's focus of attention. Assuming the child is not already overstimulated by its stimulus-seeking behavior, offering a new and interesting attraction can help dissolve the situation. Pain and anger disappear in the blink of an eye. Parents need to adopt a stance toward their child and develop ways to solve conflict situations. Therefore, parents are strongly advised to take an anticipatory approach to the ever-recurring conflict situations.

7.1.5 Aspects Requiring Particular Attention in the Parent Interview

A healthy curiosity about boundary experiences can also help parents. If they are able to see the positive aspect of their toddler's excessive defiance as a demonstration of power, they are better equipped to withstand greater strain.

An interest in the "major emotions" such as pride and anger also helps during stressful and burdensome phases in the relationship.

7.1.6 Pitfalls

It is important for parents to understand that their infant's defiant behavior does not represent rejection. The 2- to 3-year-old toddler can and wants to do much more now, until it realizes that it is not able to do everything after all, nor is it able to do things as it would like to. It lacks, moreover, the stamina and patience, despite already being able to do so much.

The defiant toddler loves its parents and wants to feel accepted by them even in its "temper tantrum" with its strong, uncontrolled, and sometimes even furious emotions. Defiance is clearly distinct from disobedience in this respect. Normal defiance is not associated with attention deficit/hyperactivity disorder (ADHD).

7.2 Excessive Defiance and Persistent Temper Tantrums

Case Report

Mrs. F. sought help due to her 20-month-old son Julian's recurrent "fits." These were occurring two to three times per day, usually triggered by trivial events. He simply didn't want to do what she wanted him to do. If she insisted for instance that it was time to eat, but he wanted to continue playing, he would fly into a rage. He would throw things about in his room and hit the wall or door with his fists and feet. When she tried to get closer in order to soothe him, he would hit her too, saying: "Go away!" He would then slowly calm down in his room on his own. Going to sleep at night was particularly problematic: Julian would only go to sleep in a parent's arms in a protracted ritual accompanied by screaming. Only then could he be settled in his bed. When Julian had one of his "fits," the mother would get so angry that she frightened herself. This was the principal reason why she had sought help. Although she had always managed as yet to "swallow" her anger and powerlessness, she now felt she had reached the end of her tether.

Definition

Disproportionately frequent, protracted, and intense defiance, sometimes taking the form of a temper tantrum, puts a strain on parents as well as infants. The toddler is highly aroused, angry, and tends toward aggressive, (auto) destructive behavior during a temper tantrum. The child is "beside itself" and incapable of self-pacification. "Problem children" are often referred to our outpatient department following aggressive acts toward objects or, more frequently, people. For instance, the toddler bites another child at the daycare center or never misses an opportunity to push or kick its younger sibling. Some children hit their heads against the wall or floor as an act of self-destructive behavior. This form of aggressive behavior is seen in almost all children during the defiant phase and initially worsens before finally abating.

Excessive defiance is not necessarily pathological. However, if the parents fail in their attempts to emotionally regulate their toddler, maladaptive interaction will persist. This bears the risk of excessive defiance evolving into oppositional behavior at some later point.

7.2.1 Prevalence

Excessive defiance and regular, protracted temper tantrums are the commonest causes for parents of toddlers aged between 15 and 30 months to seek professional advice. Of those parents visiting the parent–infant/toddler clinic at the Heidelberg University Hospital (see Cierpka 2012, Chap. 30), 27 % attend with their toddler due to excessive defiance and regular, intense temper tantrums. Needlman et al. (1991) found excessive defiance (defined as at least three temper tantrums per day lasting at least 15 min) in 6.8 % of 3-year-olds investigated. Rates lay between 5 and 20 % in other studies (Chamberlin 1974; Macfarlane et al. 1954; Richman et al. 1982). Boys in this age group exhibit excessive defiance more frequently compared with girls (Ounstedt and Simons 1978).

If defiance and temper tantrums persist, they are usually associated with oppositional behavior. Papoušek and von Hofacker (2004) rightly point out that this aggressive behavior is not intended to be destructive in the narrower sense. The toddler does not wish to cause injury, but attract instead its caregiver's attention and get its own way. It is not the emergence of aggression in the second year of life that is problematic, but rather the factors that contribute to aggressive behavior persisting and being increasingly instrumentalized by the toddler. If no boundaries are set, the infant quickly learns that its aggressive behavior can bring advantages.

7.2.2 Severity, Risk Factors, and Prognosis

Papoušek and von Hofacker (2004) put the behavioral abnormalities of excessive defiance on a continuum with regulatory disorders of infancy. As with excessive crying, excessive defiance is an extreme variant of emotional behavioral regulation. In particular its persistence—as opposed to its emergence—can become problematic.

- Excessive defiance can also be described in terms of a symptom triad (see Chap. 1) if one considers the side of both the toddler and the primary caregiver, as well as the interactional and relational structure between these two (Papoušek 2004):
- The symptom triad of excessive defiance as an early childhood regulatory disorder includes:

1. The child's difficulty(ies), in the context of an early childhood adjustment and developmental task, in achieving emotional regulation of intense affects (disappointment, anger), particularly following frustration.

2. Psychophysical overload syndrome in the mother/father/both parents in dealing with a "difficult," defiant toddler; strains caused by their own difficulties in dealing with power and powerlessness, control and submission, boundary setting, and/or with their own intense affects may compound the situation.
3. Dysfunctional behavioral patterns in their direct dealing with the child's abnormal behavior, which in turn perpetuate or worsen the behavior and result in escalation. These interactional difficulties between parents and child can be described in terms of the "weighing scale" model of autonomy and attachment.

7.2.3 Diagnosis

One approach to assessing a defiant child lies in observing it play during the initial interview. The type of communication, as well as the relationship between parents and infant, can be assessed by observing interaction between parents and infant in the consultation room. The parents' child-rearing skills can also be assessed from how they deal with their infant. From a psychodynamic perspective, transference and countertransference dynamics quickly emerge in the interview setting. The therapists' own feelings of powerlessness reflect the parents' and infant's feelings. Their own emerging feelings of aggression and thoughts of boundary-setting can be harnessed for their work with the family. There is usually no shortage of scenes permitting unconscious scenic understanding.

Prognosis depends on the extent to which the child's level of functioning is impaired. The child's temperament, as a constitutional factor, also impacts defiant behavior. Children with greater affective reactivity exhibit higher arousal intensity and a tendency toward impulsivity (Rothbart et al. 1994). The subgroup of particularly defiant children seen in the context of the Munich Program differed from other toddlers in this age group most notably on the "fussy/difficult" temperament scale. Mean differences were also seen in 2-year-olds on the "stubbornness" and "problems with social contact" scales.

An assessment of the child's level of speech development is also important. If the child's expressive language is limited, it is unable to express its needs adequately and hence experiences frustration more rapidly. Forced speech development and a predominantly verbal child-rearing style on the part of the parents can overtax the child; both can contribute to increased defiance.

Moreover, the severity of excessive defiance depends on the duration of current and previous regulatory disorders (persistence). As with the severity of regulatory disorders in infancy, the seriousness of the problem correlates with the number of disordered domains (pervasiveness). The problem is more serious when sleep initiation and maintenance disorders (see "Case study") are additionally involved.

Rapidly overstrained parents can only contribute to the emotional regulation of their infant's crises to a limited extent. Overstrained mothers of boys appear to show a particular tendency toward aversive behavior (Calkins 2002). The behavior of these parents is generally impulsive and uncontrolled, or permissive "for the sake of peace," and hence inconsistent and inconsequential in terms of behavioral responses. Consensus on a child-rearing style is lacking within the partnership. Authoritarian/controlling fathers only contribute to a worse prognosis in cases where the mothers also subscribe to this child-rearing style (Belsky et al. 1996). It is important to note in this context that research on the father's contribution is lacking.

If the child's ability to self-regulate is limited to an extreme extent, this can put excessive strain on the parents in terms of their intuitive communication skills and the self-regulation aides at their disposal. The least favorable prognosis is seen in children readily prone to affective arousal and with a tendency toward frequent temper tantrums, particularly in combination with parents that have scant resources at their disposal due to their own strained biography, poor capacity for emotional modulation, limited child-rearing skills, serious partnership crises, and current risk factors. A favorable prognosis is assumed in cases where parents have managed to cope successfully with earlier regulatory disorders in their child's infancy. A long-term study of "defiant children" up to adolescence (Olson et al. 2000) revealed the best predictors that externalizing behavior would not develop to be: parents not feeling rejected by, as well as managing to maintain a warm, emotionally positive relationship with, their child.

7.2.4 Therapeutic Approaches

In our therapeutic model (Cierpka and Cierpka 2000, see below) we see *autonomy/detachment* and *intimacy/attachment* as the two sides of a weighing scale on which the parents distribute weights with their conscious and unconscious expectations and projections, thereby affecting the balance of the scale.

With its tendency toward autonomy or attachment, a child pulls on one side of the scale from below, thereby pulling it down. In Fig. 7.1, the child and its parents pull and push equally on the weighing scale of autonomy and attachment (the vectors are equal in length). In the vast majority of cases, however, the two sides of the scale are at different levels and the vectors differ in length. Parents, with their own early negative experiences that compelled them to forced independence, may press down on the scale through their (unconscious) expectations of their child. Children with a "novelty seeking" temperament (Kagan 1997; see also Cierpka 2012, Chap. 3) may also have a tendency toward autonomy, thereby pulling down on the left side of the scale. On the other hand, parents that were anxiously attached to their own parents may expect attachment from their child, thereby pushing down on the right side of the scale. However, even a child's relatively inhibited behavior ("novelty inhibited") can pull on the right side of the scale. Disruption of the equilibrium between autonomy and attachment and a tipping of

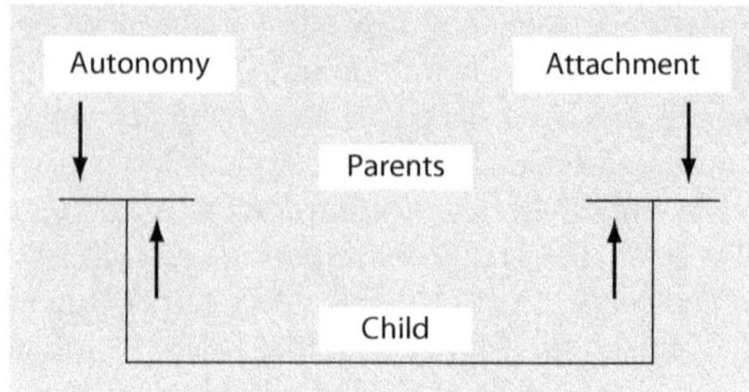

Fig. 7.1 Ideal balance between autonomy and attachment in the parent–toddler relationship

the scale to one side will trigger separation anxiety or loss-of-self anxiety in the child. It then runs the risk in the closeness/distance conflict of either losing the object through forced autonomy, or merging with the object through excessive attachment and losing the self.

Approaches to providing information, counseling, and psychotherapy need to be tailored not only to the currently burdened situation, but also geared to preventing the persistence of defiant behavior and its evolution into aggressive/oppositional behavior. Therapeutic support follows a stepwise approach according to the duration and intensity of the problem and ranges from providing information to counseling or psychotherapy.

Detailed *parent information and developmental psychological counseling* aim to instill the parents with a positive, supportive attitude and approach to their child (see above). It is important for parents to understand that the issue in moments of high tension is generally not one of content to be addressed verbally, but rather a question of them maintaining their composure, finding ways out of the situation, and keeping communication clear and unambiguous.

Some examples of what a therapist may say to parents:

- It's not about who's the strongest. Your child has trouble coping with the situation!
- His conduct is not directed against you!
- You mustn't let the child's anger be projected onto you. Let off steam, but not with your child!
- Have you been able to identify the situations in which your child does not tend toward defiance?

Psychosocial counseling becomes necessary when the "pleasant moments shared between parents and child" have receded into the background and negative experiences have come to the fore. Where this is the case, the entire family system is generally already significantly burdened. The primary goal of psychosocial counseling is to formulate solutions together with the parents that are aimed at promoting developmental and relational aspects for parents and child. A relatively modest number of sessions is often sufficient if short-term, symptom-centered counseling appears feasible. The focus here is on discussing and practicing changes in interaction between parents and child with the aim of reducing the frequency and intensity of defiance and temper tantrums. The child's linguistic competence plays a prominent role here. Karp and Spencer (2004) focus on the as yet poor linguistic skills of toddlers. The parents should mirror their toddler's emotions and put them into words. They contribute in this way to the toddler's ability to better articulate its needs and thus avoid frustration. However, parents should not overtax their toddler with attempts at verbal explanations and discussions on content. A child under the age of 3 years requires, in its toddler's experiential world, parents that will guide and show it what they do and do not want of it.

7.2.5 Aspects Requiring Attention During Parent Interviews

When dealing with temper tantrums, parents can be counseled in such a way that they are able to act preemptively to avoid trigger situations.

The following questions are helpful in this regard:

- How and in what form does defiance manifest? On what occasions? In the presence of whom? Is there a trigger? Are there exceptions?
- Where does defiance occur? Are there any recurring situations that result in escalation?
- What are the parents' theories on their toddler's defiance?

During an emotional crisis, bridges can be built for the child in the form of distraction, shifting the focus of attention, or changing the context. Parents are advised that—assuming their child's safety is not at risk, as is the case in the vast majority of instances—they should consistently ignore autoaggressive behavior. This ensures that the child's negative behavior is no longer rewarded by the parents' increased attention in such situations. Instead, one can consider together with the parents which positive aspects of behavior they could encourage in their child at that moment in order to dissuade it from self-destructive actions. The goal of the intervention is to encourage desired behavior and ignore undesired behavior.

7.2.6 Pitfalls in Practice

Aggressive behavior toward others needs to be addressed immediately: "No, Julian, I don't want you to bite me. That hurts!" Coming down to the child's eye level and establishing eye contact in order to give these words more emphasis is recommended. Attempts should be made to create a positive relational experience for the child following the crisis situation as an opportunity to praise the child's positive behavior accordingly. It is important to impress upon parents that aggressive behavior does not improve from one moment to the next. Change can only be achieved by them maintaining a consistent attitude toward their child.

Interaction sometimes escalates so sharply that the risk of abuse makes it essential for distance to be immediately created between parents and child. It sometimes help for the mother or father to leave the room in order to let affects abate and to regain self-control. Only once calm has been restored is it possible to seek alternative solutions for gridlocked situations.

The now-entrenched escalating cycles of negative interaction can be discussed during counseling. Working with video and using video feedback of a play scene between parents and child can be extremely helpful here (see Chap. 10). After a consideration of successful scenes, dysfunctional scenes can be watched and analyzed together. Becoming aware of their own feelings (anger, powerlessness, grief, disappointment) generally helps parents to reflect on their (unconscious) expectations of their child. They often also see their child's helplessness in the video feedback, which helps foster a different, more positive and supportive attitude and reduce negativism.

While on the one hand psychodynamic therapists remain mindful of their own transference and countertransference feelings in order to better empathize with both child and parents, they refrain from using these feelings in an interpretative or construing manner.

Due to frequent and severe couples' conflicts, there is often no consensus between parents on child-rearing behavior. Structured parent courses can help promote parental skills as a means of primary prevention. A Dutch group elaborated on a video feedback-based course for 1- to 3-year-olds, which they then investigated in a comparative study (Van Zeijl et al. 2006). The authors propose six sessions in the family home. Their study shows that this approach can significantly improve interactional behavior between parents and child.

Long-term *parent–child psychotherapy* is most commonly indicated when the counseling "dose" is too low to bring about changes in parental attitudes, child-rearing skills, and maladaptive interactional patterns. In such cases, parents are generally not capable of sustainably implementing the solution-oriented approaches proposed in counseling due to their own (early) childhood experiences. Either they are so preoccupied with themselves or their partnership that their view of the child and its needs has become obscured, or they perceive their child's behavior in such a distorted way due to their own experiences that they interpret its signals inappropriately and thus respond inadequately. Most importantly, parental emotional experiences, as well as affects triggered by the child's temper tantrums, are worked through. Attention needs to be paid to learned (dysfunctional and distressed) conflict-solving patterns, which are often associated with experiences of violence.

7.3 Aggressive Behavior in Toddlers

Toddlers can exhibit aggressive behavior as early on as the age of 2 or 3 years, e.g., if they regularly hurt themselves or others, find it difficult to comply with parental rules, and start giving the impression of being "naughty." After the age of 3 years, this behavior may be defiant and provocative, in which case one refers to oppositional behavior. The diagnosis of "aggressive/oppositional behavior" in toddlers, however, is premature.

Mrs. U. gave Paul's aggressive behavior as the reason for referral. She had been avoiding the playground ever since Paul, after not getting the toy he wanted, had bitten a 2-year-old on the cheek. She could no longer cope with her 2.2-year-old son. The mother reported how she was "no longer in control." Sometimes he did the complete opposite to what he was told to do. If she told him to tidy up, he would take things off the shelf and throw them about. If he didn't get his own way, Paul would start screaming and try to hit or kick her. The least little frustration would cause him to throw himself on the floor and bang his head on the ground to the point of inflicting bumps and bruises. In Mrs. U.'s experience, she was able to pacify Paul only after a certain period of time, once he was exhausted and sought intense physical contact. Recently, Mrs. U. had been responding to Paul's tantrums extremely tensely and aggressively. She also slapped him, "but not on the face," she hastened to emphasize. She felt sure that this did him no harm. He needed to feel that there were limits. These situations continued into the night, during which Paul would wake up (as often as five times per night), start crying, and sometimes lash out. In tears, Mrs. U. described how the frequent conflicts with Paul were affecting her nerves and making normal daily life virtually impossible. What was more, she had absolutely no help from anyone!

Paul had already been a "cry baby" in the first months of life. The mother reported how sleeping had always been a problem and how she had found his nighttime crying a great strain on her right from the beginning. During the day, however, Paul had also been a "sunny" baby to a certain extent. He was always smiling at her and wanting to play "silly games." In recent months, Paul had been less good-tempered. He hardly ever smiled at her and was predominantly in a bad mood and demanding.

Definition
Aggressive behavior is defined as various forms of aggressive and oppositional behavior:

- Aggressive behavior toward siblings within the family and peers outside the family.
- Temper tantrums and aggressive behavior toward parents or other adults (generally in the case of limit-setting).
- Early noncompliance with rules and limit-setting.

The parents' main focus is on their child's disobedience. However, disobedience is distinct from defiance in that the "disobedient" child conveys the impression that, although it could behave differently, it does not wish to. It is postulated that the child intentionally chooses to put up resistance. A power struggle between parents and child often ensues when parents construe defiant and aggressive behavior as disobedience. They have the impression that their child "is walking all over them." The parents then assume that the "disobedient" child wants to impose its own will on them.

Differentiating between early and late defiance can help in the interpretation of aggressive behavior among children in this age group. Early defiance is not a means to an end—it is the child's attempt to regulate its tension. The child is not capable of behaving differently during this developmental phase. Late defiance is a mixture of negative and aggressive behavior deployed intentionally by the child in order get what it wants.

▶ Aggressive behavior is not per se pathological. In the majority of 2- to 3-year-olds, it is transient, phase-typical behavior. The "intention" component in the definition of aggression in under-3-year-olds is controversial, since most children in this age group are not yet able to fully understand their aggressive actions. The decisive factors, therefore, include persistence, pervasiveness, and most notably the strain on parents and child when they fail to break the prevailing maladaptive cycles of interaction.

7.3.1 Diagnosis

DC:0-3 (Zero-to-Three 2005) does not list a diagnosis corresponding to oppositional behavior disorder, since this diagnosis is only meaningful in children from the age of 3 years. After this age, a diagnosis can help to identify a group of high-risk children whose marked aggressive behavior is highly likely to persist if the children and their parents do not receive help.

7.3.2 Prevalence

Prevalence rates for behavioral abnormalities in 2- to 3-year-old toddlers obtained using the Child Behavior Checklist/2-3 (CBCL/2-3) stand at around 12 % (2.3 % of which exhibit aggressive behavior) in the US (Achenbach 1992), the Netherlands, as well in Germany (Fegert 1996). As was to be expected, the prevalence rate in the Mannheim Longitudinal Study of Children at Risk is higher at 19.1 %: 23.8 % in boys and 15.4 % in girls (Laucht 2002). The gender ratio was confirmed in the study conducted by Rockhill et al. (2006) and stands at 2:1. What is important is that prevalence rates evidently decline to 2–3 % in older children (Rockhill et al. 2006).

7.3.3 Risk Factors and Prognosis

As with excessive defiance, there are numerous prenatal, perinatal, and postnatal organic and psychosocial stressors (Rockhill et al. 2006) that contribute to the impairment of self-regulatory skills in the child with aggressive behavior.

Data (Shaw et al. 2000; Crockenberg and Leerkes 2000) show that, in addition to gender (male), insecure attachment behavior (type D), and “difficult” temperament, primarily psychosocial risk factors such as dissocial behavior in the father, depression or other mental illnesses in the mother, couples’ conflicts, difficult social environment, the child’s exposure to violence, and/or a disorganized attachment style cause and perpetuate persistent aggressive and oppositional behavior. Recent study results on the risk factors for children in families with multiple stressors (see Cierpka 2012, Chap. 7) show that environmental conditions contribute to supposed constitutional biological factors, such as temperament or disordered serotonin levels, as early on as in the prenatal period. Aggressive behavior appears to be predominantly caused by environmental conditions, most notably dysfunctional interaction between parents and child. Externalizing behavior develops in toddlers as young as 2 years significantly more often in high-risk families (Sidor et al. 2013). The toddler’s attempts to self-regulate its strong negative emotions and its aggression fail within the context of the relationship with the primary caregiver. This assumption is further supported by the results of a study conducted by Papoušek and von Hofacker (2004): although the authors found higher values on the temperament “fussy/difficult” scale in the subgroup of defiant toddlers compared with a nonclinical control group, similar results could not be seen in the subsample of aggressive/oppositional children. Environmental conditions carry significantly more weight in this latter group from an etiological perspective.

Children with aggressive/oppositional behavior have a worse prognosis in terms of socioemotional development compared with other children, since they suffer long-term effects that can lead to impairment on all levels. Approximately 60 % of these children also continue to exhibit abnormal behavior in later childhood (Campbell 1995; Laucht 2002). Therefore, early support and therapeutic measures aimed at prevention are essential.

7.3.4 Interventional Approaches

There is no indication for the use of psychotropic drugs in children in this age group. Only psychotherapeutic approaches promise success. The following interventional options are used predominantly in children aged over 3 years; however, with appropriate modifications, they may also be applied in children from the age of 2 years.

7.3.4.1 Behavioral Therapy

One often sees a vicious circle of negative reciprocity in interaction, which Patterson (1982) described as a "coercive cycle."

- The child's aversive behavior spawns a laissez-faire attitude in the parents.
- Until the parents can no longer control their pent-up anger.
- They then punish and threaten their child, forcing it into submission.
- This again triggers aversive behavior and serves to escalate the situation.

Modifications in parental behavior can break this pattern of dysfunctional communication. The therapeutic aim is to achieve the following behavioral modifications:

- Encouraging and supporting prosocial behavior.
- Clear and friendly limit-setting in the case of aggressive behavior and guidance on prosocial behavior.
- An understanding of the child's negative affects and acceptance of the child, while at the same time unequivocally rejecting its aggressive behavior.
- Desisting from harsh verbal or physical parental disciplinary behavior, since this serves as a negative model for the child's behavior.
- Encouraging and supporting the child's feelings of self-efficacy and self-worth.

In addition to McDonough's behavioral therapy for toddlers (McDonough 1995; see Chap. 9), there are numerous parent training programs (overview of parent training programs in: Sonuga-Barke et al. 2006; Steinhoff et al. 2006; Greenhill et al. 2008), such as parent–child interaction therapy (PCIT according to Hembree-Kigin et al. 1995). This program comprises 10–15 short but comprehensive coaching sessions for parents of 2- to 7-year-olds during which parents learn through psychoeducation and by practicing more functional behavior how to alter their child's social behavior. The focus of these programs is more on discipline, rules, and limit-setting. The evidence base for this approach is strong and studies show good effect sizes (Thomas and Zimmer-Gembeck 2007; Larsson et al. 2009).

7.3.4.2 Family Therapy

Since the immediate relational context—usually the family—influences the emergence and perpetuation of aggressive/oppositional behavior, it makes sense to address the everyday problems and daily challenges faced in family life and make targeted and concrete changes here. Numerous parenting advice centers work on this premise.

7.3.4.3 Psychodynamic Interactional Parent-Child Psychotherapy

Toddlers aged between 2 and 3 years are highly engaged participants in this approach. They actively help in shaping interaction with the parents and therapists. Not only expressive language skills, but also the ability to communicate through play opens up diagnostic and therapeutic opportunities. Therefore, many therapeutic interventions concentrate directly on the association between relationship disorders and symptoms that manifest in the here and now.

The treatment method corresponds largely to the classic psychodynamic approach, complemented by the systemic perspective and behavioral therapy strategies. Psychodynamic work on two intrapsychic and interpersonal conflicts—which also represent the "dominant theme" (see Chap. 11)—very often plays a prominent role in our treatment model for 2- to 3-year-old toddlers with aggressive/oppositional behavior. Reestablishing a balance in the conflict between *intimacy/attachment* and *autonomy/detachment*, as well as the conflict between *control/power* and *submission/powerlessness*, is crucial to the therapeutic process. As mentioned above, we see the components of conflict that create tension as the two sides of a scale onto which the parents place weights in the form of conscious and unconscious expectations and projections, thereby affecting the balance. On the basis of their own experiences, parents may encourage/hamper attachment or autonomy and control or submission inappropriately vigorously or inappropriately early. Children may compound the problem with their temperament variables if, for example, they seek autonomy or are autonomy-inhibited. This dialectical approach permits a schematic representation of different relationship patterns (Cierpka and Cierpka 2000). The following illustrates this therapeutic approach using the case example of Mrs. U. and Paul described above.

The dominant themes, defined as the representations that determine relational dynamics, were enacted in the initial interview with Mrs. U. and Paul. While the 35-year-old mother was complaining about Paul's behavior, Paul explored the room and looked at the toys. He kept returning to his mother to show her toys he had found. Linguistically, Paul still had problems making himself understood. The mother was so deep in conversation as she unburdened herself emotionally to the therapists that she did not respond to Paul. He went back to her a few minutes later and pulled on her to make her go with him. He obviously wanted her to get a toy down from a shelf or play with him. She responded with a harsh "Let go of me," upon which he tried but failed to kick her. We asked Mrs. U.: "Do you have any idea what he wanted just now?" "No, I don't know." We responded: "He was pulling your arm; he must have had a reason …" "I don't know, I just don't know; he's always like that!" After pausing to think for a moment, she continued: "Maybe he wanted me to play with him. But he can see that I'm talking at the moment. He never gives up—he always has to have his own way!" Although it was unfamiliar to him, Paul explored the consulting room in a positive mood. He was used to being left alone to explore. When he became bored, he was expected to be patient.

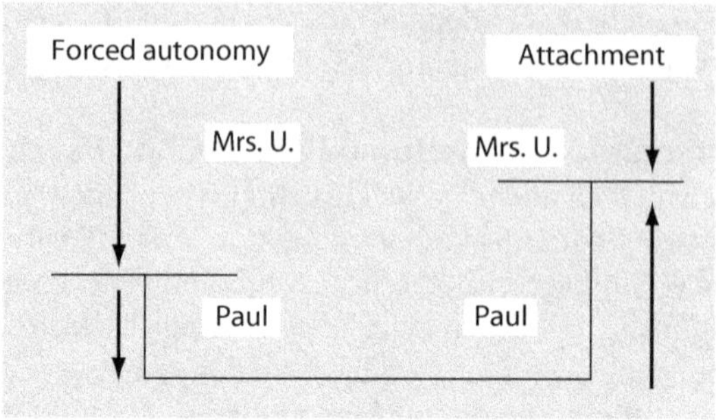

Fig. 7.2 Mrs. U. demands more autonomy from Paul, while Paul wants more attachment

Mrs. U. did not treat him like a toddler that first needs to familiarize itself with a strange environment, but more like an adolescent. She did not recognize his need for closeness when he went to her, but believed instead that he disturbed her "on purpose." This assumed intentionality, however, is not age-appropriate for a 2-year-old. The mother found it difficult to empathize with her child's needs and help him get started with a game. She was forcing his autonomy and neglecting his attachment needs. He responded with anger and attempted to get her attention by kicking her (Fig. 7.2).

Mrs. U.'s criticism of Paul continued to form the focus of the interview. As Paul became increasingly frustrated, he lay down at her feet and started to rock himself. Suddenly, he struck his head against the table leg—this gave him a fright and he had clearly hurt himself. Mrs. U. reached down—we thought she was going to console him by stroking his head, but instead she took a toy away from him. Then he really started to scream and "go berserk." He made an attempt at self-regulation by turning onto his tummy and rubbing his body on the ground, but this attempt failed. In the countertransference, we identified with Paul's pain, powerlessness, and helplessness and were able to understand his extreme anger toward his mother for not acknowledging his pain and offering consolation. Our (unexpressed) aggression toward Mrs. U. became understandable as we listened to her life story and learned of the extent to which she herself had been neglected and abused.

Mrs. U. had been physically abused as a child by her father, a heavy drinker. She described a scene in which he had beaten her black and blue for wetting her pants. She was crying as she recounted this incident and her anger and helplessness were tangible. Her mother had never come to her aid in such situations and had never protected her. She had one older and four younger brothers that had never been beaten by their father in the way she had been. She had always been seen as the "worst" of the children. During puberty, her father had called her a "slut." She would have preferred to forget her childhood altogether; she was unable to, however, since Paul kept re-evoking her feelings of powerlessness, helplessness, and anger. He was constantly reminding her of that mistreated little girl from back then. She could not allow herself to perceive his powerlessness and pain, just as her parents had not perceived hers.

Numerous expectations were made of Paul. He had been parentified; he was supposed to support her in her loneliness. The mother's yearning to be understood and accepted by a "man" did not correspond to Paul's needs. This resulted in deep disappointment and anger. She perceived Paul as an "annoying" child, as she herself had been, when he demanded her care. Mrs. U. had been a victim of violence from her previous alcoholic husband, as well as from other men since her divorce. Nevertheless, she had always wanted to become a mother. She described how looking at advertisements for baby products had made her cry, since it was her dearest wish to have a baby. When she became pregnant by a new partner, Mrs. U. and, by all accounts, also the child's father, were initially very happy at the prospect of having a baby. Due to complications in the early months of pregnancy, Mrs. U. underwent extensive medical testing and was found to be HIV-positive. Since Paul's father was not infected, this meant that she had been carrying the disease for several years without her knowledge. Paul's father had left Mrs. U. 3 days after learning of her disease. Mrs. U. had been very distressed during the pregnancy and felt entirely on her own with this huge burden. She had been extremely anxious about the health of her baby, which, to her great relief, had been born without the virus.

During the seventh month of pregnancy, Mrs. U. had been told that she was expecting a boy. She had assumed up until that point that she was expecting a girl on the basis of ultrasound images. Due to her negative experiences in the past with men, Mrs. U. feared that she may not be a good mother to a son, since a boy also had the potential to turn into a violent man in the future. Due to her fear of domination and violence, the news that she was expecting a son had come as such a shock to Mrs. U. that, for the first few days after the birth, she had not wanted to keep the child. She was clearly still ambivalent about whether to accept or reject Paul.

The goal of weekly mother–child therapy sessions over a period of 1 year was twofold: Firstly, Mrs. U. received instruction and guidance on how to interact with Paul in play, since she was "unable to play with him, just like no-one had played with her." These interventions in the play context in the here and now encouraged positive interaction and cemented Paul's attachment to his mother. Her own tension-tolerance levels progressively improved once Mrs. U. found a childminder, which meant that she was able to resume work on a part-time basis, thereby giving her "a bit of space to breathe." Secondly, Mrs. U.'s traumatic experiences were worked through on a deep psychological level and Paul's parentification dissolved. The divide between her "abuser" and "abused" behaviors and between control and submission formed the particular focus of this borderline-specific psychodynamic therapy (Pedrina 2010).

7.3.5 Typical Aspects in Everyday Practice

It is particularly important to provide the parents of children exhibiting aggressive behavior with psychotherapeutic support in order to prevent these children from remaining compromised in the long-term as a result of their aggression. The age span between 1 and 3 years is a particularly sensitive timeframe for both the development and the control of aggressive behavior and should be given greater consideration in regard to preventive approaches.

7.3.6 Pitfalls in Practice

Since many parents have themselves experienced abuse and neglect, often associated with violence, there is a second scale made up of the two scale pans "abuser/power" and "abused/powerlessness." The power/powerlessness dynamics superimposed onto closeness/distance conflicts often lead to an escalation in parent–child dynamics. The main therapeutic goal is to work through parents' separation or loss-of-control anxieties originating in their prior histories.

7.4 Conclusion

Toddlers between the ages of 13 and 36 months become ever more autonomous. As they discover themselves as independent individuals, they increasingly come into conflict with the rules of their social environment (Emde 1984). Resistance to their parents' wishes and demands, as well as their growing use of the word "no," calls for novel responses from the parents. If parents are to meet this challenge in a respectful manner, they need to weigh up how permissive or domineering their response to the child's defiant "no" is going to be. If parents and their defiant toddler succeed in accomplishing this new family—and individual—developmental task, all parties will enjoy new scope and developmental opportunities. Seen from this perspective, defiance and temper tantrums are a transitory phenomenon. When children comply with their parents' rules and limit-setting, they are increasingly making the adults' goals into their own. The calmer and more consistent the delivery of these requests and demands to the child, the easier this is to achieve. Ultimately, children internalize the values and standards of their family.

This chapter presents a step-by-step concept representing not only a dimensional explanation of but also a treatment concept covering normal defiance, excessive defiance, and aggressive behavior. It focuses on the emotional regulation of the child and its primary caregivers. In this continuum—and in the sequence of sections in this chapter going from normal to dysfunctional interactional behavior—the parents become increasingly unable to provide the child with the interpersonal emotion regulation it needs to deal with its negative emotions. The defiant child's interactions with its parents center around an aggressive self-development that is usually accompanied by strong affects. To control these strong affects, the child requires interpersonal boundaries and containment within the relationship in order to be able to increase its capacity for emotional self-regulation.

References

Achenbach TM (1992) Manual for the child behavior checklist/2-3 and 1992. Department of Psychiatry, University of Vermont, Burlington, VT

Belsky J, Woodworth S, Crnic K (1996) Trouble in the second year: three questions about family interactions. Child Dev 67:556–578

Bhatia M, Dhar N, Singhal P, Nigam V (1990) Temper tantrums: prevalence and etiology in a non-referral outpatient setting. Clin Pediatr 29:311–315
Bischof-Köhler D (1998) Zusammenhänge zwischen kognitiver, motivationaler und emotionaler Entwicklung in der frühen Kindheit und im Vorschulalter. In: Keller H (ed) Lehrbuch Entwicklungspsychologie. Hans Huber, Bern, CH, pp 325–377
Calkins SD (2002) Does aversive behavior during toddlerhood matter? The effects of difficult temperament on maternal perceptions and behavior. Infant Mental Health J 23:381–402
Campbell SB (1995) Behavior problems in preschool children: a review of recent research. J Child Psychol Psychiatr 36:113–149
Chamberlin R (1974) Management of preschool behavior problems. Pediatric Clin North Am 21(1):33–47
Cierpka M, Cierpka A (2000) Beratung von Familien mit zwei- bis dreijährigen Kindern. Prax Kinderpsychol Kinderpsychiatr 49:563–579
Cierpka M (2012) Frühe Kindheit 0 - 3 Jahre. Beratung und Psychotherapie für Eltern mit Säuglingen und Kleinkindern. Springer, Berlin Heidelberg
Crockenberg S, Leerkes E (2000) Infant social and emotional development in family context. In: Zeanah CH Jr (ed) Handbook of infant mental health. The Guilford Press, New York, NY
Dionne G, Tremblay R, Boivin M, Laplante D, Pérusse D (2003) Physical aggression and expressive vocabulary in 19-month-old twins. Dev Psychol 39:261–273
Emde RN (1984) The affective self: continuities and transformations form infancy. In: Galenson E, Tyson RL (eds) Frontiers of infant psychiatry. Basic Books, New York, NY
Fegert J (1996) Verhaltensdimensionen und Verhaltensprobleme bei zweieinhalbjährigen Kindern. Prax Kinderpsychol Kinderpsychiat 45:83–94
Fouts HN, Hewlett BS, Lamb ME (2005) Parent-offspring weaning conflicts among the Bofi farmers and foragers of Central Africa. Curr Anthropol 46:29–50
Fullard W, McDevitt S, Carey WB (1984) Assessing temperament in one- to three-year-old children. J Pediatr Psychol 9:205–297
Greenhill LL, Posnerk K, Vaughan BS, Kratochvil CJ (2008) Attention deficit hyperactivity disorder in preschool children. Child Adolesc Psychiatr Clin N Am 17(2):347–366
Hembree-Kigin TL, McNeil CB, Eyberg S (1995) Parent-child interaction therapy, 1st edn. Springer, New York, NY
Johnson A (2003) Families of the forest: the Matsigenka Indians of the Peruvian Amazon. University of California Press, Berkeley, CA
Kagan J (1997) Temperament and the reactions to unfamiliarity. Child Dev 68:139–144
Karp H, Spencer P (2004) The happiest toddler on the block: the new way to stop the daily battle of wills and raise a secure and well-behaved one- to four-year-old. Random House, New York, NY
Larsson B, Fossum S, Clifford G, Drugli MB, Handegård BH, Mørchm WT (2009) Treatment of oppositional defiant and conduct problems in young Norwegian children: results of a randomized controlled trial. Eur Child Adolesc Psychiatry 18(1):42–52
Laucht M (2002) Störungen des Kleinkind- und Vorschulalters. In: Esser G (ed) Lehrbuch der klinischen Psychologie und Psychotherapie des Kindes- und Jugendalters 102–118
McDonough SC (1995) Promoting positive early parent-infant relationships through interaction guidance. Child Adolesc Clin North Am 4:661–672
MacFarlane J, Allen L, Honzik MP (1954) A developmental study of the behavior problems of normal children between twenty-one months and fourteen years. University of California Press, Berkeley, CA
Metzger W (1972) Frühkindlicher Trotz. S. Karger, Basel
Needlman R, Stevenson J, Zuckerman B (1991) Psychosocial correlates of severe temper tantrums. Dev Behav Pediatr 12(2):77–83
Olson SH, Bates JE, Sandy JM, Lanthier R (2000) Early development precursors of externalizing behavior in middle childhood and adolescence. J Abnorm Child Psychol 28(2):119–133
Österman K, Björkquist K (2010) A cross-sectional study of onset, cessation, frequency, and duration of children's temper tantrums in a nonclinical sample. Psychol Rep 106(2):448–454

Ounsted MK, Simons CD (1978) The first-born child: Toddlers' problems. Dev Med Child Neurol 20(6):710–719

Papoušek M (2004) Regulationsstörungen der frühen Kindheit: Klinische Evidenz für ein neues diagnostisches Konzept. In: Papoušek, M., Schieche, M., Wurmser, H. (eds) Regulationsstörungen der frühen Kindheit. Frühe Risiken und Hilfen im Entwicklungskontext der Eltern-Kind-Beziehungen. Hans Huber, Bern, pp 77–110

Papoušek M, von Hofacker N (2004) Klammern, Trotzen, Toben—Störungen der emotionalen Verhaltensregulation des späten Säuglingsalters und Kleinkindalters. In: Mechthild Papoušek, Michael Schieche, Harald Wurmser (eds) Regulationsstörungen der frühen Kindheit: Frühe Risiken und Hilfen im Entwicklungskontext der Eltern-Kind-Beziehungen. Hans Huber, Bern, CH

Patterson GR (1982) Coercive family processes. Castalia, Eugene, OR

Pedrina F (2010) Mütter mit Persönlichkeitsstörungen und ihre Kinder: frühe psychotherapeutische Interventionen. Frankfurt, 16. Wissenschaftliche Konferenz der VakJP

Potegal M, Kosorok M, Davidson RJ (2003) Temper tantrums in young children: 2. Tantrum duration and temporal organization. J Dev Behav Pediatr 24:148–154

Potegal M, Davidson RJ (2003) Temper tantrums in young children: 1. Behavioral composition. J Dev Behav Pediatr 24:140–147

Richman N, Stevenson J, Graham P (1982) Pre-school to school: A behavioral study. Academic, London, UK

Rockhill CM, Collett BR, McClellan JM, Speltz ML (2006) Oppositional defiant disorder. In: Luby JL (ed) Preschool mental health: A guide for practitioners. Guilford Press, New York, NY

Rothbart MK, Derryberry D, Posner MI (1994) A psychobiological approach to the development of temperament. In: Bates JE, Wachs TD (eds) Temperament: Individual differences at the interface of biology and behavior. American Psychological Association, Washington, DC

Shaw DS, Gilliom M, Giovanelli J (2000) Aggressive behavior disorders. In: Zeanah CH Jr (ed) Handbook of infant mental health. The Guilford Press, New York, NY, pp 397–411

Shaw DS, Owens EB, Giovanelli J, Winslow EB (2001) Infant and toddler pathways leading to early externalizing disorders. J Am Acad Child Adolesc Psychiatry 40:36–43

Sidor A, Fischer C, Cierpka M (2013) Early Regulatory Problems in Infancy and Psychopathological Symptoms at 24 Months: A Longitudinal Study in a High-risk Sample. J Child Adolesc Behav 1:116

Sonuga-Barke EJS, Thompson M, Abikoff H, Klein R, Brotman LM (2006) Nonpharmacological interventions for preschoolers with ADHD: the case for specialized parent training. Infants Young Children 19(2):142–153

Steinhoff KW, Lerner M, Kapilinsky A (2006) Attention-deficit/hyperactivity disorder. In: Luby JL (ed) Handbook of preschool mental health. The Guilford Press, New York, NY

Stern DN (1992) Die Lebenserfahrung des Säuglings. Klett-Cotta, Stuttgart

Thomas R, Zimmer-Gembeck MJ (2007) Behavioral outcomes of parent-child interaction therapy and triple P-positive parenting program: a review and meta-analysis. J Abnorm Child Psychol 35(3):475–495

Tomm K, Suzuki K (1990) The Kan-No-Mushi: an inner externalization that enables compromise? Aust New Zeal J Fam Ther 11:104–105

Trad PV (1993) Short-term parent-infant psychotherapy. Basic Books, New York

Tremblay RE, Japel C, Perusse D, McDuff P, Boivin M, Zoccolillo M, Montplaisir J (1999) The search for the age of onset of physical aggression: Rousseau and Bandura revisited. Crim Behav Ment Health 9:8–23

Van Zeijl J, Mesman J, Van Ijzendoorn MH (2006) Attachment-based intervention for enhancing sensitive discipline in mothers of 1- to 3-year-old children at risk for externalizing behaviour problems: a randomized controlled trail. J Consult Clin Psychol 74(6):994–1005

Wurmser H, Papoušek M (2004) Zahlen und Fakten zu frühkindlichen Regulationsstörungen: Datenbasis aus der Münchner Spezialambulanz. In: Papoušek M, Schieche M, Wurmser H (eds) Regulationsstörungen der frühen Kindheit. Hans Huber, Bern

Zero To Three (2005) DC:0-3R. Diagnostic Classification of Mental Health and Development Disorders of Infancy and Early Childhood: Revised Edition. Zero To Three Press, Washington

Disinterest in Play in Infancy: Problems in the Regulation of Attention and Play

8

Mechthild Papoušek

8.1 Clinical Picture of Disinterest in Play in Infancy

Example 1

Fabian (17 months) attended a specialist outpatient clinic with his mother because of a sleep onset and maintenance disorder, eating problems, excessive clinginess, and defiance. He was extremely restless during the day ("ants in his pants"), fidgety, and incapable of occupying himself alone for any length of time, clinging instead "with incredible tenacity" to his mother or whining permanently for her attention and a varied entertainment program, all the while wandering around bored, aimless, and fussy. When the mother managed, despite her exhaustion, to bring herself to play with Fabian, he was unable to concentrate, became quickly frustrated, and would walk away. He was also described as stubborn, defiant, and provocative against his parents or his 2-year older brother Ben.

The mother's pregnancy had been complicated by an accident, extreme insomnia, as well as multiple family stress factors. Due to premature closure of the fontanelles, torticollis, neuromotor immaturity, early sucking weakness, failure to thrive, sustained loss of appetite, and persistent crying, the mother had perceived Fabian already early on as a problem child that constantly aroused new fears in her and needed protection, particularly from his "difficult," jealous, and often physically aggressive brother. The mother

(continued)

M. Papoušek, M.D. (✉)
Institute for Social Pediatrics and Youth Medicine, University of Munich,
Am Gries 39, 83026 Rosenheim, Germany
e-mail: mechthild@papousek.de

M. Cierpka (ed.), *Regulatory Disorders in Infants*,
DOI 10.1007/978-3-319-43556-5_8

appeared tired, anxious, tense, and irritable. She felt helplessly overstrained and reproached herself for failing as a mother and always losing her temper. The father, himself a "restless creature" as a child with suspected ADHD, was only available to a limited extent, felt as helpless as her, and only worsened the situation with his occasional bad-tempered intervention. As a result of escalating partnership conflicts, family harmony was impaired.

Fabian suffered from a pervasive regulatory disorder involving persistent crying, sleeping, and feeding disorders combined with excessive clinginess, social anxiousness, and defiance. In addition, he exhibited the clinical picture of abnormal disinterest in exploration and play, which is associated with dysphoric mood, persistent and aimless motor restlessness, and problems of attention regulation in the form of sensation seeking, distractability, and poor endurance. These abnormalities, which are suggestive of precursors of ADHD, alarm many similarly affected parents, and prompt some physicians to make a precocious diagnosis of ADHD or even to prescribe stimulant therapy.

8.1.1 Parent Complaints: Aspects of Patient History Requiring Attention

Parents of infants complain that their baby refuses to be put down even for a moment, is constantly unhappy and fussy, and cries to be picked up. Although he signals a need for closeness, he does not snuggle up to his parents and settles only when the parents carry him about in their arms with a free view of its environment. The parents of toddlers complain that their child is incapable of occupying himself alone even for a short time, is bored and cranky, and always clinging onto their legs demanding attention and varied entertainment. New toys rapidly lose their appeal. Playthings are simply pulled out of the cupboard and thrown about. The only activities offering any lasting appeal include watching TV and exploring all things forbidden, such as computers, plug sockets, or remote controls, usually with provocative intent in order to gain the parents' attention. The idea of playing quietly is inconceivable. Playing together brings little reward: The infant is passive and listless, cannot sit still, shows little interest in stimulation, and is easily distracted or frustrated.

This leads to disinterest in play in the parents as well. Due to their sheer exhaustion, they often find it difficult to gather their strength to play with their infant. They feel uninspired, burnt out, empty, and lacking motivation, driven by restlessness themselves, and unable to cope with their infant's temperament and hyperactivity—and often feel that "the ceiling is falling in" at home. The parents feel under pressure not to miss any of the numerous programs aimed at advancing their infant's development, even when the calendar is filled with new attractive activities every day. A remarkable number of mothers and fathers have (or make) no time to play with their child, attribute no importance to play, or are unable to recall ever having themselves played in their childhood. A considerable number of parents fear a hereditary risk on the basis of the mother, father, or other family member having been dubbed "a fidget" or indeed treated for ADHD as a child.

8.1.2 Conditions of Origin in the Context of Pervasive Regulatory and Relational Disorders

The clinical syndrome described for "disinterest in play" emerges mainly in the context of persistent and pervasive regulatory disorders beginning in infancy. Based on own investigations of 590 infants and toddlers consecutively referred to and treated in the Munich Program for Fussy Babies for regulatory disorders between the ages of 4 and 30 months, the syndrome of disinterest in play was seen in 35 % of cases; these proved to be the most seriously affected cases in terms of persistence, pervasiveness, and degree of burden on the parents (Papoušek 2008). Over 90 % of the children in this subgroup had already cried excessively in the first months of life. Depending on age at referral, disinterest in play was associated with long-standing sleep disorders in 80–90 %, persistent feeding and eating disorders in 40 %, as well as—in toddlers—with a high rate of defiance and aggressive/oppositional behavior.

Overall, the subgroup of regulatory disordered infants and toddlers exhibiting disinterest in play differed from the rest of the clinical group by a concurrence of particularly strong constitutional risk factors in the area of arousal control and sensory processing, more frequent and severe problems of the mother's mental condition, a higher rate of family conflicts, and, depending on the child's age, increasing rates of perturbed and disordered mother–child relationships. Whether and how some of these individual factors contribute to sensation-seeking/restless exploration and play behavior in the child, to dysfunctional communication patterns in parent–infant play or to a striking lack of positive play experiences, needs to be elucidated in individual cases.

8.2 Normal Developmental Course of Play and Attention

8.2.1 Infant Needs of Play and Self-Efficacy

Ever in the shadow of attachment research, play has received remarkably little attention in clinical and theoretical concepts of developmental psychopathology. Like attachment, play is one of the basic psychobiological needs of young children and embodies their elementary way of life, taking up the majority of their waking time from infancy onwards. Infants—in a state of alert wakefulness, under stress-free conditions, and driven by intrinsic motivation and own initiative without external purpose—follow their need to become familiar with their social and physical environment, to comprehend it and gain some control over it, to discover its regular and predictable aspects, and to assimilate these experiences (Papoušek et al. 1987). Children's play behavior is conceived as self-regulated implicit learning (Largo and Benz-Castellano 2008). Play enables children from early on to practice their maturing sensorimotor, cognitive, and integrative skills and to construct their inner world of experiences and concepts. Driving forces include their intrinsic biological motivations, beginning with curiosity about everything that is new, unknown, or unfamiliar and offers stimulation for their attention, their early needs for self-initiated activity, self-efficacy, self-agency, and exploration, and, in the course of further motor and cognitive development, their pleasure on success, and mastery motivation (Heckhausen 1973).

8.2.2 Regulation of Play and Attention

Playful dialogues, solitary play, and joint play interactions represent the most important early childhood learning contexts (Ruff and Rothbart 1996) for the development of attention regulation during the phase of neurobiological maturation of the attention systems (Spitzer 2002).

During the first weeks of life, attention as a state of general vigilance is primarily controlled by the basal regulation of arousal and quieting and the organization of behavioral states (Papoušek 2008). States of alert wakefulness are still rare and transient. The parents' repertoire of intuitive behavior during playful dialogues with their infant contains abundant behavioral patterns, the intensity and variability of which are attuned to the infant's signals of alertness, fatigue and tolerance limits and which stimulate and modulate the infant's attention. Thanks to the parents' regulatory support, the infant learns to focus and maintain his visual attention and to regulate his level of arousal by means of gaze allocation and aversion.

Active, attentive waking states increase in number and stabilize in the course of a first developmental spurt in the third month. The development of selective attention begins in the form of the so-called orientation response (OR) (Sokolov 1960). Triggered by anything entering the visual field that is new or that deviates unexpectedly from the familiar, the orientating response functions like a spotlight, focusing sensory perception and integrative processes on the new stimulus (Spitzer 2002), while general arousal and spontaneous motor activities are inhibited and the heart rate drops measurably. As soon as the stimulus loses its novelty value and habituation takes place, competing stimuli are able to divert attention. However, if the orientation response abates without there being something new within eyeshot, a state of low-intensity arousal arises, that may be perceived as unpleasant or boring.

Maturing brain functions deploy more effective regulatory aids for the activation and maintenance of attention as early as in the second 3 months of life. Development of grasping enables the infant to discover new characteristics and details of objects during manual, oral, and visually coordinated exploration. In addition, cognitive incentives come increasingly into play, such as the discovery of regularity, as well as the rediscovery of the familiar, of expectations, and of anticipation (Papoušek et al. 1987). As Watson's (1972) experiments with mobiles show, sustained attention is achieved by experiencing self-efficacy and related intrinsic motivation processes. Self-efficacy as a motivating experience apparently deactivates the mechanism of habituation and appears to protect against distraction through associated inhibitory processes.

Other maturational and developmental stages in play begin hand-in-hand with the capacity for intentional focused action, action planning, and performing sequential actions. The attention span required for this needs effective inhibitory control functions that inhibit premature habituation of stimuli relevant to the goal on the one hand, while on the other they block possible orientation reactions to distracting endogenous and exogenous stimuli, as well as to disruptive affective and motor impulses. These functions come into play with the beginning of neurobiological maturation of the prefrontal attention system and its networks (Spitzer 2002). The driving forces of attention regulation are once again intrinsic motivations: The need for self-efficacy in realizing own action goals; the need for and expectation of reward, striving after success and mastery, as well as needs for social acceptance.

8.2.3 Parent–Infant Communication in Joint Play

Given the significance of the infant's self-efficacy in play, the parents' primary role is to create a safe, stimulating, and explorable environment with age-appropriate stimuli to attract the infant's attention and promote self-initiated activity in solitary play, as well as to protect the infant from overstimulation, excessive demand, and physical hazards. Successful communication plays a key role in joint play by making it possible to provide the infant with a responsively attuned framework for his self-initiated activity—a framework in which the infant can try out and practice his maturing skills in a self-efficacious manner. The parents' repertoire of intuitive communication skills, with its intrinsic playful elements and regulatory support, comes into play here (Papoušek M 2008, 2011).

A prerequisite of successful communication, however, is the parents' willingness to engage in their infant's play initiatives and current experiential world with their undivided attention and emotional availability, and to let themselves be intuitively guided by the infant's signals and reactions that provide the parent with information on the infant's receptivity, tolerance limits, over-/underload, focus of attention, play themes, affective experience, motivation, skills, and difficulties. Affective attunement, the use of referential language, and small regulatory aids in appropriate measure and at the right moment foster self-efficacy and endurance in play. Mutual agreement on a joint focus of attention enables the parent and infant to: convey and share their intentions, interests, and feelings; cooperate in play; make reference to activities or objects; experience the significance of these and symbolize them in words; and, in this way, build up a common experiential background to support speech comprehension and vocabulary development.

As such, joint play assumes a central role in the development of intersubjective emotional relatedness, shared intentionality, social cognition, and empathy. In the long term, joint and solitary play form a resource on which to build sound parent–child relationships and foster the infant's resilience (Papoušek 2011). Moreover, the developmental shift toward symbol and role play relate to upcoming developmental and relational issues in the frame of self development (Oerter 2003; Papoušek 2003), while the developmental shift toward collaborative play with other children fulfills important tasks in terms of building prosocial, impulse-inhibiting, empathetic, and self-reflexive skills (Panksepp 2007; Renz-Polster 2011).

8.2.4 Play and Attachment Security

The motivation and capacity of an infant to engage in exploration and play presume physical and mental wellbeing, feelings of safety and emotional security (Largo and Benz-Castellano 2008). Thus, play and attachment needs are fundamentally intertwined (Grossmann and Grossmann 2004): If the attachment system, with its needs for closeness and emotional security, is activated by hunger, fatigue, insecurity, anxiety, separation, or other emotional stressors, the exploratory system will be simultaneously inhibited. Curiosity, as well as the desire for exploration and activity will not evolve until the infant's needs for closeness and security are satisfied. Insecure/ambivalent or disorganized attachment representations impair the infant's capacity for both solitary and joint play and have a long-term impact on endurance and task orientation in the further course of development (Crockenberg and Leerkes 2000). Conversely, successful joint play contributes to building a positive attachment relationship.

8.2.5 Regulatory Developmental Tasks in Play, 0–3 Years

- Regulation of sensory input and sensory processing
- Grasping, as well as manual, oral, and visual exploration
- Regulation of selective, focused attention
- Sustained attention during play
- Self-efficacy, self-agency
- Intentional, targeted action
- Joint attention, intentions, feelings, cooperation
- Building an intersubjective, meaningful experiential background

8.3 Diagnostic Assessment of Disinterest in Play: Observation of Solitary and Joint Play

Standardized and validated procedures for the clinical assessment of self regulation, play motivation and attention in early childhood are not yet available. Standardized questionnaires on infant temperament (Bates et al. 1979) and behavioral checklists for the 1½- to 5-year age range provide information in terms of type and severity of an infant's constitutional regulatory problems, as well as clinically relevant early symptoms of externalizing and internalizing behavioral problems (CBCL/1½–5, Döpfner et al. 2000). Although methods to systematically measure sensory reactivity and sensory processing in relation to the individual sensory modalities are of scientific interest, they are not feasible in the consulting practice because of time and complexity—except as a basis for sensory integration therapy in an occupational therapy practice.

Incidental and structured observations of exploratory and play behavior in solitary play, communication in joint play, as well as an analysis of the mechanisms and processes that trigger, perpetuate, or exacerbate the disorder in everyday life form the core of play-related diagnosis. They make it possible to identify specific starting points for play-centered therapeutic counseling, interaction guidance, and psychotherapy.

8.3.1 Incidental Observations During Counseling Sessions

Incidental observations of an infant's exploratory and play behavior, as well as the parents' distribution of attention during patient-history taking and conversation with the therapist provide initial information.

Example 1, Continued

After a short warm-up phase, Fabian began to restlessly explore the toy-filled shelves and indeed the entire consulting room during patient-history taking. After a cursory inspection of the toys, he threw them on the floor, opened cupboards and doors out of curiosity, and climbed on chairs and benches—behavior that prompted the mother's keen vigilance. After about 15 min, his enthusiasm waned, he became bored, and began to whine and cling to his mother, demanding her attention by tugging at her and fidgeting about on her lap fussing. The mother tried in vain to detach her attention from Fabian's demanding behavior and to pacify him by stroking him half-heartedly, all the while oscillating ambivalently between solicitude, growing anger, and her urgent need to tell the therapist about her difficulties. Interactions between Fabian and his mother revealed a rather close, but tense relatedness with neither at ease during contact.

Fabian's problems of motor restlessness and superficial, curiosity-driven sensory hunger, which would turn into listless boredom after a while and prompt him to restlessly demand his mother's attention, had already been apparent during the first appointment. The mother's temporary detachment behavior was insecure/ambivalent; she was unable to clearly focus her attention on the interview and trust Fabian to play alone at her side for a while.

8.3.2 Structured Video-Supported Observation

Video recordings during a specially scheduled joint diagnostic/therapeutic play session with mother (or father) and child have proved to be effective for in-depth diagnostic assessments and treatment. The play situation follows a three-step sequence, with each sequence lasting 10 min at the least: (1) Free joint play involving mother and child; (2) timed solitary play while the mother, still in the same room, detaches herself—as in urgent, unavoidable situations at home—to perform tasks requiring her full attention (e.g., filling out a questionnaire); (3) joint play is resumed. Recordings are used (preferably at the follow-up appointment) for video feedback sessions with parents on previously selected sequences, as well as for the subsequent therapy (see Chap. 10).

8.3.3 Aspects Requiring Attention During Joint Play and Solitary Play

Behavioral analysis of the joint-play and detachment-situation focuses on identifying, on the basis of infant and parental behavioral characteristics, at least one sequence showing successful communication, as well as sequences highlighting dysfunctional communication.

Example 2

The mother of 9-month-old Lea sought help due to an escalating problem with crying and clinginess. Although Lea was able to sit on her own, she had not as yet shown any signs on a motor level of exploratory behavior and crawling; she cried and clung instead to her mother as soon as the latter detached herself for even a moment from her and permanently demanded attention and passive entertainment. The mother, meanwhile exhausted, was at her wits end; the crying had become intolerable—a complete nightmare ("It drives me crazy; by the evening I'm absolutely fuming!").

Video-Supported Observation: In joint play, the mother turned in a kindly manner towards her daughter, who was seated in front of her on a play mat, with a mirror in the background; Lea was interestedly trying to pick up and explore the few toys that lay around her one by one. Positive communication with visual contact only occurred in one moment when the mother joyfully responded to Lea's candid gaze in the mirror and commented happily. Apart from that, the mother pursued her own ideas for play, without paying attention to Lea's initiatives. She removed a picture book out of Lea's focus of attention, rolled a ball towards her, and spun one object after the other on the floor in quick succession, until Lea looked around confused, her hands filled with toys, but her needs for self-efficacy unfulfilled. In the detachment situation,

(continued)

the mother sat Lea on the play mat facing toward the mirror, caringly moved the toys to within the infant's reach, crouched behind her ready to stand up any moment, and encouraged her to play. Lea promptly turned toward her mother, clung tightly to her clothes, and cried. The mother initially attempted to detach herself in a kindly way, at which Lea protested screamingly; the mother finally freed herself and, with a loud and angry "Now play!," sat heavily in the chair 2 m away from Lea. The infant's crying escalated to the point that the mother could bear it no longer and, frustrated, sat back on the playmat. Lea's crying stopped as if by the flip of a switch and she was once again ready to be entertained.

8.3.3.1 Observations in the Context of Persistent Crying

Unable to satisfy her need for self-efficacy in play with her mother, Lea achieved this instead with her disproportionate, instrumentally demanding crying and clinginess, which were a mixture of passive helplessness and loud protest. The mother fluctuated ambivalently in her immediate reactions between warm empathy and escalating frustration, until her anger and harsh rebuff finally broke through.

The early regulation of sensory input and sensory processing is generally hampered in infants with persistent crying (Papoušek 2008; Rothbart et al. 1994). Fussy, overwrought states predominate, while quiet alert waking states are only rarely achieved following sleep and, at best, in an upright position—the position that activates the vigilance system and provides a view of varying visual stimuli. If problems with crying persist beyond the age of 3 months, the infants keep demanding with their fussing and crying to be held in a vertical position and carried around passively with a free view of their environment, to sit or stand on a caregiver's lap, and to let themselves be entertained and kept busy with ever new stimuli. However, these infants miss out on the positive experiences of self-efficacy to be had from the self-efficacious grasping and exploration of objects with their hands, mouth, and eyes while lying in a relaxed position on their back or tummy and putting their maturing motor skills to the test. Self-initiated movement and exploration by means of turning, crawling, and pulling themselves up may thus be delayed in the further course.

In contrast, these infants make negative experiences of self-efficacy with their tried and tested instrumental crying, to which the parents (for whom the crying has long since become a nightmare) react by immediately picking them up ("for a bit of peace") and, irritated, carry them about, force them to sit prematurely, and constantly offer new toys and distractions. The pattern tends to continue as soon as the infants learn to move about on their own, follow their parents' every step, pull themselves up on their parents' legs, and demand entertainment with their fussing.

8.3.3.2 Observations in Restless/Sensation-Seeking Toddlers

In the course of this type of vicious cycles, some toddlers previously prone to persistent crying acquire their own strategies to overcome dysphoric/restless affective states and boredom by stimulating themselves with ever new arousing attractions (sensation seeking), and by demanding diversified passive entertainment (e.g., watching TV). Such forms of intense, yet generally short-lived stimulation trigger neurophysiological orienting responses that temporarily put the infant in a positive state of focused attention which, however, as a result of habituation, quickly reverts back to a state of bored fussiness. In the long term, the quality of play remains on a superficial level of curiosity-led sensory processing. These toddlers have just as little scope to experience trying out and practicing their self-efficacy and more mature play motivations as they have to learn regulating their attention and persistence at a developmental stage when the anterior attention systems begin to mature.

As seen in the video-supported diagnostic assessment of Fabian and his mother, the problem behavior is perpetuated by dysfunctional communication patterns in joint play and solitary play.

Example 1, Continued

During *joint play*, Fabian and his mother initially played a coordinated game with a stacking pyramid for a short period. Fabian, from a standing position, took the rings offered him by his mother, who was sitting on the floor, and put them on the pyramid in a random order, which his mother commented on with kind affection. However, when he picked up the full pyramid at the end of the game, turned it upside down, let the rings fall off, bit into one of the rings, and walked away, the mother responded with disappointment: "Oh, now you've broken it all." The mother tried to get Fabian's attention several times by calling him over to her in a kind tone, showing him how to do things, and holding out the rings for the stacking pyramid. Driven by his restlessness and curiosity, Fabian was exploring the room without lingering on any one object; he finally stumbled listlessly across the pyramid, kicked it, and threw the rings his mother gave him about the room. With resignation, his mother asked him to gather the rings. Instead, Fabian took hold of the pyramid and banged it against the mirror. The mother called him back, shaking her finger sternly and exclaiming a firm "No," upon which Fabian continued to bang the mirror unperturbed. A second, more half-hearted "No" also failed to elicit a reaction. During the entire play situation, the mother showed subdued kindness and helpless attempts at boundary setting, yet appeared to be largely emotionally absent and barely noticeable to the child, responding to Fabian's restless and provocative behavior with resignation and disappointment and ultimately letting him do what he wanted.

During the requisite solitary-play situation, the mother tried to concentrate her attention on the questionnaire; this, however, aroused Fabian's curiosity. The mother's renewed requests for him to continue playing on the play mat fell on deaf ears. Fabian began fussing and sought contact and closeness by repeatedly banging his head against his mother's lap. Closer scrutiny of the mother's nonverbal requesting behavior clearly showed her growing ambivalence: Bending forward, she pointed with her outstretched finger to the play mat, while at the same time putting her other arm around him and pulling him toward her. With sudden—but ineffectual—determination, she finally put him back on the mat and sat ostentatively back on her place. Fabian thereupon began to entice his mother out of the detachment situation with his provocative behavior (i.e., banging the mirror while looking at his mother). Indeed, the mother stood up twice, scolded him, and put him back on the mat. When she remained seated, clearly resigned to the situation, Fabian tried to drag her from her seat with his pitiful crying, until she finally took him on her lap and comforted him gently in her arms.

8.3.3.3 Observations in Hypersensitive Toddlers Unable to Filter Stimuli

Example 3

Florian (18 months) exhibited entirely different behavior: Alert and in good spirits, he explored all the new objects in the room with keen interest, took hold of several toys at once to investigate them, followed what was going on in the room with his eyes, while at the same time engaging in contact with his parents and the therapists; however, all of this he did with great restlessness, as if driven, and breathless with excitement. Moreover, he was simultaneously alert to every noise in the corridor or on the street. To help Florian calm down, the mother provided regulatory support by sitting on the mat with him, thereby enabling him to become engrossed in a prolonged solitary game.

The parents, who had sought help for Florian's sleep and feeding disorders, as well as states of extreme arousal with vomiting, attested to their infant's hypersensitivity to noise and reported how he would respond to physical constraint with screaming resistance, e.g., during diaper changing or when put in his carseat. He had never been a typical "cry baby," but rather a "ray of sunshine." However, he would cry and vomit whenever his feelings overwhelmed him and in response to all forms of excitement, both when crying and when happily enthusiastic and laughing. He would run away on the street as if in a trance, unstoppable in his eager excitement.

Thanks to insightful and sensitive regulatory support (focusing on only one toy at a time, clearing away distracting objects), Florian was perfectly capable of playing enthusiastically for a prolonged period of time with his mother or father, as well as for short periods on his own. The mother took care to ensure regular breaks in a soothing "timeout corner" equipped with cushions, soft toys, and a pacifier. The parents no longer visited other families or made trips to the grandparents, since Florian would invariably become overwrought, have trouble falling asleep in the evening, and wake up repeatedly at night with nightmares after the excess of new impressions. Both parents had remarkable intuitive skills at their disposal and provided flexible closeness–distance regulation in their relationship with Florian.

Like Florian, some children stick out through abnormally pronounced hyperexcitability and hypersensitivity to stimuli from infancy onward as a manifestation of generally heightened excitability or lowered sensory thresholds in one or more sensory areas (touch, restriction of motion, noises, odors). Striking for their marked alertness, they are highly curious, "wide-eyed" children that perceive their environment as if with fully extended antennae—no movement in a room or background noise escapes their attention. Since they are incapable of filtering out, habituating, and deactivating unimportant stimuli, they are highly prone to distraction, quickly reach their tolerance thresholds, and respond to a glut of new impressions in an unfamiliar environment or an excess of toys by becoming extremely overwrought, throwing tantrums, and developing sleeping problems up into toddlerhood. In order to be able to selectively focus their attention, they need a soothing environment and special regulatory support ("timeout corners"), which Florian's parents were able to deploy skillfully and effectively thanks to their sensitive insight into their infant's problem.

8.3.3.4 Observations on Communication in Joint Play and Detachment

Despite their exhaustion, most mothers give in to their infant's continual demands for activity; they neglect the housework, as well as their own needs, to instead carry their infant about for hours on end or try to keep him happy and entertained with all manner of toys. Often their only aim here is to finally put a stop to the now unbearable crying and fussing that makes them confront their failure ad nauseum and elicits feelings of hurt, helpless subjection, anxiety, or even powerless rage. Neither the initial carrying around nor the time spent playing together are able to satisfy the infant in the way desired, nor are they perceived by the mother as fulfilling or gratifying. The infant remains passive, fussy, easily bored, and constantly craving ever new stimuli. In addition, busy daily schedules, overfilled playrooms, and the TV constantly on in the background afford neither infant nor parents any peace—rest periods and sleep are in short supply.

A lack of successful communication and positive emotional relatedness in play ensues and is compounded by the infant's behavioral problems, as well as the

Table 8.1 Aspects requiring attention in joint parent–infant play and solitary play

Infant behavior	Parental behavior
Joint play (Note: *positive characteristics are given in italics*, dysfunctional characteristic in normal type)	
Sensory excitability and sensory processing	***Expressivity of intuitive communication***
Receptivity	*Undivided attention*
Self-regulation: aversion from overstimulation	*Emotional availability*
Overstrain, hypersensitivity, hyperreactivity	*Motherese, mirroring facial expressions,* etc.
Sensation-seeking	*Speech accompanying joint focus of attention*
Motivation to play and play behavior	*Affective attunement to infant signals* of:
Self-efficacy, self-agency	Fatigue, overstimulation, overload
Self-initiated exploratory play	Initiative, self-agency, self-efficacy
Intentional, goal-oriented action	Focus of attention
Passivity	Emotional experience, joy, pleasure of success
Boredom, listlessness, aimlessness	Developmental stage, skills
Giving up early	Difficulties, asking for help to help himself
Emotionality	**Attunement problems**
Enjoyment of play, concentrated earnestness and eagerness	Competing own agenda
Undue earnestness, anger, frustration	Pressure to train/force infant competence
Resignation, disappointment	Overstimulation
Motor organization	Overprotective interference
Motor restlessness, fidgeting	Directive controlling behavior
"Ants in the pants," inability to sit still	Intrusiveness
Hyperactive craving for stimulation	Distorted perception
Attention	**Problems of expressivity**
Receptivity	Distress
Endurance, persistence	Depressive inhibition
Selective, focused attention	Blockage
Distractability, fluctuating attention	Inauthentic, exaggerated, forced
	Stereotypical facial and vocal behavior
Solitary play during the detachment situation	
Motivation to play, endurance	*Visual and physical alignment with:*
Self-initiated exploration and play	*The task, the infant*
Contact-seeking behavior with mother	*Unambiguousness of messages for the infant*
Attention-seeking behavior	*In response to infant contact-seeking behavior*
Attachment behavior: crying, clinginess	Alternating/ambivalence between:
Angry/aggressive behavior	Overprotective care
Provocative behavior	Anger, strictness, rejection
	Yielding/permissive behavior, resignation, laissez-faire

parental stressors in various facets (Table 8.1, Examples 1 and 2). The parents' intuitive communication, as well as their emotional availability are blocked or inhibited: They appear tense, listless, burnt-out, themselves uninspired and bored, or covertly hostile; their kindliness sometimes seems unnaturally stereotypical or false, or they lapse into silence, absorbed by their worries and unsolved conflicts. All this results in a lack of responsive, contingent attunement to the infant's real play needs, his signals, and his regulatory problems.

Exhausted, many parents fail to notice their infant's subtle signs of pleasure and satisfaction even in positive moments; they are unable to either perceive or appreciate what is motivating their infant, his eagerness to play, intense earnestness, desire to move, and inevitable disappointment at little failures and setbacks, as well as subtle signs of delight and pride in success. In this way, they deprive not only themselves but also the infant of a source of positive relational experiences.

If the parents fail to attune themselves to their infant's receptivity and tolerance limits, signs of fatigue and overexcitability, a dysfunctional pattern of overstimulation, overload, and infant resistance emerges. —Allowing the infant to take any initiative becomes problematic for parents with high expectations of their infant's achievements or strong tendencies to control their infant. They follow their own agenda, tend toward directive/controlling behavior, thwart the child in his goal-oriented, self-directed activities, only to respond to the child's withdrawal or resistance by being intrusive and overbearing.—Insecure parents in particular allow their play agenda be guided more by age norms, parenting manuals, the toy market, or the developmental status of children of the same age rather than by their own child's spontaneous interests and feedback signals; this approach can quickly lead to the infant being over- or underchallenged.

If parents follow their own agenda during joint play without taking their infant's focus of attention and play intentions into consideration, the child becomes discouraged, loses the desire to play, withdraws back into a passive role (Example 2) or walks away bored. In other cases an escalating conflict ensues that ends in an impulsive temper tantrum (Example 1).—Other infants are denied the experience of self-efficacy and success if overprotective or impatient parents preempt their success in play by intervening prematurely or providing unsolicited undue support. Their attention is interrupted and the children, discouraged or frustrated, give up.

The different dysfunctional patterns described above inhibit an infant's intrinsic motivations to play in a variety of ways and lack intuitively attuned parental support of self-efficacy, goal orientation and sustained attention, and incentives to explore, succeed or gain new skills.

8.4 Counseling and Therapy in Routine Practice

The multifactorial emergence of "disinterest in play" in the context of pervasive regulatory disorders calls for an integrative developmental, dynamic, and systemic therapy concept and a stepwise treatment plan that covers all domains of regulatory impairment (The Munich Model, Wollwerth de Chuquisengo and Papoušek 2008).

The goal of play-related developmental counseling, play-focused guidance in parent–infant communication, and psychodynamic communication-centered relational therapy is threefold: (1) To reinforce the infant's self-agency, incentive to play, and endurance in play; (2) to create scope for the infant to have positive relational experiences in order to build-up and reinforce a secure attachment relationship; and (3) to give the parents emotional and mental access to their infant's experiential world and enable them to perceive, understand, and empathetically share it with their infant (Wollwerth de Chuquisengo and Papoušek 2008).

A therapeutic relationship and attitude based on empathy and respect provide a supportive framework and secure basis for the parents and infant and are essential for providing a stress-free space in which the parents and infant can communicate intuitively and engage in experiencing positive reciprocity and emotional relatedness (Papoušek 2011).

8.4.1 Play-Related Developmental Counseling

Developmental counseling is primarily aimed at fostering the parents' understanding of: the significance of play for their infant, as well as the infant's need for self-agency and -efficacy; joint play as a source of positive relational experiences; and the importance of play in attention regulation (see Sect. 8.2). Counseling is oriented to the infant's developmental stage and his individual strengths and difficulties.

The central theme here is the daily routine to which the parents' complaints relate and for which the following recommendations (and their implementation) are specifically discussed with the parents.

Counseling topics

- Structuring of daily routines to provide sufficient sleep, regular rest periods, a joint "cozy corner" to act as a "timeout island," and plenty of motor activity in fresh air.
- Practicing short joint play periods with undivided attention alternated with periods of solitary play.
- In the context of persistent crying (Example 2): Avoiding automatically picking the infant up, as well as distinguishing between his need for closeness and his need for stimulation. Making a lying position on the changing table or floor mat playfully attractive through physical games, or fostering self-efficacy offering toys for grasping and exploration. Engaging in communication while carrying the infant about and discovering the environment together.
- In the case of fussiness that is inappropriate to the situation and parental difficulties with detachment: Practicing reasonable, short episodes of solitary play while the mother concentrates on an everyday task within view of the infant, followed by playing with the infant with mutually focused attention.
- Counteracting restless sensation seeking behavior (Example 1) or extreme hypersensitivity to stimuli (Example 3) by protecting the infant from sensory overload and overstimulation; creating a play area with sparse toys (alternating the toys that are available, tidying up together every evening).
- Given the fast pace of modern life and social pressure to achieve: Freedom from the pressure to keep the infant entertained and provide constant activity programs.
- Making time to relax and fulfill basic parental needs.

8.4.2 Play-Focused Guidance in Parent–Infant Communication and Psychodynamic Communication-Centered Relational Therapy

In cases in which parents fail to implement counseling advice in everyday domestic life, feel unable to play, or have reservations about being videotaped, time is made for joint play on the play mat (floortime) in order to experience and appreciate play in the here and now (Papoušek and de Chuquisengo 2006). The mother receives support to engage in joint play with her infant and devote her undivided attention and emotionality to the game, while allowing herself to be led by the infant's initiatives. The therapist, in his/her role as a participating observer, picks up on emotionally responsive, spontaneous episodes of the infant's self-efficacy, positive reciprocity, and affective attunement. He/she attempts to open the mother's eyes to: her infant's endearing qualities, skills, need to play, and difficulties, as well as to moments of intuitive emotional relatedness. In this way, the therapist reinforces the mother's self-confidence in her own intuitive competence, as well as her confidence in her infant.

Where this fails, the mother—on the play mat together with the therapist for support—can initially adopt the "watch, wait, and wonder" approach, whereby the focus of the intervention is put on the infant's spontaneous activity (Cohen et al. 2003; see Chap. 9). This approach aims to enhance the mother's sensitivity to her infant's signals and help her recognize, understand, and appreciate her infant's motivations, preferences, interests, strengths, and developmental advances. It is important to discuss emerging negative maternal affective states openly and address any potentially pent-up negative affects and neglected basic needs.

Despite this level of support, mothers with severe psychosocial stressors or depression, are often unable to engage emotionally in play with their child. This is the point at which psychodynamic communication-centered relational therapy starts, its goal being to dissolve parental inhibitions and blocks, and to create access to and self-confidence in their hidden intuitive playful competence (Papoušek 2011). The play context, in particular, offers a welcome interface between observable parent–infant interaction and the parent's representation, between the here and now and the past. It offers starting points to address disturbing affects and impulses, stressful recollections, and mental images, and to identify infant behavior that acts as a trigger, in order to gain insight into distorted perceptions, projected negative attributions, and unconscious reenactments—the "ghosts" from the parent's previous relational history. The aim of relational psychotherapy is to support the parents' self-reflexive functions and mentalization in relation to the real child and his current needs. Thus, play situations in the here and now provide concrete starting points for psychodynamically oriented discourse in the context of relational therapy.

8.4.3 Video-Supported Guidance in Play and Psychodynamic Relational Therapy

The use of video feedback has proved to be highly effective in play-focused guidance and psychodynamic communication-centered play and relational therapy (Papoušek 2000; Wollwerth de Chuquisengo and Papoušek 2008; see Chap. 10). It offers a unique way to: relive and reflect, from the safety of the therapeutic relationship, the successful and dysfunctional play and detachment scenarios; spend time considering (and reconsidering) moments of positive relatedness and return to these at any time; give time and space to feelings (including those of ambivalence), mental images, and recollections that emerge; anchor positive experiences in the parent's awareness; alternate sensitively between the infant's and the parent's perspectives; reveal distorted perceptions and projected attributions, resolve these with back-reference to the real child, and thus initiate mentalization processes.

A three-step approach has proven valuable—always beginning with a positively attuned sequence, followed either immediately or in a subsequent session (depending on time and parental resilience) by a therapeutic working-through of a dysfunctional sequence, and culminating with a rerun of the positive sequence and an anchoring of feelings of positive emotional relatedness in the parents' awareness.

8.4.4 Indications for Individual Psychotherapy and Occupational Therapy

Play therapy-based communication and relational therapy cannot and does not replace individual psychotherapy or couple therapy in the case of parental psychological disorders requiring treatment. However, if play therapy succeeds in stimulating the parents' self-reflexive functions and mentalization, it may motivate the affected parent to undertake individual psychotherapy, or both parents to undertake couple therapy, with the aim of dispelling the "ghosts… to their subterranean dwelling place" durably and preventing them from intruding anew into the nursery (Fraiberg et al. 1975).

Supplemental occupational therapy to promote sensory integration has proven effective in pronounced problems of infant sensory perception and sensory processing, for infants with extreme hypersensitivity to stimulation, (Example 3), as well as for infants with restless sensation-seeking behavior (Example 1).

8.5 Pitfalls in Practice

8.5.1 Problems in the Treatment Plan

Formulating a stepwise plan may prove challenging in the context of pervasive regulatory disorders. The cumulative sleep deficit associated with pronounced sleep disorders may impair the infant's as well as the parents' well-being during waking hours, their regulatory capacities, and willingness to play to such an extent that treating the sleep disorder takes priority. On the other hand, however, parent–child relations may be so strained and conflict-laden that it appears more reasonable to begin with play-oriented communication and relational therapy, which not only helps overcome disinterest in play, but also provides scope to experience positive relatedness; moreover, it makes it easier to resolve existing sleep problems and detachment or limit-setting conflicts.

8.5.2 "No Time to Play"

Feeding disorders and failure to thrive may dominate everyday life around the clock to such an extent that there is literally no time left for play activities. However, precisely in order to defuse generally highly charged feeding interactions, attention should be steered toward the infant's play needs, and the treatment of feeding interaction complemented by communication and relational therapy on the joint-play level.

8.5.3 Headwinds Driven by Social Trends

"No time to play": independent of clinically relevant disorders, the phenomenon of early childhood disinterest in play appears to be widespread and promoted by social factors. American authors (e.g., deGrandpre 2002) talk of a "rapid-fire culture" and "high-speed society" of the postmodern era. By this they refer to: our fast-paced and hectic way of life with its busy schedules, action-packed free time, and lack of leisure and relaxation; the flood of media information with its sensational stimuli and the rapid feed of information that can be only poorly integrated; the children's rooms filled to bursting with toys designed to evoke intense but short-lived stimulation; changing family structures with an abundance of "how-to manuals" and parenting programs; new forms of rapid, superficial communication and information processing, as shaped by TV, the internet, and cell phones, that produce "fast-food brains" and compromise parent–child communication during family mealtimes and joint play activities.

8.6 Disinterest in Play in Infancy and Developmental Psychopathology of ADHD

Disinterest in play, dysphoric fussiness, and hyperactivity deserve our full attention and careful treatment, given the significant psychological strain these problems place on the infant, the parents, and their relationship. Furthermore, specific prospective long-term studies are needed to establish whether or not these problems next to a lack of positive play experiences carry any specific predictive value in relation to ADHD (Wolke et al. 2002). Three clinical aspects in particular suggest developmental psychopathological links: firstly, a surprisingly corresponding multifactorial genesis of both disinterest in play and ADHD involving similar emphasis on neurobiological, constitutional, psychosocial, and relational factors (Carey 2002; Döpfner et al. 2000; Laucht et al. 2004; Moll and Rothenberger 2001); secondly, the striking relationship between behavioral problems in the domains of attention, motor activity, and affect/impulse regulation (Papoušek 2008); and thirdly, the anticipated effects of a lack of age-appropriate play experience (e.g., Crockenberg and Leerkes 2000; Panksepp 2007).

8.7 Conclusion

The aim of the present chapter is not to pathologize the phenomenon of early childhood disinterest in play and label infants with a psychiatric diagnosis of early-onset attention-deficit hyperactivity disorder (EOADHD; Dunitz-Scheer et al. 2001). It aims far more to give professionals and parents an understanding of the adaptive functions of play as a factor of resilience in infant development and parent–child relationships (Papoušek 2011). The most important prerequisites of play, both on the part of the parents and the child, are increasingly threatened by influences of the zeitgeist, as well as in the context of early childhood regulatory disorders. Young children that are disinterested in play often lack a sense of security, leisure time, and protective space, as well as an environment in which the parents manage to engage in play with undivided attention, emotional availability, and intuitive responsive communication with their potentially "difficult" infant and his intrinsic motivations for self-initiated joyful play activities. The earlier one manages to identify the conditions conducive to the emergence of disinterest in play and fussiness, the more effectively it can be prevented—in the present and, presumably, also in the long term—through counseling and therapy on the level of joint play.

References

Bates JE, Freelan CA, Lounsbury ML (1979) Measurement of infant difficultness. Child Dev 50:794–803

Carey WB (2002) Is ADHD a valid disorder? In: Jensen PS, Cooper JR (eds) Attention deficit hyperactivity disorder: state of the science; best practices. Civic Research Institute, Kingston, NJ

Cohen NJ, Muir E, Lojkasek M (2003) "Watch, Wait and Wonder"—ein kindzentriertes Psychotherapieprogramm zur Behandlung gestörter Mutter-Kind-Beziehungen. Kinderanalyse 11:58–79

Crockenberg SU, Leerkes E (2000) Infant social and emotional development in family context. In: Zeanah C (ed) Handbook of infant mental health, 2nd edn. The Guilford Press, New York, pp 60–90

DeGrandpre R (2002) Die Ritalin-Gesellschaft. Beltz Verlag, Weinheim

Döpfner M, Lehmkuhl G, Heubrock D, Petermann F (2000) Diagnose psychischer Störungen im Kindes- und Jugendalter. Hogrefe, Göttingen

Dunitz-Scheer M, Schein A, Fuest B, Oswald Y, Scheer P (2001) EOADHD; Early onset attention deficit disorder. Elterninformationsbroschüre der Univ, Klinik Graz, Graz

Fraiberg S, Adelson E, Shapiro V (1975) Ghosts in the nursery: a psychoanalytic approach to the problem of impaired infant-mother relationships. J Am Acad Child Psychiatr 14:387–422

Grossmann KU, Grossmann KE (2004) Bindungen—das Gefüge psychischer Sicherheit. Klett-Cotta, Stuttgart
Heckhausen H (1973) Entwurf einer Psychologie des Spielens. In: Flitner A (ed) Das Kinderspiel. München, Piper, München, pp 133–149
Largo RH, Benz-Castellano C (2008) Critical moments in child development: the Zurich fit model. In: Papoušek M, Schieche M, Wurmser H (eds) Disorders of behavioral and emotional regulation in the first years of life: early risks and intervention in the developing parent-infant relationship. ZERO TO THREE, Washington, DC, pp 1–12
Laucht M, Schmidt MH, Esser G (2004) Problems of behavioral and emotional regulation: precursors to psychiatric disorders in later childhood. In: Papoušek M, Schieche M, Wurmser H (eds) Disorders of behavioral and emotional regulation in the first years of life: early risks and intervention in the developing parent-infant relationship. ZERO TO THREE, Washington, DC, pp 299–316
Moll GH, Rothenberger A (2001) Neurobiologische Grundlagen: Ein pathophysiologisches Erklärungsmodell der ADHD. Kinderärztliche Praxis: Soziale Pädiatrie und Jugendmedizin 72:9–110
Oerter R (2003) Als-ob-Spiele als Form der Daseinsbewältigung. In: Papoušek M, von Gontard A (eds) Spiel und Kreativität in der frühen Kindheit. Pfeiffer bei Klett-Cotta, Stuttgart, pp 153–173
Panksepp J (2007) Can play diminish ADHD and facilitate the construction of the social brain? J Can Acad Child Adolesc Psychiatr 16:57–66
Papoušek H, Papoušek M, Harris BJ (1987) The emergence of play in parent-infant interactions. In: Görlitz D, Wohlwill JF (eds) Curiosity, imagination, and play. On the development of spontaneous cognitive and motivational processes. Erlbaum, Hillsdale, NJ, pp 214–246
Papoušek H (2003) Spiel in der Wiege der Menschheit. In: Papousek M, von Gontard A (eds) Spiel und Kreativität in der frühen Kindheit. Pfeiffer bei Klett-Cotta, Stuttgart, pp. 17–55
Papoušek M (2000) Einsatz von Video in der Eltern-Säuglings-Beratung und-Psychotherapie. Praxis der Kinderpsychologie und Psychotherapie 49:611–627
Papoušek M (2008) Dyphoric fussiness and disinterest in play in infancy: precursors or early manifestations of ADHD? In: Papoušek M, Schieche M, Wurmser H (eds) Disorders of behavioral and emotional regulation in the first years of life: early risks and intervention in the developing parent-infant relationship. ZERO TO THREE, Washington, DC, pp 317–344
Papoušek M (2011) Resilience, strengths, and regulatory capacities: hidden resources in developmental disorders of infant mental health. Infant Mental Health J 32(1 Special Issue):29–46
Papoušek M, Wollwerth de Chuquisengo R (2006) Integrative kommunikationszentrierte Eltern-Kleinkind-Psychotherapie bei frühkindlichen Regulationsstörungen. Prax Kinderpsychol Kinderpsychiatr 55:235–254
Renz-Polster H (2011) Menschen-Kinder. Kösel, München
Rothbart MK, Derryberry D, Posner MI (1994) A psychobiological approach to the development of temperament. In: Bates JE, Wachs TD (eds) Temperament: individual differences at the interface of biology and behavior. American Psychological Association, Washington, DC, pp 83–116
Ruff HA, Rothbart MK (1996) Attention in development. Oxford University Press, Oxford
Sokolov EN (1960) Neuronal models and the orienting reflex. In: Brazier MA (ed) The central nervous system and behavior. J Macy jr. Foundation, New York
Spitzer M (2002) Lernen. Spektrum Akademischer Verlag, Heidelberg
Watson JS (1972) Smiling, cooing, and „the game". Merrill-Palmer Q 18:323–339
Wolke D, Rizzo P, Woods S (2002) Persistent infant crying and hyperactivity problems in middle childhood. Pediatrics 109:1054–1060
Wollwerth de Chuquisengo R, Papoušek M (2008) Integrative communication-centered parent-infant counseling and psychotherapy. In: Papoušek M, Schieche M, Wurmser H (eds) Disorders of behavioral and emotional regulation in the first years of life: early risks and intervention in the developing parent-infant relationship. ZERO TO THREE, Washington, DC, pp 245–272

Treatment Approaches for Regulatory Disorders

9

Manfred Cierpka

9.1 Early Childhood Interventions Using a Stepwise Treatment Concept

9.1.1 Providing Parents with Information

Providing parents with information plays an important role in the spectrum of interventions in early childhood (and early interventions) and is therefore mentioned here by way of introduction. Parents address their questions before and after the birth of their infant to a multitude of experts; the midwife, the gynecologist, and, following birth, the pediatrician are their most important points of contact. Problem-oriented information can serve to reassure parents and allay their concerns and fears about their infant.

By providing information, the numerous experts that come into contact with parents in the context of childbirth can help ensure that the parents nourish their infant correctly, follow the necessary hygiene steps, stabilize their infant's sleep–wake rhythm, and, despite caring around the clock for the new arrival, keep themselves and their partnership in mind. In order to be able to find help within their social network, new parents need to be informed about the support options on offer. The pediatrician-based, early preventive medical checkups introduced, e.g., in all German federal states in 1991, play a central role here. The pediatrician is usually the first point of contact for parents and, as such, an interface to the network of early interventions.

It may well be that parents today are in actual fact more insecure than they were in the past. The reasons for this are undoubtedly diverse (see Cierpka 2012, Chap. 8). Whatever the case may be, the quest for security is behind the success enjoyed by a multitude of parenting manuals. Expert-based parenting manuals, such as the parent folder "Growing-Up Healthy" (*Gesund groß werden*) published by the German

M. Cierpka, M.D. (✉)
Institute for Psychosocial Prevention, University Hospital Heidelberg,
Bergheimer Str. 54, Heidelberg 69115, Germany
e-mail: manfred.cierpka@med.uni-heidelberg.de

M. Cierpka (ed.), *Regulatory Disorders in Infants*,
DOI 10.1007/978-3-319-43556-5_9

Federal Centre for Health Education (Bundeszentrale für gesundheitliche Aufklärung, BZgA), are recommended. The folder is issued to parents at the time of their infant's birth. It is intended as a supplement to the preventive medical check-ups performed by the pediatrician between the ages of 0 and 6 years. The parent folder tells parents everything they need to know about their infant at various ages. The BZgA website (http://www.kindergesundheit-info.de) and the National Center for Early Intervention website (*Nationales Zentrum Frühe Hilfen*, http://www.fruehehilfen.de) also provide parents with a wealth of information.

Being familiar with the spectrum of what constitutes normal development is essential for the identification and treatment of mental disorders. It becomes apparent during discussions with parents seeking advice that there are gaps in their knowledge about the various causes of their infant's age-appropriate symptoms. Providing information about child development can help to reassure a high percentage of parents by enabling them to see their infant's behavior as a completely normal variant on the spectrum of possible behaviors.

Providing information also plays a significant role in the context of counseling and frequently also in psychotherapy. Providing answers to questions is particularly important in the case of highly strained parents or mentally unstable parents.

Parent Information

Parent information relates to the following four domains:

- Infant development
- Infant behavior
- Mother–infant interaction
- The parent's partnership

Advice on how to deal with their infant is particularly welcome. It is possible to maintain an infant-centered perspective by focusing on behaviors that promote maturation and development.

Example

Advice on alternative ways of holding the infant during nursing not only makes breastfeeding easier for the infant—the parents' modified response to their infant's hunger also helps to better satisfy its needs and thereby ensure better attachment security.

Support should be tailored to the family's needs as well as to the capacity of the support provider. It is worthwhile building on the resources of the typically young families in order to reinforce their sense of self-efficacy. The following rule of thumb therefore applies: "As little as possible, but as much as necessary"—which also satisfies economic considerations.

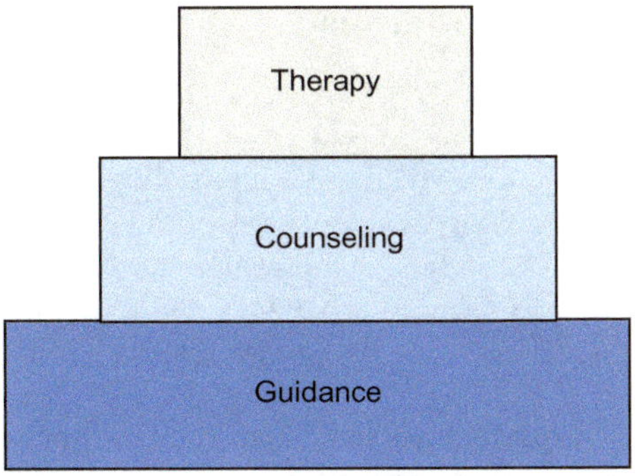

Fig. 9.1 The three-tiered treatment concept (according to GAIMH 2000 guidelines)

While elaborating standards for training and continuing education (http://www.gaimh.de/publikationen/standards.html), a working group of the German-speaking Association of Infant Mental Health (GAIMH) differentiated and defined early intervention measures for the purposes of guidance, counseling, and psychotherapy and developed a multitiered treatment concept. The three modules (see Fig. 9.1) complement one another to create a concept of early intervention (Fig. 9.1).

Standards and recommendations on content have been elaborated for all three modules of early intervention. During training and continuing education, professionals have the opportunity to gain specific qualifications to work with parents and infants or toddlers. The separate formulation of standards for each module takes into account the fact that counseling tasks can differ widely between the different groups seeking help. The core competencies of the different professional groups involved (social educators, teachers, social workers, midwives, pediatric nurses, physicians, psychologists, etc.) also vary.

9.1.2 Guidance

Guidance

According to the GAIMH definition, guidance should be low-threshold and tailored to coping with everyday life without a specific problem necessarily being present. Guidance can begin in the prenatal context, e.g., in the form of prenatal classes, and can cover, for instance, postnatal parenting courses, care services for children, and early remedial education. Guidance should be preventive in function by providing helpful information, activating available resources, using existing networks, and creating new networks.

Guidance is frequently indicated in families under strain in order to offer them support in times of crisis and is often necessary only in the short term. Precisely for these families, which are often unable to organize external support themselves, specific forms of intervention are required. Early interventions to support families are discussed in detail in (see Cierpka 2012, Chap. 38). The following sections focus primarily on counseling and psychotherapy.

9.1.3 Counseling

Counseling
The GAIMH defines counseling as a process of jointly formulating solutions to support development and relationships in a wide variety of strained or critical situations. Counseling should be task-, solution-, and resource-oriented. Brief, symptom-focused counseling is often sufficient for many families.

Counseling is indicated when information and instruction provided to the parents fail to bring about change, thereby making additional, more direct measures aimed at the parent–infant relationship necessary. The focal point of counseling is an intervention aimed at promoting development; moreover, counseling needs to be tailored to the infant's developmental phase. Stern (1998) rightly points out that, depending on the infant developmental tasks at hand, a variety of problems arise that point to particular counseling topics. These may be topics relating to the motherhood constellation (see Cierpka 2012, Chap. 9), or to the developmental steps in the first 3 years of life (Stern 1998, pp. 90–98; see also Cierpka 2012, Chap. 2).

A specialist book on developmental counseling written by Ziegenhain et al. (2004) is used by many German professionals in the context of early intervention. Dysfunctional interaction sequences can be addressed in the counseling context.

▶ Interaction-centered counseling based on sound developmental psychology is indicated in regulatory disorders of short duration (of no longer than 3 months' standing) that do not affect more than one domain and exhibit no relevant relational pathology.

In many cases, it is possible to help parents of excessively crying infants within only a few sessions by counseling them on alternative behaviors that are more suited to their infant (see Chap. 3). For example, once parents have been made aware of their infant's irritability and low sensory threshold and are able to perceive these more readily, they attempt to try out strategies that are more soothing and low-stimulus.

Developmental counseling is very much tailored to the perception and appropriate interpretation of infant signals. When parents see their infant as already "older" or "more mature," they are often overestimating its competencies. The infant then becomes hyperresponsive and is unable to settle or fall asleep due, for example, to a deluge of information or severe fatigue. Perceiving infant signals appropriately can be practiced with parents during "reading-your-baby" sessions (Barth 2000).

It is important to create a sustainable relationship with the parents, since only by so doing will they feel they can turn to the counselor at times of crisis. The mother's own need to be "mothered," as well as conflicts relating to autonomy and independence, etc., can be discussed and worked through in the context of "good grandmother transference" (Stern 1998). "Good-grandfather" therapists are helpful in the counseling of fathers.

Sessions can take the form either of therapeutic discussions (with the mother, father, or both parents) in the presence of the infant, or of joint play during which the infant is sheltered by the therapeutic relationship (e.g., in the case of a blockage of intuitive skills). Between 50 and 90 min should be allocated for each session. Therapy sessions once or twice weekly are generally sufficient; however, depending on the specific case, therapy can also take the form of a high-frequency crisis intervention or of low-frequency guidance sessions (GAIMH guidelines, http://www.gaimh.de/publikationen/standards.html).

Parent–infant counseling is predominantly case-related work in an institutional setting. An expertise on the status of psychosocial prevention/early intervention in Germany compiled on behalf of the BZgA (Cierpka et al. 2007) identified 355 contact points altogether in Germany; however, these showed widely varying characteristics in terms of structural quality (e.g., institutional features relating to service providers, billing modes, services on offer, collaborative structures, target group characteristics), process quality (e.g., reasons for registration, annual throughput, treatment modalities, interventions), and quality of outcome. This expertise shows that a wide range of psychologists, physicians, teachers, and social educators are able to maintain a sustainable infrastructure of low-threshold support in Germany. Services are provided by highly qualified professionals. However, since statutory financing is lacking, institutions of this kind are still few and far between.

Counseling interventions, which are constantly growing in importance, are also performed in the context of parenting courses offered by a variety of providers. Modern concepts focusing on parent behavior are based primarily on attachment theory. Promoting sensitivity (“parental sensitivity”) is an intermediary goal. The assumption is that the internal working models of the parents’ attachment strategies alter as a result of improved sensitivity, thereby leading to more functional parent–infant interaction. Parenting courses of this kind take a wide variety of forms (see Cierpka 2012, Chap. 37). In their meta-analysis, Bakermans-Kranenburg et al. (2003) summarize the studies based on attachment theory concepts and their impressive results. Although courses aimed at improving parental sensitivity are predominantly offered for parents of infants, there is a growing number of courses on offer for parents of toddlers (van Zeijl et al. 2006).

9.1.4 Psychotherapy

Psychotherapeutic Treatment

The GAIMH defines the psychotherapeutic treatment of infants and toddlers aged up to 3 years and their parents/primary caregivers as a process that serves to improve not only the infant’s psychological and/or somatic functional disorders, but also the quality of the infant–caregiver relationship. Psychotherapy in early childhood can begin with treating the parents during the pregnancy.

In Germany, the psychotherapy of parents with infants and toddlers is offered as part of the national framework of psychotherapeutic health care. It is performed by approved child and adolescent psychotherapists, child and adolescent psychiatrists, as well as adult psychotherapists as a service provided by the statutory health care system (despite repeated attempts by the various statutory health insurances to trim services). A diagnosis according to ICD-10 is mandatory in order for this service to be covered by the statutory health insurance (see Chap. 2).

Parents and their infant are generally experiencing a significant crisis when they attend counseling or psychotherapy. The latter is an indication established following an initial consultation, which comprises providing information to the parents as well as developmental counseling. Parent–infant psychotherapy should be considered in cases where these initial interventions prove insufficient.

Sameroff et al. (2004) described three goals of psychotherapy (the "three Rs"): "Remediation" refers to the rapid stabilization of an infant affected by a disorder or symptom; "redefinition" aims to alter the parents' perception of and attitude toward their child; "re-education" attempts to modify the parents' behavior toward their child. Parent–infant/toddler psychotherapy generally achieves stabilization within only a few sessions (between five and ten).

Indications for Parent–Infant/Toddler Psychotherapy (Papoušek et al. 2006)
Long-term parent–infant/toddler psychotherapy is indicated when:

- Developmental psychological counseling fails to achieve a significant improvement of symptoms.
- The infant disorder is already of long standing (more than 3 months).
- The infant disorder affects multiple interactional and regulatory domains and is associated with maladaptive interaction patterns or even a risk of neglect or abuse.
- Maternal/parental perception and interpretation of infant behavior (e.g., due to postnatal depression, neurotic or other mental disorders) is markedly impaired or distorted and/or intuitive parenting skills are severely impaired.

Additional individual or couples therapy should be considered in the case of psychological/psychiatric comorbidity in one or both parents.

Particular attention should be paid during history-taking to early childhood neglect, experiences of parental separation and loss, exposure to violence, as well as unresolved transgenerational trauma and relational conflicts.

Psychotherapeutic treatment can be conducted either in an individual or in a group setting. In the vast majority of cases, between one and two therapists treat one set of parents and their infant. Group therapy approaches have been described in recent years in particular in relation to maternal or paternal personality disorders. Pedrina (2000, 2006; see also Cierpka 2012, Chap. 36) describes group therapy involving mothers with postnatal depression.

The Circle of Security™ is an evidence-based therapeutic approach that aims to enhance attachment security between parents and infant. Developed by Marvin et al. (2002) in the USA as an attachment-based psychoanalytic therapy for parents with children aged between 0 and 5 years, it is a group-therapy approach comprising 20 weekly sessions of 90 min each involving groups of six parents. A diagnostic assessment is made of the attachment strategy of each parent–child dyad prior to therapy. This enables the therapists to define the personal strengths and (clinically) relevant attachment and caregiving difficulties of the individual parents while taking the infant's attachment and exploratory systems and needs into consideration, and to formulate an individualized treatment protocol for each mother/father in the group. Video interaction analysis and reflective dialogue within the group form the core elements of this attachment-based approach (see Chap. 10). The Circle of Security™ is currently undergoing clinical evaluation in German-speaking countries for mothers with postnatal mental illness and their infants (Ramsauer et al. 2010).

9.2 Treatment Modalities

The goal of all psychotherapeutic methods, as with counseling concepts, is to achieve attachment security and embed the infant in an environment that is as conducive to its development as possible. However, this can be achieved in a variety of ways. Treatment techniques differ according to the levels of psychotherapeutic approach chosen:

- Primarily behavior-centered approaches, with their focus on the interactional sequences between parents and infant, tend to address the changes in interaction between parents and infant and aim to alter parental behavior. Interactional approaches attempt to interrupt dysfunctional interactions. They promote parental skills in a more structured approach and, via the parents, more functional interaction on the part of the parents with the infant.
- Psychodynamic approaches focus above all on the mostly subconscious expectations and attitudes (representations) of the parents and on the relational patterns these give rise to. These approaches are concerned with how the parents perceive, experience, and understand their infant. Due to negative parental experiences in the family of origin, their relationship to their own infant may be disordered.
- Many therapists attempt to combine these approaches.

9.2.1 Focusing on Parental Behavior

Behavior-oriented concepts focus on observable interaction and attempt to influence the structure of this by directly addressing interaction processes. The aim here is to modify parental behavior, without taking parental fantasies about the child into consideration.

Interaction guidance therapy (McDonough 1993) involves the therapist visiting the family at home. The concept was originally developed for families under severe strain for whom other therapies were ineffective or unacceptable. A prerequisite here is that consent is obtained from the mother/father to discuss interaction sequences prior to initiating therapy. The method is geared toward parental behavior, which is recorded by video camera. The therapist then works with positive interaction sequences between the mother/father and infant in order to avoid further undermining the self-confidence of the already highly insecure parent(s) with critical comments. Explicit emphasis is put on the well-being and happiness visible in the interaction between mother/father and infant. The therapist then takes the caregiver—either live in the here and now or via video feedback—to recorded interaction sequences containing particular infant signals and discusses these signals, as well as the interactional behavior they trigger, with the mother/parents. Thus, the infant's involvement in the therapy process is minimal.

Therapy generally comprises between 10 and 12 weekly sessions. Each session follows roughly the same procedure. In a first step, a play scene between the mother/father and infant lasting approximately 6 min is recorded by video camera; the therapist and caregiver then watch and discuss a positive interaction sequence in the video; the session is rounded up with a summary of the results. Barth (2000) refers to these guided practice sessions with mother/parents and infant as "reading-your-baby" sessions. The sessions involve practicing together with the mother/parents to "read" their infant's signals, i.e., receive and label the signals with a meaning in the sense of "decoding" them. Only once parents are capable of understanding what their infant is trying to tell them are they able to react appropriately. "Intuitively" understanding and responding to infant signals is particularly challenging in the case of restless, hypersensitive infants.

One great advantage of this method is that, by virtue of the supportive therapeutic relationship within which it is conducted, it generally succeeds in steering the parents' attention to functional (and later also dysfunctional) interaction with their baby. The parents see the therapist's careful consideration of interaction not as criticism, but rather as extremely helpful. In this way, it is possible to largely avoid offensive confrontations and interpretations (see Chap. 10 on the advantages of video analysis). Naturally, this technique can also be used in psychodynamic therapies, most notably in the case of parents with structural deficits in mental functioning.

Interaction Guidance Therapy (McDonough 1993) Summarized

- Uses video-supported techniques.
- Recordings are watched together with the mother/parents.
- Supports the caregiver by identifying positive, caring behavior.
- Reviews problematic interaction sequences, revealing possible maternal misperceptions of infant signals.
- Proposes possible alternative interpretations of infant behavior.
- Reinforces positive interactions by means of encouragement and praise.
- Focuses on the "here and now."
- No attention is paid to the caregiver's past or to projection processes.

9.2.2 Focusing on Representations

Psychodynamically oriented therapy aims to address the unconscious conflicts in the parents' unresolved biographical past. Past experiences, as well as unresolved relationship conflicts with the family of origin, are internalized by the parents as representations and influence relationships in their current family. The parents' unresolved biographical past reemerges in the relationship with their infant. This can result in the parents being unable to understand or "empathize with" their infant's emotional state or communicative expressions, or indeed misperceiving them, since these are superimposed with the parents' projected attributions of significance. The focus of treatment is placed on the parents' relational disorders.

In psychoanalysis, representations are regarded as affectively charged internal notions. They comprise traces of remembered self-perceptions and object perceptions. Representations are formed by recurrent experiences, often brought about by interaction with significant others, e.g., at meal times or during play. However, rarer processes that are of great subjective significance also result in representations. According to Stern (1998), a representation develops as a result of these frequently recurring experiences of subjective interpersonal processes. The manifestation of significant interpersonal experiences should not be equated with events taking place in external reality, since these events are worked through subjectively. Thus, current experiences with one's own baby become interwoven with previously significant relational experiences as a baby or child with one's own parents. Intersubjective experience is also at the core of Stern's concept. Representations are formed on the basis of a "schema-of-being-with-another" and the associated sensations, perceptions, affects, thoughts, motivations, contextual elements, etc. (Stern 1998).

Once representations have formed, they go on to initiate behaviors and influence perceptions, feelings, and the way in which relationships are interpreted. The reason it is so important to focus on representations is that these internalized parental experiences are able to explain the parents' behavior toward their infant. The psychodynamic cognitive process taps into them and makes them accessible.

The "dominant theme" (Stern 1998) is well suited to gaining access to the mother or father's representational world in the interview setting. It takes up a considerable amount of time and space in the parents' representational world and is highly relevant in terms of behavior and experience. The theme can be based on unconscious intrapsychic parental conflicts or may be a manifestation of coping with serious family crises or traumas (Fraiberg et al. 1975). Searching for the dominant theme offers an extremely helpful starting point for a more differentiated psychodynamic diagnostic assessment (see Chap. 8). The dominant theme is identified on three relational levels, which can be superimposed onto one another like relationally dynamic transparencies. Indicators are gleaned from:

- The relational system observed between infant and parents in the interview setting
- The multigenerational relational patterns described by the parents
- The relationship that forms between the therapist and the family system

Parent–infant psychotherapy is characterized by a number of important differences that make it distinct from the classic psychoanalytic setting: The parents introduce their infant's problem while the infant is present during the session and interacts with the caregiver; in this way, the parents' internalized relational experiences are reenacted in the here and now (see Cramer and Palacio-Espasa 2009).

The treatment procedure largely corresponds to the classic psychodynamic approach. The therapists become involved in the interaction pattern as part of the dialogical process and encounter the parents' expectations and notions (including those relating to the infant). At the same time, the parents describe their relationship with their infant. They also relate how the child has altered their relationship as a couple and how it currently affects that relationship.

There are a number of different "ports of entry" (Stern 1998) providing access to the therapist–family system in order to psychodynamically work through and modify parental representations (Stern 1998; Dornes 1999; Hirschmüller 2000; von Klitzing 1998; Windaus 2007; Cramer and Palacio-Espasa 2009).

9.2.2.1 Parental Representations as the Starting Point

The authors of these psychoanalytic approaches follow Selma Fraiberg's concept to a greater or lesser degree and develop it further. Fraiberg, the pioneer of parent–infant therapy, worked in San Francisco together with a number of social workers; the aim of her work visiting homes ("psychotherapy in the kitchen") was to prevent infants being taken into care (Fraiberg et al. 1975). Fraiberg (1980) described how "ghosts in the nursery," the ghosts from the family's past, are present as "uninvited guests" in every nursery. Counseling experience shows that these "ghosts" are not easily banished. They interfere in the "dialogue" between parents and infant and may cause sustained perturbation on this level. Spirals of dysfunctional interaction ultimately lead to symptom formation in the infant.

The conflict-laden relationship with the infant, which is generally caused by maternal/parental projections onto the infant, is worked through during therapy sessions. A distinction is made between two types of projections ("ghosts"):

- Projection of self-representatives: Parents describe their child as though it is or feels precisely as they do.
- Projection of object representatives: Parents describe their child as though it feels or thinks like a significant figure in the parental past.

One finds not only the maternal representatives of the infant at the center of this dialogue, but also the symptomatic interaction between mother and child that accompanies them. It is assumed that the mother's internal working model is modified by gaining insight into the dynamic causes of her perturbed relationship with her child. The main work is done in the interplay between therapist and mother. Often, the infant is only indirectly involved, e.g., if its activity or play is interpreted as a scene. As in psychoanalytic therapy, Fraiberg focuses on understanding as a motive for maternal change. However, greater sensitivity in the perception of her child's qualities and better responsivity to these also modifies the mother's internal working model. This promotes the differentiation of the child from the mother, and thus a more objective perception of the child's behavior—resulting in modified interactions.

Lieberman and Pawl are Selma Fraiberg's direct successors. In their concept of child–parent psychotherapy (CPP), they place emphasis on the "corrective attachment experience of the therapeutic relationship" (Lieberman and Pawl 1993, p. 430). Like Fraiberg, they also worked with a group of mothers of low socioeconomic status (single mothers, drug-addicted mothers, mothers belonging to minorities or known to the authorities, etc.). Since these mothers are often negatively disposed toward counseling and support, particular attention is paid to creating a workable therapeutic alliance and acceptable transference–countertransference conditions. Lieberman and van Horn (2004) expanded CPP methodology to include therapeutic work with early-childhood experiences of loss and violence. The final volume by Lieberman and van Horn (2011) also describes the use of this treatment approach with less structurally disturbed mothers.

The approach adopted by the "Geneva school" (Cramer and Palacio-Espasa 2009) is also based on Fraiberg's work. Like Lebovici (1980, 1983), Cramer and Palacio-Espasa are seen as proponents of the brief mother–infant psychotherapy developed in France. Their approach differs from that of Lieberman and Pawl in that they place more emphasis on interpretation than on intervention in the therapeutic process. The mother's self-representation and how it evolves in the relationship with the therapist is the preferred clinical focus here.

9.2.2.2 From Infant Behavior to Parental Representation

The Boston pediatrician, Terry Brazelton, proposed making infant behavior the starting point from which to modify the maternal/parental representation of herself/themselves or of her/their infant (Brazelton 1984,1992). It is sometimes necessary for a mother or father to first develop a "baby representation." A teenage mother that, to all intents and purposes, rejects her baby and does not wish to engage in a relationship with it may be able to start building a relationship by observing her child. It is not the observed behavior that takes center stage with this method, as in McDonough's approach (see above), but rather the mother/father's representation of the infant. The infant's behavior can be observed in numerous examination situations, e.g., during preventive medical checkups. The therapist talks to the mother/father about the observed behavior during the examination. This approach, therefore, is particularly suited to implementation in a pediatric medical practice.

A method of psychotherapeutic practice, "Watch, Wait and Wonder" (WWW), was described by Cohen et al. (1999). WWW focuses on infant behavior and parental representations and is ideally initiated in infants aged between 4 and 6 months. Parents are encouraged to let themselves be led by their infant in the therapeutic setting.

During the first half of the session ("watch"), they observe their infant's self-initiated activity and only respond at their infant's initiative ("wait"). They should be physically available; when this is the case, the infant will involve them in the relationship. The authors based this approach on concepts of attachment theory.

They emphasize the importance of the mother/father's attentive physical presence while the infant plays.

The mother/father's observations and experiences are discussed with the therapist ("wonder") in the second half of the session. The therapist provides a safe, familiar environment and atmosphere for this discussion. Thus, the parents gain insight into the interrelationships and problems caused by their efforts to follow their infant's lead. Exploring their own mental models enables the mother/father to review the internal working models they have of themselves in relation to their infant. This results in a modification to maternal/paternal representations and, in turn, to an internal working model with a secure attachment style in the infant/toddler.

9.2.2.3 Mentalization-Based Parent-Infant Psychotherapy

Mentalization-based psychotherapy (MBT; Bateman and Fonagy 2008) has also become established as a parent–child psychotherapeutic approach in recent years. The authors seize on results from theory-of-mind research, which, e.g., investigates how an infant discovers that it and its caregiver are beings with mental states. How does an infant learn the mental act of imagining why someone feels and acts in one way rather than another? The aim of MBT in parent–infant psychotherapy is to enable parents to better understand their own as well as their infant's wishes, thoughts, and perceptions, thereby contributing to the further maturation of their mentalizing ability. Understanding the crying infant as an infant reacting emotionally to a previous action of the parents is, e.g., a step in this direction.

The mentalization-promoting technique is particularly suited to treating disorders in parents with inadequate structural abilities and skills in cases where these cannot be achieved by means of classic work on representations. MBT is particularly helpful when interpretation or the use of empathy is ineffective in patients with disorders of affect regulation, alexithymia, or autistic symptoms. The aim is always to improve the parents' reflective functions (Slade et al. 2005). The expressed wishes, intentions, and communicative messages of the parents, usually the mother, are discussed during the therapy session. An affect-focused questioning technique supports the mentalization process. The therapist serves as a model and is relatively active and verbal in the process in order to help the mother/father "learn" to mentalize about their infant.

From a historical perspective, the use of parent–child psychotherapy is based on the findings of Winnicott (1974), who referred to the significance of maternal mirroring in the development of a mentalized sense of self. He underlined that the psyche does not develop independently from inside outwards, but much more from outside inwards. Infants discover their psyche in the psyche of the caregiver. By mentalizing their interaction with their infant, the parents contribute to the infant acquiring a capacity for mentalization.

Following in Winnicott's footsteps, Thompson-Salo et al. (1999) focused on direct psychoanalytic work with very small infants, particularly those of parents with limited capacity to reflect on their infant. The therapists have no qualms about taking the infant and talking or playing with it. The actions become a model for parental mentalization.

Mentalization-based group therapy for parents has proved beneficial for mothers and fathers attending the Heidelberg parent–infant/toddler clinic (Bark 2013). Both closed and open sessions generally involving three to five mothers are held regularly. The general procedure prior to group therapy includes conducting an individual interview and establishing the indication. A video recording of play interaction between mother and infant is made after the first or second group session, once the mothers have gained confidence in the setting. Working with video feedback in the group has proven extremely helpful and is also essential to the subsequent dissemination of this therapeutic approach by providing video-based teaching material.

9.2.2.4 Access via Therapist Countertransference

In this approach, the therapist's countertransference provides access to the psychodynamic level (see also Windaus 2007). This concept assumes that the therapist is able to make himself aware not only of his own countertransference feelings, but rather he needs to have learned (generally through self-analysis) how to distinguish between his own countertransferences and the feelings elicited in him by others (the infant, the parents). The myriad identifications with the infant and its parents, which remind him of his own childhood and his experiences with his own parents, make this a challenging task that can only be accomplished through practice.

Child and adolescent psychotherapists learn this during their training according to the model formulated by Esther Bick (1964): Students undertake to find an infant that they will visit at home over a 1- to 2-year period, starting shortly after birth. The therapist observes the mother in her relationship with the infant, while at the same time paying heed to his own "subjectivity" and feelings of countertransference. All observations are protocoled and subsequently presented in a group seminar. The (presumed) infant representations can be inferred from the transference–countertransference dynamics. How must he feel at that moment? What could be going on in his mind?

During infant observation, the participating students remain distanced from the mother and infant and do not intervene in their interaction. They practice their analysis of countertransference dynamics. However, it is assumed that the mother identifies with the therapist's observant/reflective stance, thereby reinforcing her mentalizing, reflective competencies. The mother's representations of her infant can be modified in this way.

Countertransference feelings can also be used as the port of entry for psychodynamic analysis in parent–infant psychotherapy. In psychotherapy, not only the parent's representations, but also the infant's emotions can be inferred from the transference–countertransference feelings.

The psychoanalytic concept is based in part on Bion's conceptualization of the mother–infant or therapist–mother relationship as a container–contained relationship (Bion 1963; see Cierpka 2012, Chap. 6), in which the mother "digests… raw" (poorly differentiated) feelings and affects for her child and mirrors them (in a more differentiated form), much like the therapist picks up on the mother's feelings, as mediated via his countertransference feelings, and returns them to her "digested." Whether this process is suited as a concept to psychoanalytic therapy in very early developmental disorders (Israel 2007) has not yet been proven.

Kleinian psychoanalysis traditionally uses the infant's representations as a starting point (see Cierpka 2012, Chap. 6). According to Melanie Klein, the disappointment associated with weaning, the "loss" of "bodily substances" (feces, urine), and being excluded from the parental primal scene gives rise already in early infancy to fantasies about the "good" and the "bad" breast or the "good" and the "bad" penis (Klein 1932). The French child psychotherapist, Dolto (1971), followed this tradition by putting the infant's presumed experience and expectable fantasies into words addressed to the infant. The therapist's words are intended not only for the infant, but also for the parents. However, the therapist also assumes that these verbal interpretations are understood by the infant. Windaus (2007, p. 16) doubts, and rightly so, that the infant is able to understand the content of the therapist's comments. He suggests that the therapist achieves part of the therapeutic effect by treating the infant in the presence of its primary caregivers, as a result of which the session increases the infant's containment. This can have an effect on how the parents deal with their infant.

9.2.2.5 Mother/Father–Infant Interaction as a Starting Point

Most concepts use mother/father–infant interaction as the starting point for and access to the psychodynamic level. It is assumed that parental representations are reenacted in the interaction between parents and infant. In terms of focus, the representations of the parent figure influence the recorded interactional dynamics significantly more than do those of the infant. Stern (1998) paid close attention to the parent's and infant's way of being together. He suggested that the evolving way of being together is internalized by the infant as a representation and can be essential in terms of the subsequent object choice.

Psychodynamically oriented psychotherapists are accustomed to watching out for relevant events and interesting new interaction sequences between therapist and patient. Access to childhood experiences can be gained through the observation and analysis of interaction. The option to capture, so to speak, particular interactional sequences between parents and child (e.g., by means of video recordings) and work through these scenes is novel. The interaction sequences are identified and, where videotaped, analyzed scene by scene (see Chap. 10). It initially feels unfamiliar to the psychoanalyst to look at the scenes together with the parents on the monitor, thereby leaving the familiar context; however, viewing specific interaction sequences enables an immediate and very direct diagnosis of the different representations activated in the parents. These activated representations trigger conscious and unconscious memories in the parents of their own experiences, which are often highly affect-laden and could provide the key to understanding distorted perceptions in relation to their infant. For this reason, interactive reality has taken on greater importance in parent–child psychotherapy compared with intrapsychic processes.

As in family therapy, brief psychotherapeutic interventions are more common in psychodynamic parent–child psychotherapy. Numerous authors report that more than 50 % of cases ultimately proved to be counseling cases (e.g., Cramer and Palacio-Espasa 2009) and that psychotherapy can be described as short-term psychotherapy (mostly even <12 sessions). This makes it possible to treat a particular topic or psychodynamic focus over a certain period of time, followed by an analysis of what has been achieved. This approach focuses on family resources and reinforces self-regulatory strengths. Our focus-oriented psychoanalytic parent–infant psychotherapy, which also uses parent–infant interaction as a port of entry, is discussed in detail in Chap. 11.

9.2.3 The Integration of Approaches

Interventional concepts in parent–infant counseling and psychotherapy differ from other psychotherapeutic methods in children, adolescents, and adults in terms of their strongly integrative approach. Most approaches attempt to use and integrate cognitive behavioral, interactional, systemic, and psychodynamic methods and techniques. This is chiefly due to the fact that the "presenting problem" (Wynne 1988) responsible in the majority of cases for the "sick" child's referral has multiple determinants. In the case of persistent symptoms, causes are often found not only in the infant, but also in the parents and in the relationships of the burdened families with their infant.

Multi-method interventions targeted at different levels of the system (individual person, partnership, family, social milieu) are called for in order to help the family in crisis as quickly and effectively as possible. In a spirit of pragmatism, one seeks points of departure for interventions that will stabilize and modify the parent–infant relationship as rapidly as possible.

This multimodal approach is intended in particular for the 3–8 % of families classified as high-risk according to a UNICEF Report (2005).

Results from the growing body of empirical research (see Cierpka 2012, Chap. 36) also suggest that there should be no school-oriented "either/or." Clinical windows should permit a view not only of parental and infant behavior, but also of their internalized representations and internal working models.

Greater therapeutic flexibility makes different starting points for interventions possible. One gains better access to the psychodynamic level when different ports of entry (Stern 1998) are used, e.g., not only via the analysis of transference–countertransference dynamics, but also via interaction analysis. With the "presenting problem" and their search for help, the family invites the therapist to establish a relationship, and by accommodating the needs of the family, the therapist reinforces the therapeutic alliance from the outset.

Integrative approaches generally put parent–child interaction at the center of the clinical focus. As the key element, it first needs to be analyzed and understood in order for the therapist to be able to consider, in a further step, the possibilities for modification. A communication-centered method was developed by an interdisciplinary team of pediatricians and psychologists led by Mechthild Papoušek in the 1990s, and has since undergone continuous further differentiation (Papoušek et al. 1994; Papoušek 1998; Wollwerth de Chuquisengo and Papoušek 2004). Its roots lie in H. Papoušek's research work over many years into the early development of the infant's integrative skills, as well as in coauthored works on intuitive early parenting in the context of pre-verbal communication (see Cierpka 2012, Chap. 5).

This integrative concept is tailored to the family's current needs. Parent–child communication in day-to-day interactions, with its stress points in soothing, nursing/feeding, settling to bed, diaper changing, and in dialogue or play with the infant, forms the focus here. Communication and relational therapy includes not only the level of observable interactions, but also the psychodynamic aspects that impair intuitive parenting skills and imperil the early development of communication, attachment, and relationships.

In an integrative approach, additional modules—depending on the severity of the disorder, the individual needs of the infant and its parents, and the crisis at hand—are integrated into the treatment in order to achieve a comprehensive improvement as rapidly as possible. Promoting parental sensitivity through parenting courses, psychotherapy geared to parental behavior, or mentalization-based psychotherapy sometimes need to precede psychodynamic conflict-oriented psychotherapy in cases where the parents lack the structural capabilities needed to pick up on pointers relating to their projections. In this respect, concepts that raise the parents' mentalization level and increase their reflective competence in a first step (Fonagy 1991; Fonagy et al. 2004) are an extremely helpful supplement in the spectrum of interventions.

In cases where one parent suffers from severe trauma in their own childhood or from a posttraumatic stress disorder (PTSD), e.g., triggered by the birth of their own child (see Thiel-Bonney and Cierpka 2004), trauma therapy approaches should be considered. One must assume that these traumas crucially affect interaction. In such cases, one might consider eye movement desensitization and reprocessing (EMDR) therapy in the mother or father prior to initiating parent–infant psychotherapy. In the course of the SAFE (Secure Attachment for Education) program (Brisch 2010), expectant mothers may find themselves confronted with their own traumas, for which they should subsequently receive therapy. PTSDs in infants and toddlers are currently under discussion and the first standardized treatment methods have been described (Hensel 2010). It remains to be elucidated whether trauma therapy techniques are appropriate at such an early age.

Daniel Schechter attempts to combine trauma therapy techniques with psychodynamic parent–infant psychotherapy. He found that the biographies of many of his New York patients included experiences of abuse and violence in early childhood, experiences that are linked to mental disease in adulthood, such as PTSD, personality disorders, and chronic depression. Although the traumatized mothers wanted to be good mothers, they had great difficulties "reading" their infant's signals. Schechter identified a tendency in these mothers to misattribute their infant's intentions (Schechter et al. 2003, 2005). As a result, the infant frequently adopts the misattribution and behaves accordingly in order not to imperil attachment to the caregiver. These children are often also in a state of hypervigilance, meaning that a traumatization-tinged intersubjectivity emerges and is maintained between mother and child (Schechter et al. 2007). These factors can ultimately lead to transgenerational transfer of trauma.

Schechter developed a therapeutic approach designed to modify the mother/father's representations of their infant, the clinician assisted video feedback exposure sessions (CAVES). Using the interaction guidance method described above as a model (see also Chap. 10), he shows the parents video clips of play situations with the infant, but concentrates in particular on separation and other stressful situations. The therapist asks the mother or father to reflect on what she/he as mother/father, as well as what the infant felt and thought in a specific situation. The technique fosters mentalization and emotional regulatory competence in the traumatized parent. The method integrates elements of trauma exposure therapy (Foa et al. 1999), since, in considering the situation that is stressful to the infant, the primary caregiver is also exposed to stress over a prolonged period.

Conclusion

Parent–infant/toddler counseling and psychotherapy have evolved in recent decades to become an integral component of the psychotherapeutic spectrum and health care concept to treat mental disorders in early childhood. Methods have become more differentiated and can be adapted in line with differential indications to meet the needs of those seeking help. Since families often come to us when they are in an acute crisis situation, the somatopsychological recovery of the still fragile infant or toddler takes precedence.

Given that they permit several levels to be addressed simultaneously, integrative approaches have proven their value by virtue of their pragmatic and flexible implementation in family crisis situations. Video recordings and video feedback often make up an integral part of interventions. There has been a growing call in recent years for greater inclusion of fathers in the counseling concept and psychotherapeutic process in order to better understand and use triadic dynamics (Bürgin 1998; von Klitzing et al. 1999; see Cierpka 2012, Chap. 10). All methods attempt to influence parent–infant interaction in such a way that the child can achieve secure attachment and grow up and mature in the best possible environmental conditions. Studies on intervention efficacy show that these methods are effective (see Cierpka 2012, Chap. 36). When a multigenerational perspective is taken, therapy can succeed in interrupting the transgenerational transfer of trauma and other severe conflicts. Thus, the psychotherapeutic treatment of parents with infants and toddlers serves a preventive function (see Cierpka 2012, Chap. 38).

References

Bakermans-Kranenburg MJ, van Ijzendoorn MH, Juffer F (2003) Less is more: meta-analysis of sensitivity and attachment interventions in early childhood. Psychol Bull 129(2):195–215

Bark C (2013) Mentalisierungsbasierte Mutter-Kind-Therapie in der frühen Kindheit. Psychotherapeut 58:388–394

Barth R (2000) Baby-Lese-Stunden für Eltern mit exzessiv schreienden Säuglingen. Prax Kinderpsychol Kinderpsychiatr 8:537–549

Bateman W, Fonagy P (2008) Psychotherapie der Borderline-Persönlichkeitsstörung. Ein mentalisierungsgestütztes Behandlungskonzept. Psychosozial-Verlag, Gießen

Bick E (1964) Notes on infant observation in psycho-analytic training. Int J Psychoanal 49:484–486

Bion WR (1963) Elements of psycho-analysis. Heinemann, London

Brazelton TB (1984) To listen to a child. Addison-Wesley, Reading, MA
Brazelton TB (1992) Touchpoints. Guilford Press, New York
Brisch KH (2010) SAFE©—Sichere Ausbildung für Eltern. Sichere Bindung zwischen Eltern und Kind. Klett-Cotta, Stuttgart
Bundeszentrale für gesundheitliche Aufklärung (BZgA) (2009) Elternordner Gesund groß werden. BZgA, Köln
Bürgin D (1998) Triangulierung. Der Übergang zur Elternschaft. Schattauer, Stuttgart
Cierpka M, Stasch M, Groß S (2007) Expertise zum Stand der Prävention/Frühintervention in der frühen Kindheit in Deutschland. BZgA, Köln
Cierpka M (Hrsg) (2012) Frühe Kindheit 0-3 Jahre. Springer, Berlin
Cohen NJ, Muir E, Parker CJ, Brown M, Lojkasek M, Muir R et al (1999) Watch, wait, and wonder. Testing the effectiveness of a new approach to mother-infant-psychotherapy. Infant Mental Health J 20:429–451
Cramer BG, Palacio-Espasa F (2009) Psychotherapie mit Müttern und ihren Babys: Kurzzeitbehandlungen in Theorie und Praxis. Psychosozial-Verlag, Gießen
Dolto F (1971) Psychanalyse et pédiatrie. Édition du Seuil, Paris
Dornes M (1999) Die Entstehung seelischer Erkrankungen: Risiko- und Schutzfaktoren. In: Suess GJ, Pfeifer WKP (Hrsg) Frühe Hilfen. Die Anwendung von Bindungs- und Kleinkindforschung in Erziehung, Beratung, Therapie und Vorbeugung. Psychosozial-Verlag, Gießen
Foa EB, Dancu CV, Hembree EA, Jaycox LH, Meadows EA, Street GP (1999) A comparison of exposure therapy, stress inoculation training and their combination for reducing PTSD in female assault victims. J Consult Psychol 67(2):194–200
Fonagy P (1991) The role of the dyad and the triad in coming to understand mental states: clinical evidence from the psychoanalytic treatment of borderline personality disorder. International Symposium on the Theme of the Phenomena of the Transition in Child and Adolescent Psychiatry 1, Basel, Switzerland
Fonagy P, Gergely G, Jurist E (2004) Affektregulierung, Mentalisierung und die Entwicklung des Selbst. Klett-Cotta, Stuttgart
Fraiberg S (1980) Clinical studies in infant mental health. Basic Books, New York
Fraiberg S, Adelson E, Shapiro V (1975) Ghosts in the nursery. A psychoanalytical approach to the problems of impaired infant-mother relationships. J Am Acad Child Adolescent Psychiatr 14:387–422
GAIMH (2000) Fort- und Weiterbildungsstandards für Begleitung, Beratung und Psychotherapie für Kinder von 0 bis 3 Jahren mit ihren Eltern und anderen Bezugspersonen, http://www.gaimh.de/publikationen/standards.html
Hensel M (2010) Posttraumatische Belastungsstörungen bei Säuglingen und Kleinkindern. Prax Kinderpsychol Kinderpsychiatr 57:247–263
Hirschmüller B (2000) Von der Säuglingsbeobachtung zur analytischen Psychotherapie von Müttern mit Säuglingen und sehr kleinen Kindern. Analytische Kinder- und Jugendlichen-Psychotherapie 31:419–450
Israel A (ed) (2007) Der Säugling und seine Eltern: die psychoanalytische Behandlung frühester Entwicklungsstörungen. Brandes & Apsel, Frankfurt a.M
Klein M (1932) The psycho-analysis of children. Hogarth, London
von Klitzing K (1998) Psychotherapie in der frühen Kindheit. Vandenhoeck & Ruprecht, Göttingen
von Klitzing K, Simoni H, Amsler F, Bürgin D (1999) The role of the father in early family interactions. Infant Mental Health J 20:222–237
Lebovici S (1980) Névrose infantile, névrose de transfert. Rev Fr Psychanal 5–6:743–857
Lebovici S (1983) Le nourisson, la mère et le psychanalyste: Les interventions précoces. Le Centurion, Paris
Lieberman AF, Pawl JH (1993) Infant-parent psychotherapy. In: Zeanah C (Hrsg) Handbook of infant mental health. Guilford Press, New York, S427–S442
Lieberman AF, van Horn P (2004) Don't hit my mommy: a manual for child-parent psychotherapy with young witnesses of family violence. Zero To Three Press, Washington

Lieberman AF, van Horn P (2011) Psychotherapy with infants and young children: repairing the effects of stress and trauma on early attachment. Guilford Press, New York
Marvin R, Cooper G, Hoffman K, Powell B (2002) The Circle of Security™ Project: Attachment-based intervention with caregiver-pre-school child dyads. Attach Hum Dev 4:107–124
McDonough S (1993) Promoting positive early parent-infant relationships through interaction guidance. Child Adolesc Psychiatric Clin N Am 4(3):661–672
Papoušek M (1998) Das Münchner Modell einer interaktionszentrierten Säuglings-Eltern-Beratung und -Psychotherapie. In: Klitzing K von (Hrsg) Psychotherapie in der frühen Kindheit. Vandenhoeck & Ruprecht, Göttingen, S88–S118
Papoušek M, von Hofacker N, Malinowski M, Jacubeit T, Cosmovici B (1994) Münchner Sprechstunde für Schreibabys. Erste Ergebnisse zur Früherkennung und Prävention von Störungen der Verhaltensregulation und der Eltern-Kind-Beziehungen. Sozialpädiatrie in der Pädiatrie 16:680–686
Papoušek M, Rothenberger S, Cierpka M, von Hofacker N (2006) Regulationsstörungen der frühen Kindheit. CD-basierte Fortbildung. Stiftung Kindergesundheit, München
Pedrina F (2000) Gruppentherapie mit Müttern und Babys in postpartalen Krisen. Ausschnitte aus der qualitativen Auswertung eines Pilotprojekts. Analytische Kinder- und Jugendlichen-Psychotherapie 31:469–484
Pedrina F (2006) Mütter und Babys in psychischen Krisen. Forschungsstudie zu einer therapeutisch geleiteten Mutter-Säuglings-Gruppe am Beispiel postpartaler Depression. Brandes & Apsel, Frankfurt a.M
Ramsauer B, Lotzin A, Gehrke J, Romer G, Powell B (2010) A German evaluation of an attachment-based group intervention program ("Circle of Security") for women with mental illness and their infants (RTC). Infant Mental Health J 31(Suppl 3):286
Sameroff AJ, McDonough S, Rosenblum KL (eds) (2004) Treating parent-infant relationship problems. Strategies for intervention. Guilford Press, New York
Schechter DS, Kaminer T, Grienenberger JF, Amat J (2003) Fits and starts: a mother-infant case study involving pseudoseizures across three generations in the context of violent trauma history (with commentaries by RD Marshall, CH Zeannah, T Gaensbauer). Infant Mental Health J 24(5):510–528
Schechter DS, Coots T, Zeanah CH, Davies M, Coates SW, Trabka KA et al (2005) Maternal mental representations of the child in an innercity clinical sample: violence-related posttraumatic stress and reflective functioning. Attach Hum Dev 7(3):313–331
Schechter DS, Zygmunt A, Coates SW, Davies M, Trabka KA, McCaw J et al (2007) Caregiver traumatization adversely impacts young children's mental representations of self and others. Attach Hum Dev 9(3):187–205
Slade A, Sadler L, De Dios-Kenn C, Webb D, Currier-Ezepchick J, Mayes L (2005) Minding the baby: a reflective parenting program. Psychoanal Study Child 60:74–100
Stern D (1998) The Motherhood Constellation. Karnac Books, London
Thiel-Bonney C, Cierpka M (2004) Die Geburt als Belastungserfahrung bei Eltern von Säuglingen mit Selbstregulationsstörungen. Prax Kinderpsychol Kinderpsychiatr 53:601–622
Thompson-Salo F, Paul C, Morgan A, Jones S, Jordan B, Meehan M et al (1999) Free to be playful: therapeutic work with infants. Int J Infant Observation Appl 3:47–62
UNICEF-Report: Progress for Children (2005) A World Fit for Children. Statistical Review, New York
Windaus E (2007) Behandlungskonzepte der tiefenpsychologisch fundierten und analytischen Psychotherapie im Säuglings- und Kleinkindalter. In: Hopf H, Windaus E (Hrsg) Lehrbuch der Psychotherapie: Psychoanalytische und tiefenpsychologisch fundierte Kinder- und Jugendlichenpsychotherapie, Bd 5. CiP-Medien, München, S3–S20
Winnicott D (1974) Reifungsprozesse und fördernde Umwelt. Kindler, München
Wollwerth de Chuquisengo R, Papoušek M (2004) Das Münchner Konzept einer kommunikationszentrierten Eltern-Säuglings-/Kleinkind-Beratung und -Psychotherapie. In: Papoušek M, Schieche M, Wurmser H (Hrsg) Regulationsstörungen der frühen Kindheit. Hans Huber, Bern, S281–S309

Wynne L (1988) The "presenting problem" and theory-based family variables: keystones for family therapy research. In: Wynne L (Hrsg) The state of the art in family therapy research. Family Process Press, New York, S89–S108
van Zeijl J, Mesman J, van Ijzendoorn MH, Bakermans-Kranenburg M, Juffer F, Stolk MN et al (2006) Attachment-based intervention for enhancing sensitive discipline in mothers of one- to three-year-old children at risk for externalizing behavior problems. A randomized controlled trial. J Consult Clin Psychol 74:994–1005
Ziegenhain U, Fries M, Bütow B, Derksen B (2004) Entwicklungspsychologische Beratung für junge Eltern. Juventa, Weinheim

10 Video and Video Feedback in Counseling and Therapy

Consolata Thiel-Bonney

10.1 Introduction

Video-supported behavioral observation has been expanding our knowledge in the field of developmental psychological research since the early 1970s. Video documentation and behavioral microanalysis have made a crucial contribution to the international surge in infant and toddler research. The research efforts in Germany of Mechthild and Hanuš Papoušek based on the microanalysis of recorded interaction sequences opened up direct, empirical access to intuitive behavioral forms stored in the implicit procedural memory that encompass broad sections of preverbal communication between parents and infant (Papoušek 1994, 2000, 2004).

Human behavior in the context of relationships and social communication is a "highly volatile phenomenon" that only exists as long as it is taking place (Thiel 2003), that alters constantly in its great complexity, and which, by its very nature, is "singular and unrepeatable, often subtle and individually unique" (Papoušek 2000). Interaction partners are capable of perceiving, understanding, working-through, and responding to the behavior observed in their counterpart largely unconsciously. Events of this kind can only be perceived subjectively and "stored" as partial aspects and individual images by the interaction partners themselves or by an observer. This takes place against the backdrop of the individual's cognitive system and under the influence of their previous biographical experiences, culture and world view, theories and concepts, attention to particular aspects of communication, as well as their affects and emotional state at that moment. Thus, human behavior defies objective comprehension and is subject to methodological and epistemological limitations (Thiel 2003).

C. Thiel-Bonney, M.D. (✉)
Center for Children, Adolescents and Families, Hospital Hochried, Hochried 1-12, Murnau 82418, Germany
e-mail: cthiel-bonney@gmx.de

M. Cierpka (ed.), *Regulatory Disorders in Infants*,
DOI 10.1007/978-3-319-43556-5_10

Video techniques have made it possible to extend the boundaries of our perceptual and cognitive faculties. Images afford the viewer distance both from the event and from themselves. By means of for example repetition, slow motion replay, and still frames, the rapid succession of interaction sequences is slowed down—interactional processes can be captured in the millisecond range and later reflected upon.

The recognition of dynamic interdependencies in early communication clearly demonstrate that the behavior of the young child cannot be considered separately from parental intuitive and co-regulatory skills, the parent–child relationship, parental representations, and the social context in which the family lives. The active contributions of both the infant and its caregivers in terms of structuring relationships and communication are concretely depicted in their interaction. This insight has furthered the development of therapeutic techniques that focus on the interaction and quality of the early parent–infant relationship and take both partners into consideration: the infant *and* its parents. As such, video documentation and behavioral (micro)analysis have afforded not only new insights in infant research (e.g., Beebe et al. 2010; Fivaz-Depeursinge 2009), but have also become an increasingly important instrument in diagnostic assessment (see Cierpka 2012, Chaps. 33 and 34), prevention (Juffer et al. 2005; Ziegenhain et al. 2004; see Cierpka 2012, Chap. 38), as well as the counseling and treatment of families with young children (see overviews in Rusconi-Serpa et al. 2009; Fukkink 2008; see also Cierpka 2012, Chap. 30). Video clips and video feedback are used today in a variety of contexts: In home visit-based work among families with particularly high levels of psychosocial risk factors (Klein Velderman et al. 2006), in the context of parent–infant/toddler counseling and psychotherapy (Papoušek 2000; Papoušek and Wollwerth de Chuqisengo 2006; Zelenko and Benham 2000; McDonough 2004), and in bringing research and counseling together, e.g., the still-face paradigm (Weinberg and Tronick 1996; Reck et al. 2001) and the Lausanne trilogue play (Fivaz-Depeursinge and Corboz-Warnery 2001; Fivaz-Depeursinge et al. 2004; Borchardt et al. 2010; see also Cierpka 2012, Chap. 34).

10.2 Counseling and Therapy Concepts Using Video Feedback

Video-supported interventions are anchored in various theories (social learning theory, communication theory, attachment theory, psychodynamic/psychoanalytic and systemic theory), all of which emphasize the importance of mother/parent–infant interaction for infant development in the socio-emotional and cognitive domains (Fukkink 2008; Bünder et al. 2009). A number of approaches in prevention programs (see Cierpka 2012, Chaps. 37 and 38) and counseling (e.g., McDonough 2000; Kalinauskiene et al. 2009) are guided more closely by concrete interaction and by behavior; psychodynamic therapy concepts, on the other hand, aim to understand and work through not only the observable interaction between family members as a reflection of the their relationship in the present, but also the parents' representations of their own biographical experiences (Beebe 2003; Zelenko and

Benham 2000; overview in Rusconi-Serpa et al. 2009). The video helps the parents to “see” and “remember,” and connect the “story” of the presenting symptoms, the “story” observed in concrete interaction, and the “story” of the parents’ own childhood experiences in a psychodynamic process (Beebe 2003). In this way, the videotape grants unparalleled and immediate access to the infant’s current situation within the family, to feelings, perceptions, fantasies, and to the parents’ own early memories. It raises awareness of unconscious, ongoing communication patterns between the involved partners and enables them to reflect, in equal measure, on the levels of concrete behavior/interaction, emotional regulation, and relationship regulation (Papoušek 2000; Thiel-Bonney 2002; Thiel-Bonney et al. 2005). The “directness” and immediacy of what is observed represents a chance—particularly for parents who have difficultly engaging in the interview context or who ward off psychodynamic aspects of interaction and relationship regulation with their infant—to feel that their own point of view, as well as their resources, weaknesses, and difficulties, are being taken seriously. In our work, we experience again and again how viewing video feedback acts as a “door opener” to the young family’s internal perspective; the parents are able to *see*, *experience*, and *reflect on* themselves and their infant in the observed interaction and, as a result, participate henceforth as active partners in the therapeutic process (see also McDonough 2000, 2004).

Attachment-based counseling concepts use video feedback as an opportunity to sensitize the parents to their infant’s signals, reinforce their parental sensitivity, and foster a secure attachment relationship (Bakermans-Kranenburg et al. 2003; Kalinauskiene et al. 2009). Ziegenhain and colleagues (2008) developed a brochure for professionals designed to provide guidance on the observation of sensitive, interactive behavior. Like other working groups (overview in Fukkink 2008), the “Munich Model” (Papoušek 2000), “video microanalysis therapy” (Downing 2003), and the strategy adopted at our parent–infant/toddler outpatient clinic (Thiel-Bonney 2002; Borchardt et al. 2010) attempt to combine approaches on the concrete-observable-behavior level with those on the representational level. Working with video-supported techniques has come to be seen and used as an important module in the developmental- and family-centered psychodynamic-interactional treatment of early childhood disorders of behavioral regulation and, as such, is integrated in the training of fellow experts (see Chap. 28 in Cierpka 2012).

10.3 Videotaping and Video Feedback

10.3.1 The Videotaping Context

Videotaping and therapeutic work with this medium can only take place within a diagnostic and therapeutic alliance based on trust. Videotaping mother/father–infant interactions encroaches on the clients’ private sphere. Most people find it strange to see themselves on video. Parents may feel embarrassed or alarmed at seeing themselves communicating with their infant, particularly in the case of obviously dysfunctional interaction. Moreover, since the situation is “committed to videotape,” it can be replayed and, in principle, viewed by outsiders. It is therefore understandable that some parents initially respond with misgivings to the proposal of videotaped counseling; families should be informed about each step of the videotaping and video feedback process, as well as about the therapists' duty of confidentiality. We request parents to provide written consent prior to videotaping; we also ask whether they consent to video material being used for research and/or training purposes. There are (a few) families who refuse outright to work with video-supported techniques; when this is the case, their refusal should be accepted without need for qualification.

The validity of videotaping is constantly called into question, and justifiably so. Critical voices refer to the shortness of sequences usually comprising not more than a few minutes, the unfamiliarity of the environment to both parents and infant, and the possible "demonstration effect" that occurs during videotaping in an outpatient department, as confirmed in a study conducted by Field and Ignatoff (1981). This effect can be compensated for, however, by home videos filmed by the parents themselves in the family's usual domestic surroundings and extended to include interaction sequences in various contexts (e.g., mealtimes, diaper changing, and play). In our experience, when parents are asked whether what they just experienced with their infant is, in their view, typical of everyday life at home (Papoušek 2000), they usually answer in the affirmative; the infant's presence seems to rapidly activate "schemas-of-being-with-another" (see Stern 1998) that the interaction partners have already experienced together on numerous previous occasions.

10.3.2 The Therapist's View of Parent–Infant Interaction and Videotaping

In social interaction, according to Beebe et al. (2010), the infant experiences attunement with its partner: on a *physical level* (e.g., facial expression, as well as head and body posture); *in the time course* of interaction (sequence, frequency, rhythm, and tightness of contingency in behavioral patterns; see also Hedenbro et al. 2006); in the *spatial organization* of interaction (e.g., mutual approach or avoidance/withdrawal); in *affect* (shared affect, affect attunement, matching); in the correction of discrepancies (interactive repair), the *transformation of affect* through the involvement of the partner; in *attention* (joint/shared attention to the same object at the same time); and in arousal patterns. Experiencing contingency and intersubjectivity is seen as the foundation of early experiences of relationship between the self and the other (see Chaps. 5 and 6 in Cierpka 2012). Beebe and colleagues (2010) discuss the emergence of secure or insecure attachment based on a dyadic system of co-construction in which interactive contingency between mother and child, but in particular the manner in which mother and infant regulate their *own* behavior (self-contingency), are relevant.

Video-supported counseling in our outpatient department usually involves recording a short sequence (5–15 min) of mother/father–infant interaction (e.g., during mealtime or joint play). After videotaping, the therapist selects one or two sequences showing positive interaction patterns, which he/she then discusses with the parents during the following session.

In line with research results from studies in recent years, therapists observe events in the video according to the interaction parameters mentioned in the first paragraph of this section and bearing the following aspects in mind (see also Downing 2002; Raudzus Groden 2008; Beebe 2003; Bünder et al. 2009; Favez et al. 2011; Drawert 2010):

What form does emotional contact between parents and infant take (eye contact, verbal, facial expression, posture of the mother/father and infant)?

What level of willingness to interact does the infant show (e.g., active, alert and attentive, passive, tired, hyperaroused, stressed)? Does the infant take initiatives? What self-regulatory/self-soothing skills does the infant possess? Are these supported by the parents?

To what extent is intuitive parental behavior contingent on the infant's level of willingness to interact (adequate, over-regulating, under-regulating, appropriate to age and developmental stage)? How do the parents co-regulate the respective affective state of their infant?

How do the partners manage to maintain communication? Who takes the initiative? Who follows? To which signals does the partner respond—and how? How is the infant involved? What form does verbal exchange take (e.g., "descriptive" or "prescriptive language")?

How do the partners show mutual closeness? Do they have physical contact? How do the parents respond to their infant's desire for closeness?

In what way do the parents support their infant's initiatives and autonomy (e.g., waiting for the infant to take initiative or interrupting it, "turn-taking")? Is the support (e.g., in exploration/short separations) developmentally appropriate?

How do the parents and infant deal with conflict?

Spatial and temporal organization: Are the participants facing one other on a physical level? Do they exclude one another? How do the parents and infant structure the course of an interaction sequence, e.g., in play (beginning, high point, end, general speed)? Do parents and infant share a joint focus of attention and do the partners work together on the action level? Who leads and who follows?

What form do transitions between individual interaction sequences take? Does the form of the transition promote predictability for the infant and cater to its need for security?

How do the family members approach a task on a practical level? How are roles distributed? What shape do the resources and problem-solving skills of the family members take?

10.3.3 Video Feedback

Finally, parents are shown a short selected scene, which they discuss with the therapist during the video feedback session. Ideally, the parents view the video without their infant present in order to be able to become fully involved in the images and emotional events. Before viewing the video, the parents are asked whether the scene represents a typical family situation or whether it was different to similar situations at home. Was there anything that surprised the parents during filming? How did the parents feel about the interaction with their infant during videotaping? How did the mother and father perceive events themselves?

The following procedure has proven helpful during video feedback sessions (see also Downing 2003):

10.3.3.1 Part 1: Positive Scene

Showing a ***positive***, successful scene that is mutually rewarding initially, even if this is an exception in the video sequence as a whole.

Replaying a scene: This enables parents to re-live and appreciate more keenly a sequence of successful communication and positive emotional relatedness in dialogue and in play (even if this is merely a still frame of eye contact or a moment of shared happiness); by replaying a scene, the therapist allows the caregiver time to perceive their own feelings and needs for closeness and to empathize with their infant's experience and perspective.

Close *observation of positive reciprocity* between the partners: The therapist emphasizes how parents and infant manage to successfully structure an encounter in play and communication, how both partners take the initiative, and what response the parents receive from their infant in the form of feedback in the interaction so that a positive reciprocity emerges. As a result, the parents feel reinforced in their own intuitive competence and self-confidence and gain confidence in their infant's abilities. This helps them to develop positive relationship representations.

Addressing the parents' *emotional reaction* to the viewed scene: How did the parents fare as they watched the video? How did they feel as parents and how do they think their infant felt? What physical reactions did they experience during the interaction (Downing 1996)? Intrusive negative emotions can be discussed and resolved where necessary.

What *impact* do the viewed scenes have on the parents and on their being together with the infant, as well as in the family?

Inquiring about *memories of own childhood*: Do the parents remember scenes of this kind from their own childhood? What do they feel reminded of?

Do the parents perhaps require additional information following the microanalysis session, e.g., relating to *developmental psychological issues*.

10.3.3.2 Part 2: Negative (dysfunctional) sequences

Negative (dysfunctional) communication sequences can be addressed if the therapeutic alliance is sufficiently robust. Viewing a negative film clip can be introduced as follows, for instance:

> *Now we could have a look at a play scene that didn't work out quite so well; we can think together about what contributed to that and how you could manage taking more pleasure in playing with your infant. Would you be willing to do this?*

Assuming there is sufficient time and the infant's caregiver feels secure enough, a short dysfunctional sequence can then be viewed following a positive scene; alternatively, it can form part of a subsequent counseling session:

Close *joint observation* of the infant's triggering and feedback signals, as well as identification of negative reciprocity with back reference to parental behavior.

Addressing the *feelings* that influence parental behavior, the intrusive affects and impulses, stressful memories, internal images and "ghosts from the past," as well as possible triggering moments in the infant's behavior.

Revealing and *resolving distorted perceptions and projected attributions* and referring back to the real infant in the "here and now" in the video sequence.

Promoting the parents' self-reflective functions and mentalization in relation to the real infant (in the video).

10.3.3.3 Part 3: Anchoring feelings of positive emotional relatedness

The process of re-living and consciously **anchoring feelings of positive emotional relatedness** serves to round-off the session and promote the successful translation of these interactions into everyday life:

- *Reviewing* and re-experiencing positive play sequences.
- Preparing for their *translation into home life*: Have positive play experiences occurred hitherto at home, under what conditions, and, if not, what could be standing in their way? How can the parents do more of what it is that contributes to successful communication with their infant (according to the positive scenes in the video), and how can these pleasant moments of being together become embedded in everyday life at home?

  This approach can, e.g., encourage a father who intervenes in an over-regulating manner in the interaction with his infant (who in turn responds with gaze aversion) to wait and grant his infant more time. Similarly, the therapist may ask a mother who is unable to make a significant contribution to happy joint play due to depression, to put into words and comment on what she sees and what she and her infant are currently doing. In this way, the parents manage to empathize with the feelings of their baby, that determine his behavior and needs.

- The therapist concludes the session by elaborating how parents can create stress-free time windows in their daily routine to experience positive joint play, and how they can safeguard against the renewed intrusion of biographical experiences and distorted perceptions in the interaction with their infant.

10.3.4 Case Studies

10.3.4.1 Case Study 1

Distraught, the mother of Paulina (5 months) contacted our outpatient clinic by telephone: She urgently required an appointment, since her infant was rejecting her and she was seriously considering entrusting her daughter's care to someone else in order to avoid doing the infant further harm. At the initial interview, the mother reported Paulina's sleeping problems, which had persisted since birth. She woke at 1- to 2-h intervals during the night and needed to be soothed with nursing. She napped only rarely during the day, was grumpy and fussy, and could barely occupy herself alone for a moment. The mother needed to distract and cajole her daughter all day long in order to keep her happy and make her smile. She would carry Paulina about almost from morning till night and was herself exhausted. However, the worst thing was that Paulina was increasingly avoiding eye contact; in fact, Paulina had not looked at her mother for the past 2 days. Paulina sought eye contact with her father as soon as she heard him come home from work in the evenings and greeted him happily.

Both parents came from strained families of origin. It was important to the mother to find security and happiness within her own family, in contrast to her own and her husband's experiences in their childhoods. They had assumed that their baby would be happy and "straightforward," and that she would strengthen their partnership and fit in well with the busy everyday working life of both parents. Paulina's mother had had to assume considerable responsibility in her family of origin for the wellbeing of her own mother, who had suffered from recurrent bouts of severe depression requiring inpatient treatment. She had noticed anxious, depressive mood swings in herself since Paulina's birth. She was now checking her infant constantly to see whether she detected signs of sadness in her facial expression. She was concerned that Paulina may have inherited a tendency toward depression from her family of origin. Whenever the infant was quiet, the mother perceived her as "sad" and, as a result, constantly attempted to "make her smile"; this brought the mother temporary emotional relief. The mother's dearest wish for Paulina was for her to be "a happy child."

Paulina appeared quiet and withdrawn; she showed virtually no desire to explore or any initiative to play. When the mother spoke to her, she immediately responded by avoiding her mother's gaze. Up to this point, Paulina had had little or no opportunity to find her own rhythm or experience early self-efficacy (either with regard to herself/to her environment in quiet, alert moments, or in communication with her mother). In an atmosphere of anxious tension, the mother overwhelmed her daughter in dialogue and stimulated her in even the briefest of quiet phases. Both parents were oblivious to the infant's signals of fatigue. Paulina's father did not perceive his daughter as sad; however, he too had frequently overstimulated the infant in their game as an "action man" (the father's own words).

In a video clip of dialogue with the mother, the clearly dysphoric-appearing infant did in fact make very brief but nevertheless beckoning eye contact with her mother at the end of a still-face sequence, to the therapists' relief, thereby *visibly* demonstrating to the mother her interest in contact. The mother was very moved upon viewing this short selected sequence during the second session. She finally went home with two "tasks" previously discussed with the therapist: Firstly, she was tasked with considering what could be going on in Paulina's mind when the infant was peaceful and simply looking about the room or out of the window (the mother had previously seen sadness, while the father suspected, e.g., that she was watching the clouds go by); the parents were asked to briefly discuss their various "hypotheses" with each other. Secondly, the mother was encouraged to "not do all the work" in communication with Paulina, but instead to let herself be "beckoned" a bit by her infant—as Paulina had just shown she was capable of in the video clip.

After a total of three therapy sessions, the parents perceived their infant as "completely altered": Paulina's total sleep time had increased to 15 h and she "laughed and cooed" with both parents; she also enjoyed periods of quiet solitary play, which the mother was able to grant her without stress or fear of signs of impending depression. The mother expressed her surprise at the extent to which her own previous experiences had, unbeknown to her, influenced her interaction with Paulina.

10.3.4.2 Case Study 2

Video-supported microanalysis can be deployed as a useful therapeutic instrument most notably in complex relational systems—as discerned on the multigenerational and support levels during the counseling of parents with infant and toddlers—and in the case of challenging treatment requirements (see also McDonough 2000):

Using this approach, it was possible to treat Lena (19 months) for her hitherto therapy-resistant feeding disorder and failure to thrive by offering the parents "concrete" video-supported help amid a glut of offers from the support system. At the time, both the father and mother were undergoing psychotherapeutic treatment, attending couples counseling, taking advice from their daughter's daycare facility, and taking advantage of offers to talk from an allopathic and from an anthroposophical pediatrician. The clearly weakened infant had previously been treated twice in pediatric hospitals with different areas of therapeutic specialization, with no visible success. Bearing in mind psychodynamic events on the multigenerational and couples level, in the support system, in the dyadic and triadic relationship, and in parent–infant interaction, we decided to base our approach exclusively on video-supported techniques for a period of time. Using video feedback, the parents recognized that they could trust their daughter with greater autonomy and understood how they could help her on her way to this goal. The parents were able to slowly release their infant from her role in their conflict-laden and fraught relationship. Within only a few months, Lena was able to make up for her initially delayed physical and verbal development (see Thiel-Bonney 2002 for a detailed description of this case study).

10.4 The Effectiveness of Video Feedback

Video feedback has enjoyed growing popularity in psychotherapeutic work ever since the 1950s and is used today as a therapeutic measure in a variety of fields. Experience has been garnered in parent–infant/toddler counseling and psychotherapy in the domains of, e.g., early childhood disorders of behavioral regulation (Papoušek 2000; Papoušek and Wollwerth de Chuquisengo 2006; Bünder et al. 2009; van Zeijl et al. 2006); postnatal depression, anxiety disorders (Reck 2006, 2008; Vik and Braten 2009), and psychosis (Hornstein et al. 2006); maternal eating disorders (Stein et al. 2006); insecure attachment relationships (Bakermans-Kranenburg et al. 2003; Kalinauskiene et al. 2009); young (Downing and Ziegenhain 2001) and traumatized mothers (Schechter et al. 2006); families with premature infants (Landry et al. 2006); foster and adoptive families (Juffer et al. 2005; Bünder et al. 2009); as well as families under particular psychosocial strain (Ziegenhain et al. 2004; Mendelsohn et al. 2005; McDonough 2004; Bünder et al. 2009). A meta-analysis of 29 studies of video-supported therapy programs (Fukkink 2008) revealed statistically significant effects: Video feedback had a favorable impact on parental interactional behavior (increased sensitivity, positive effects on parents' stimulating and intrusive behaviors); contributed to a more positive attitude in parents toward parenthood (reduced parental stress on the level of parent–child interaction, greater parental self-confidence); and showed positive effects in terms of infant development in the family. However, these effects were less pronounced in families belonging to high-risk groups. Bakermans-Kranenburg and colleagues (2003) investigated intervention programs focusing on parental sensitivity and infant attachment security. Their meta-analysis revealed that time-limited interventions with a clear behavioral focus on maternal sensitive behavior in interaction with her infant were the most effective. Interventions aimed at improving maternal sensitivity were more effective when video feedback was used. Although the meta-analysis was not able to include more than a handful of studies that also involved fathers, these investigations showed a significantly greater effect than did those focusing on mothers only. These results suggest that interventions should always bear the systemic character of the family in mind; considering *both* parents, as well as the entire family context, strengthens not only the mutual support within the family, but also the effectiveness of counseling.

10.5 Conclusion

A stable and supportive therapeutic relationship provides the foundation to steer parents' attention, in the context of video feedback, to functional and dysfunctional interaction with their infant. By gaining insight into the links between "before" and "now" in a viable and respectful atmosphere, parents generally do not see the therapist's careful scrutiny of their interactions as criticism, but rather as a particularly supportive form of help in the face of problems in the dyadic or triadic relationship and in the family (see also Gloger 2010). The parents' biographical experiences influence their intuitive skills in the relationship and in communication with their infant. Taking a psychotherapeutic approach to working-through video images enables "ghosts in the nursery" (Fraiberg et al. 2003) to be identified and "banished"; the parents succeed in dissolving distorted perceptions and in perceiving themselves and their infant as independent personalities. Together with the therapist, they discover resources and are able to elaborate and try out alternative communication patterns, thereby paving the way to positive relational experiences with their infant.

References

Bakermans-Kranenburg MJ, van Ijzendoorn MH, Juffer F (2003) Less is more: meta-analysis of sensitivity and attachment interventions in early childhood. Psychol Bull 129(2):195–215

Beebe B (2003) Brief mother-infant treatment: psychoanalytically informed video feedback. Infant Mental Health J 24(1):24–52

Beebe B, Jaffe J, Markese S et al (2010) The origins of 12-month attachment: a microanalysis of 4-month mother-infant interaction. Attach Hum Dev 12(1–2):3–141

Borchardt S, Schwinn L, Eickhorst A, Frey B (2010) Lausanner Trilogspiel in der Eltern-Säuglings-Beratung. Psychotherapeut 55:147–152

Bünder P, Sirringhaus-Bünder A, Helfer A (2009) Lehrbuch der Marte-Meo-Methode. Entwicklungsförderung mit Videounterstützung. Vandenhoeck & Ruprecht, Göttingen

Cierpka M (Hrsg) (2012) Frühe Kindheit 0-3. Beratung und Psychotherapie für Eltern mit Säuglingen und Kleinkindern. Springer, Heidelberg

Downing G (1996) Körper und Wort in der Psychotherapie. Kösel, München

Downing G (2002) Video-Mikroanalyse-Therapie. Seminar, persönliche Mitteilung. Universitätsklinikum Heidelberg, Heidelberg

Downing G (2003) Video-Mikroanalyse-Therapie: Einige Grundlagen und Prinzipien. In: Scheurer-Englisch H, Suess GJ, Pfeifer WKP (Hrsg) Wege zur Sicherheit—Bindungswissen in Diagnostik und Intervention. Psychosozial-Verlag, Gießen, S 51–68

Downing G, Ziegenhain U (2001) Besonderheiten der Beratung und Therapie bei jugendlichen Müttern und ihren Säuglingen—die Bedeutung der Bindungstheorie und videogestützter Intervention. In: Suess GJ, Scheurer-Englisch H, Pfeifer WKP (Hrsg) Bindungstheorie und Familiendynamik. Anwendung der Bindungstheorie in Beratung und Therapie. Psychosozial-Verlag, Gießen, S 271–296

Drawert C (2010) Marte Meo—"Aus eigener Kraft". EREV-Schriftenreihe 51(4):105–119

Favez N, Scaiola CL, Tissot H, Darwiche J, Frascarolo F (2011) The family alliance assessment scales: steps toward validity and reliability of an observational assessment tool for early family interactions. J Child Fam Stud 20(1):23–37

Field T, Ignatoff E (1981) Videotaping effects on the behaviours of low income mothers and their infants during floor-play interactions. J Appl Dev Psychol 2:227–235

Fivaz-Depeursinge E (2009) Trianguläre Kommunikation von Babys in "Zwei-für-einen"- versus "Zwei-gegen-einen"-Dreiecken. Familiendynamik 34(2):136–145

Fivaz-Depeursinge E, Corboz-Warnery A, Keren M (2004) The primary triangle: treating infants in their families. In: Sameroff AJ, McDonough SC, Rosenblum KL (Hrsg) Treating parent-infant relationship problems. Guilford Press, New York, S 123–151

Fivaz-Depeursinge E, Corboz-Warnery A (2001) Das primäre Dreieck. Vater, Mutter und Kind aus entwicklungstheoretisch-systemischer Sicht. Carl-Auer-Systeme, Heidelberg

Fraiberg S, Adelson E, Shapiro V (2003) Gespenster im Kinderzimmer. Probleme gestörter Mutter-Säuglings-Beziehungen aus psychoanalytischer Sicht. Analytische Kinder- und Jugendlichenpsychotherapie 34:465–504

Fukkink RG (2008) Video feedback in widescreen: a meta-analysis of family programs. Clin Psychol Rev 28:904–916

Gloger C (2010) Wie erleben Eltern und Kinder den Videoeinsatz im ambulant-klinischen Setting? Prax Kinderpsychol Kinderpsychiatr 59:193–206

Hedenbro M, Shapiro A, Gottman JM (2006) Play with me at my speed: describing differences in the tempo of parent-infant interactions in the Lausanne triadic play paradigm in two cultures. Fam Process 45:485–498

Hornstein C, Schenk S, Wortmann-Fleischer S et al (2006) Videotherapie bei postpartalen Störungen. Ein interaktionales Behandlungskonzept bei Müttern mit Depressionen und Psychosen. Psychotherapeut 51:363–368

Juffer F, Bakermans-Kranenburg MJ, van Ijzendoorn MH (2005) The importance of parenting in the development of disorganised attachment: evidence from a preventive intervention study in adoptive families. J Child Psychol Psychiatr 46:263–274

Kalinauskiene L, Cekuoliene D, van Ijzendoorn MH et al (2009) Supporting intensitive mothers: the Vilnius randomized control trial of video-feedback intervention to promote maternal sensitivity and infant attachment security. Child Care Health Dev 35(5):613–623

Klein Velderman M, Bakermans-Kranenburg MJ, Juffer F, van Ijzendoorn MH (2006) Effects of attachment-based interventions on maternal sensitivity and infant attachment: differential susceptibility of highly reactive infants. J Fam Psychol 20(2):266–274

Landry SH, Smith KE, Swank PR (2006) Responsive parenting: establishing early foundations for social, communication, and independent problem-solving skills. Dev Psychol 43(4):627–642

McDonough SC (2000) Interaction guidance: an approach for difficult-to-engage families. In: Zeanah CH (Hrsg) Handbook of infant mental health. Guilford Press, New York, S 485–493

McDonough SC (2004) Interaction guidance. Promoting and nurturing the caregiving relationship. In: Sameroff AJ, McDonough SC, Rosenblum KL (Hrsg) Treating parent-infant relationship problems. Guilford Press, New York, S 79–96

Mendelsohn AL, Dreyer BP, Flynn V et al (2005) Use of videotaped interactions during pediatric well-child care to promote child development: a randomized, controlled trial. J Dev Behav Pediatr 26(1):34–41

Papoušek M (1994) Vom ersten Schrei zum ersten Wort. Anfänge der Sprachentwicklung in der vorsprachlichen Kommunikation. Hans Huber, Bern

Papoušek M (2000) Einsatz von Video in der Eltern-Säuglingsberatung und -psychotherapie. Prax Kinderpsychol Kinderpsychiatr 49:611–627

Papoušek M (2004) Regulationsstörungen der frühen Kindheit: Klinische Evidenz für ein neues diagnostisches Konzept. In: Papoušek M, Schieche M, Wurmser H (Hrsg) Regulationsstörungen der frühen Kindheit: Frühe Risiken und Hilfen im Entwicklungskontext der Eltern-Kind-Beziehungen. Hans Huber, Bern, S 77–110

Papoušek M, Wollwerth de Chuquisengo R (2006) Integrative kommunikationszentrierte Eltern-Kleinkind-Psychotherapie bei frühkindlichen Regulationsstörungen. Prax Kinderpsychol Kinderpsychiatr 55:235–254

Raudzus-Groden U (2008). Die Münchner klinische Kommunikationsskala (MKK) zur Erfassung der Eltern-Säuglings-Kommunikation. Reliabilität und Validität. Dissertation, unveröffentlicht, Ruprecht-Karls-Universität, Heidelberg.

Reck C (2006) Integrative stationäre Psychotherapie für psychisch erkrankte Mütter und ihre Kinder. Psychotherapie im Dialog 7(1):53–59

Reck C (2008) Depressionen und Angststörungen im Peripartalzeitraum: Epidemiologie, Mutter-Kind-Beziehung und Behandlungskonzept. Nervenheilkunde 6:489–490

Reck C, Backenstraß M, Möhler E et al (2001) Mutter-Kind-Interaktion und postpartale Depression—Theorie und Empirie im Überblick. Psychotherapie 6(2):171–186

Rusconi-Serpa S, Rossignol AS, McDonough SC (2009) Video feedback in parent-infant treatments. Child Adolescent Psychiatr Clin North Am 18:735–751

Schechter DS, Myers MM, Brunelli S et al (2006) Traumatized mothers can change their minds about their toddlers: understanding how a novel use of videofeedback supports positive change of maternal attributions. Infant Mental Health J 27(5):429–447

Stein A, Woolley H, Senior R et al (2006) Treating disturbances in the relationship between mothers with bulimic eating disorders and their infants: a randomized, controlled trail of video feedback. Am J Psychiatr 163(5):899–906

Stern DN (1998) Die Mütterlichkeitskonstellation: Mutter, Säugling und Großmutter rund um die Geburt. In: Hildenbrand B, Enderlin R (Hrsg) Gefühle und Systeme. Die emotionale Rahmung beraterischer und therapeutischer Prozesse. Carl-Auer-Systeme, Heidelberg, S 102–118

Thiel T (2003) Film- und Videotechnik in der Psychologie. In: Keller H (Hrsg) Handbuch der Kleinkindforschung, 3. Aufl. Hans Huber, Bern, S 649–708

Thiel-Bonney C (2002) Beratung von Eltern mit Säuglingen und Kleinkindern. Videogestützte Verhaltensbeobachtung und Videomikroanalyse als Interventionsmöglichkeit. Psychotherapeut 47:381–384

Thiel-Bonney C, Cierpka M, Cierpka A (2005) Präventives Beratungsmodell für Familien mit Säuglingen und Kleinkindern. In: Cierpka M (Hrsg) Möglichkeiten der Gewaltprävention. Vandenhoeck & Ruprecht, Göttingen, S 110–138 van Zeijl J, Mesman J, van Ijzendoorn MH, Bakermans-Kranenburg MJ, Juffer F, Koot HM et al (2006) Attachment-based intervention for enhancing sensitive discipline in mothers of 1- to 3-year-old children at risk for externalizing behaviour problems: a randomized controlled trail. J Consult Clin Psychol 74(6):994–1005

Vik K, Braten S (2009) Video interaction guidance inviting transcendence of postpartum depressed mothers' self-centered state and holding behaviour. Infant Mental Health J 30(3):287–300

Weinberg MK, Tronick EZ (1996) Infant affective reactions to the resumption of maternal interaction after the still-face. Child Dev 67:905–914

Zelenko M, Benham A (2000) Videotaping as a therapeutic tool in psychodynamic infant-parent therapy. Infant Mental Health J 21:192–203

Ziegenhain U, Derksen B, Dreisörner R (2004) Frühe Förderung von Resilienz bei jungen Müttern und ihren Säuglingen. Kindheit und Entwicklung 13:226–234

Ziegenhain U, Gebauer S, Ziesel B (2008). Die Chance der ersten Monate. Feinfühlige Eltern—gesunde Kinder. Ulm: Klinik für Kinder- und Jugendpsychiatrie/Physiotherapie, Universitätsklinikum Ulm

Focus-Oriented Psychotherapy of Parents with Infants and Toddlers

11

Michael Stasch, Manfred Cierpka, and Eberhard Windaus

11.1 The "Relationship" as the Basis of Psychoanalytically Oriented Parent–Infant/Toddler Psychotherapy

The origins of infant/toddler–parent psychotherapy can be traced back to the observations and treatment of infants and toddlers by Bernfeld, Anna Freud, Burlingham, Fries, Winnicott, and Spitz, for instance (Windaus 2007a). It was already clear back then that the complex relationship and interaction system between infant/toddler, mother, and father required a specific approach. Widely varying counseling and therapeutic strategies emerged over the years (see Windaus 2007b). More recently, a working group composed of analytical child and adolescent therapists and family therapists elaborated a treatment manual for psychoanalytic focal therapy of (early) childhood regulatory disorders (Cierpka and Windaus 2007), which forms the basis for the present chapter.

In order to gain a clinical insight into relationship dynamics, one needs to make a fundamental distinction between manifest behavior and latent, unconscious underlying attitudes. While the manifest exchange between mother, father, and infant is being played out in current actions in the here and now, the underlying interaction is at the same time being shaped by the parents' latent attitude toward their infant, their psychological state, their own internal parent–child experiences, as well as by

M. Stasch, Dipl.Psych. (✉)
Private Practice, Rohrbacher Straße 22, Heidelberg 69115, Germany
e-mail: praxis@psychotherapie-stasch.de

M. Cierpka, M.D.
Institute for Psychosocial Prevention, University Hospital Heidelberg,
Bergheimer Str. 54, Heidelberg 69115, Germany
e-mail: manfred.cierpka@med.uni-heidelberg.de

E. Windaus, Dr.phil.
Private Practice, Länderweg 45, Frankfurt/M 60599, Germany
e-mail: zoubek-windaus@t-online.de

M. Cierpka (ed.), *Regulatory Disorders in Infants*,
DOI 10.1007/978-3-319-43556-5_11

the psychosocial context. If the latent background is filled with tension and conflict, the parents will not have the appropriate resources at their disposal to soothe their infant, or to stimulate it in a manner conducive to development. As a result, the parents' co-regulatory skills are inadequate and the relational disorder may cause or exacerbate a regulatory disorder in the infant.

Thus, identifying restrictive and stereotypical interaction patterns {XE "Interaction patterns, stereotypical"} forms the focus of the diagnostic process. Observing the effects of dysfunctional interactional processes on individual symptoms also has a long tradition in the field of family research. In his "system model," Beavers (1982) assumes that "healthy" (i.e., functional) relationship systems are able to respond flexibly to the needs and signals of individuals in an overall emotionally positive and respectful atmosphere. There are clear roles in the family system, which can alter appropriately according to family developmental tasks {XE "Developmental tasks, family}. "Healthy" families of this kind attend a parent–infant outpatient clinic when they encounter problems in dealing with their possibly hypersensitive infant, and when the otherwise competent parents have been made to feel insecure by a variety of parenting manuals. Providing developmental psychological information or concrete regulatory support (e.g., bedtime rituals) in such cases is often sufficient to solve the problem. As such, these are counseling cases and not ones requiring psychotherapeutic intervention. The aim is to minimize a transient, non-generalized regulatory disorder exhibiting no relationship pathology in a resource-oriented approach (Ziegenhain 2004). In contrast to clinically abnormal relationship systems, interpersonal control is not overly rigid in this case and there are no repetitive dysfunctional interaction patterns at play that have already colored the relational history, e.g., of the couple prior to the birth of their infant.

However, more advanced psychotherapeutic interventions may become necessary when parents, armed with well-meant tips, persistently fail, perhaps due to a bedtime ritual triggering separation anxiety in the parents that could be typically overcome in the parents' childless past by strong clinginess in the relationship. In cases such as these, the parents' repertoire of relational behavior is limited. However, even typically conflict-laden parents of this kind ("neurotic" family systems, according to Beavers), are by all means capable of reflecting on their own experience and behavior and of modifying this with therapeutic help.

Family systems on the "severely dysfunctional" level (according to Beavers 1982), on the other hand, are characterized by a markedly reduced capacity to regulate self and others, which manifests in impulsive behavior, acts of destruction, vague or "tyrannical" role attribution, and ambiguous communication. From a psychodynamic perspective, these family systems lack the structural skills needed to meet the requirements of their external as well as their "internal" emotional and cognitive reality.

As a result, psychotherapy with infant/toddlers and their parents needs to be tailored to the psychological framework prevailing in the respective family system. According to Beavers' model, one is able to distinguish between at least three types of family system, each with different problem areas that form the focus of counseling or therapy:

1. The functional, "healthy" family system, where the focus lies on resolving the infant's specific problem.
2. The impaired, "neurotic" family system, where the focus lies on working-through mostly unconscious interpersonal conflicts.
3. The "severely dysfunctional" family system, where the focus lies on dealing more appropriately with structural deficits in relationship regulation.

Whereas interaction processes can be observed and described, the parents' representations and unconscious attitudes toward their infant can be ascertained in the process of gaining psychoanalytic insight. Since a psychodynamic view covers both aspects, observation and interpretation are mutually enlightening. Relationship forms (e.g., contact avoidance) are based on intentions (e.g., disinterest) that can be either conscious or unconscious. Unconscious intentions relate to the object (e.g., rejection) and to the subject (e.g., feelings of overload), without this link being explicit on the action level. The parents' internal representations help to steer interactions and intentions to a great extent. Therefore, the current, observable relationship between mother and infant is associated with her earlier significant relational experiences with other objects (e.g., the mother's own parents) and herself (the baby in the mother) that have manifested as internal representations.

Example

An observable, intrusive-appearing feeding scene can stem from, e.g., the mother's intention to satisfy her infant's feared greed by means of forced and overbearing conduct in order to prevent the infant from becoming a reproachful character as the mother once was herself. Thus, the mother's own earlier mother–infant experience forms the foundation for the current mother–infant relationship. While the level of dysfunction in a feeding situation can be identified and measured through comparative observation of eye contact, gaze aversion, feeding speed, volume of food fed, and empathetic relatedness, the internal representations, projections, or childhood experiences on which this behavior is based are not observable and need to be verbalized in order to be given meaning. It is important, therefore, to choose a therapeutic approach that takes both aspects, interaction and representations, into equal consideration.

11.1.1 Access to the Psychodynamic Level via the "Dominant Theme"

In the case of "clinically striking" families, a dominant theme {XE "Dominant theme"} (Stern 1998) generally emerges in the psychodiagnostic interview situation when discussing the reason for presentation. This dominant theme is characterized by the fact that it takes up a considerable amount of time and space in the parents' representational world and is highly relevant in terms of their behavior and experience. The theme can be based on unconscious intrapsychic parental conflicts or may be a manifestation of coping with serious family crises or traumas (Fraiberg 1982). The dominant theme affects not only the parents' perception, but also how they deal with their infant and, as such, needs to be identified in relationship regulation and in the transference–countertransference dynamics {XE "transference–countertransference dynamics"} between the family and therapist systems. The heuristics of the dominant theme, therefore, forms an extremely helpful starting point for a more differentiated psychodynamic diagnostic assessment.

The concept of scenic understanding (Argelander 1970; Lorenzer 1970) involves psychoanalytic interpretation, which takes both interactional and representational aspects of the dominant theme into consideration insofar as the internal meaning contained in a scene can be inferred on the basis of observable and verbalized scenes. Since parent–infant interaction in the therapeutic setting is made up of a multitude of short scenes, the concept of scenic understanding {XE "Scenic understanding"} is particularly suited to translating observations and aspects of countertransference into a meaningful overall context.

To generate hypotheses on the psychodynamic focus, Malan (1965), as well as Menninger and Holzman (1977), used triangles that illustrate the complexity of the focus as comprehension aids in the conceptualization of the focus. These include the triangle of defense (conflict level) and the triangle of insight (life story). Klüwer (1983) added the third level, the triangle of action (subject–object action). For psychoanalytic therapy based on the manual discussed here, the following modification to the triangle concept is made (Cierpka et al. 2007) when using the focus concept:

▶ The level {XE "Defense level"} of defense
The level {XE "Relationship level"} of relationship
The level {XE "Enactment level"} of enactment (in the form of an active dialogue that takes place between the family and the therapist).

11.2 Therapeutic Foci in Psychoanalytic Parent–Infant Psychotherapy

The primary aim of psychoanalytic psychotherapy in infancy and toddlerhood is to achieve an understanding of the problem in the actualized relational disorder by linking it to the parents' childhood past in such a way that this process of understanding influences parental actions. The parents' need to be supported in their skills to withstand their infant's overwhelming affects, understand its psychological and physical needs, adjust willingly to its perspectives, and modify the external world appropriately. By working on their potentially reduced capacity for empathy, parents make gains in terms of reflectivity.

▶ A fundamental distinction is made in therapeutic work (based on OPD-2; OPD Task Force 2008) between a *conflict focus* {XE "Conflict focus"} and a *structural focus* {XE "Structural focus"}.

While a conflict focus can be attributed to neurotic processing methods within the family system, a structural focus is based on early traumatic disorders experienced in the relationship that have caused structural limitations in the parents' ego functions, in relationship regulation, and in self-perception. As such, therapeutic methods need to be adapted to the relevant level of dysfunction. Thus, the principle of identification takes the place of the principle of interpretation when working on a structural focus.

11.2.1 Conflict-Centered Therapeutic Foci

Conflict

"Conflict" in a psychoanalytic context denotes the failure to integrate conflicting intrapsychic or interpersonal motivational systems (wishes, interests, demands and their fulfillment). Conflict that exists on the unconscious level needs to be distinguished from primarily consciously experienced tension.

Long-lasting unconscious conflicts can be deduced from the clinical description of perceivable behaviors and experiences. They manifest on both the subject and the object level (intrapsychically as well as in interaction with the partner or infant) and are often associated with "lead affects" typical of conflict. The scenic enactment of relationship regulation, as well as biographical data, provides the therapist with important diagnostic information in the clinical situation (Argelander 1970; Lorenzer 1970). Particular attention is paid, moreover, to the analysis of the mother/parents' transference "readiness" {XE "Transference readiness"} and the therapist's experience of countertransference. The immediacy of a conflict often emerges from the fantasies, emotional reactions, and action impulses (enactment) elicited in the therapist.

Clinically relevant conflicts revolve around the following life-determining motivational systems inspired by the "conflict" axis in Operationalized Psychodynamic Diagnosis (OPD Task Force 2008; see also Cierpka et al. 2007 for a detailed discussion):

- Individuation versus dependency
- Need for care versus self-sufficiency
- Submission versus control
- Self-worth
- Guilt
- Oedipal issues in the sense of gender-specific role identification
- The "motherhood constellation" (Stern 1998) as an actual conflictual event

▶ In a conflict-oriented, motive-seeking approach, one looks behind the striking symptomatic features for what it is that is actually spawning the relational disorder. Work begins with the parents' resistance and their attempts to cope, in order to get to their suppressed motives and fears. A variety of techniques are used to this end, among which interpretation plays a prominent role. General conditions and interventions that involve the family in the conflict, thereby mobilizing the associated affects, are helpful in treatment.

Example
Providing therapeutic guidance to an eating disordered toddler in the context of a feeding situation during the session can be particularly lively. The therapeutic momentum leads from resistance to content and on to the affective core of the conflict. The central elements of the conflict are enacted together and recorded interpretively by the therapist. Where necessary, conflict-oriented work can also include a working-through of collusive couples dynamics or transgenerational delegation processes.

11.2.2 Structure-Centered Therapeutic Foci

In the case of a primarily low structural level in the personality development of the parents, one can assume, e.g., that their perception of the infant's affective state or their regulation of the affective relationship with their infant is dysfunctional. Due to their own misinterpretations or regulatory difficulties, they may be incapable of adequate object relations. Fonagy et al. (2002) make the emergence of the parents' distorted perceptions in the current relationship with their infant (resulting from their own conflictual childhood experiences) dependent on the functional capacity of a reflective self. A revealing and interpretive technique may overchallenge parents that have structural deficits. For this reason, work to establish structure is required in a first step, before unconscious conflict material can be addressed.

▶ Assessing the structural level is crucial to the selection of the psychodynamic therapeutic technique, particularly in terms of whether one should work with a supportive and structuring or rather an interpretive and revealing approach.

We invoke the concept of the parents' capacity for mentalization {XE "Capacity for mentalization"} to assess the structural level of a family system, since the quality of parental mentalization offers direct conclusions to be drawn about the functionality of relationship formation with the infant. Mentalizing is defined as perceiving and interpreting behavior associated with mental processes. How the parents reflect on the states of their infant and its behavior goes a long way to determining their reactions.

▶ The mother/parents' ability to form an internal image of her/their infant as an independent being with wishes, intentions, and feelings is decisive in terms of their functional level of mentalization {XE "Mentalization, functional level of"}. The parents are able to understand their infant and act appropriately on the basis of this internal representation of the infant.

11.2.2.1 Structural Level of Mentalization {XE "Mentalization"}

Fonagy and Target (2002) described a number of "structural levels" in the ability to mentalize, the identification of which appears necessary in order to be able to pursue an appropriate treatment plan tailored to the structural level.

A Good Functional Level

This describes the mother or father's ability to mitigate the infant's negative affect by producing contingent behaviors characterized by "markedness" that mirror the infant's emotions. In this way, he/she helps the infant form secondary representations of its primary emotional state. The infant introjects the marked, decoupled, affect-mirroring expressions.

Moderate Structural Level: Distorted Representation Due to a Lack of Categorical Congruence

This describes the prevalence of "marked" yet categorically distorted maternal mirroring, an over-controlling stance, and/or a defensive, distorted perception of the infant's affect by the primary caregiver. If, for example, the erotically tinged arousal of an infant resulting from physical contact with the mother triggers fear and defensive anger in the mother due to her own intrapsychic conflicts relating to physical affection, the mother may project her defensive, emotional reaction onto the infant and perceive, distortedly, its libidinal arousal as aggression. She then attempts to modulate this misperceived affect of her infant by mirroring the aggression it expresses. Probable consequences: since the mirrored affect is marked, it is decoupled from the mother. There is a sufficiently high level of contingency between the infant's—incorrectly categorized—affective state and the marked affect mirroring, such that it is referentially anchored as belonging to its primary emotional state. Since the category of the mirrored affect-expression does not correspond to the infant's true affective state, the infant produces a distorted secondary representation of its primary emotional state and will, as a result, ascribe dispositional information to itself that does not tally with its true emotional state. This results in the infant having a distorted perception of its self-state. According to Fonagy and Target (2002), this interactional mechanism is causally linked to distorted self-representations (as in Winnicott's concept of "false self"; see Winnicott 1990).

Low Structural Level: Absence of Affect-Marking

The marking of affect is lacking in the primary caregiver, who is unable to contain their infant's negative affect-expressions due to unresolved intrapsychic conflicts or structural limitations. They react to negative affect-expression by producing the same—categorically congruent—expressions of emotion in an unmarked, realistic manner. Probable consequences: Since the mirroring affect-expression is unmarked, it is not decoupled from the mother, but instead attributed to her as a genuine emotion; as a result, it cannot be anchored as belonging to the infant. As a consequence, the infant does not produce a secondary representation of the primary affective state, leading to a deficiency in self-control of affect. It experiences its negative affect as "out there," belonging to the other, and not as its own. The infant's negative affect remains unregulated and the fact that it perceives the corresponding, realistic negative affect in the primary caregiver intensifies its negative state. Traumatization ensues rather than containment {XE "Containment"}. This corresponds to the dominant form of emotional experience in borderline personalities (Gergely et al. 2003).

Implications for Therapy

In the case of structural impairments, no circumscribed conflicts have accumulated intrapsychically, and the inner psychological space in which these could occur and be reflected on is lacking. The primary goal of therapy when dealing with structurally impaired parents is *not* to understand the problem in terms of conflict dynamics and biographical contingency, but rather to modify how the problem is dealt with. Therefore, the therapeutic goal also in the parent–infant setting should be to restore lost self-efficacy (with oneself, the partner, or the infant) and reconstitute and maintain interpersonal relationships. In addition to the principle of containment, it is important to take a supportive stance that puts auxiliary ego functions (concern, affect mirroring, emotional resonance, realistic confrontations, etc.) at the parents' disposal. Rather than interpreting the structural problem in the transference—since this option would prove futile in the absence of self-reflective skills—it is analyzed together as a third-person phenomenon and concretely worked through. Since structural problems cause situations in which the parents may feel overwhelmed and fail, techniques that additionally involve and mobilize affects are contraindicated (see also Rudolf 2004).

▶ The fundamental aim of structure-centered interventions is to improve the mentalization process {XE "Mentalization"} between parents and infant. Parents should be encouraged in such a way that they are capable of mitigating their infant's negative affect by producing contingent, marked, and emotion-reflective behaviors.

On the cognitive level, a realistic perception of the self and the object take the foreground in therapeutic efforts. The goal here is to achieve stability and direction in oneself and in the external world in order to be able to better accept and consider reality. Doing perception exercises with the infant can be particularly helpful here.

On the regulatory level, the regulation of own impulses, affects, self-appraisals, and relationship desires takes precedence. The intervention should help parents adopt a detached, observant, and autonomous position, while empowering them to disentangle themselves from overwhelming, monopolizing, or void situations. Working specifically on interaction with the infant can also be helpful here.

On the emotional level, it may be a question of helping the parents to engage better with their infant and allow themselves to be emotionally accessible. The therapist can encourage parents to address emotionality also in dealing with their infant, in order to help make their resulting perturbation endurable.

On the level of internalization, parental self-regulation using internalized positive objects or external relationship resources is paramount. In his interventions, the therapist might encourage parents to take advantage of fundamentally available opportunities (in the external world, in the therapeutic situation, and in their biographical experience) or to process contradictory experiences. In some cases, it may be necessary to actively involve external support systems, e.g., socio-educational family support.

11.2.3 Mixed Forms: Conflictual and Structural Foci

In order to be able to select therapeutically relevant foci, the therapist needs to be able to form a picture of the dynamic relationships between the different focus domains. Conflictual and structural foci may be entangled and interact. Often, a problem arising superficially as a conflict issue serves, on closer scrutiny, as a mechanism to cope with another underlying conflict or structural vulnerability—the actual, or deeper, problem. In routine therapy, one sees mixed forms of this kind primarily in the form of, e.g., "purely" conflict-related problem constellations. A distinction is made between the following mixed forms according to the severity of conflict-related or structural limitations within a family system:

- Predominantly conflict-based limitations
- Predominantly structure-based limitations
- Conflict-based limitations further complicated by structural constraints

11.3 Diagnostic Questions and Clinical Synopsis

Generating clinical hypotheses before initiating therapy is intended to permit conclusions to be drawn on the general orientation of treatment as primarily conflict-centered, structure-centered, or "mixed." To facilitate and systematize the diagnostic process, the following information-gathering procedure, designed as a list of diagnostic questions and concluding with the clinical synopsis, is proposed:

- What is the reason for presentation, or what are the presenting symptoms?
- Which "dominant theme," associated in the interview situation with the description of the reason for presentation, can be identified?
- What shape does the current relationship reality between parents and infant, as well as within the partner relationship, take? (Formulated individually for each person present.)
- What transference potential can be identified in the parents? What affects does the infant induce?
- Which biographical aspects are relevant in relation to current relationship regulation?
- What form of defensive behavior does the mother, father, and infant/toddler exhibit?
- What is the issue being defended against? (Hypotheses relating to the infant should be guided by psychoanalytic developmental psychology.)

- What is the dominant fear?
- How good is triangulation within the family?
- Which scene does the therapist feel drawn into in the sense of an enactment {XE "Enactment"}? What countertransference fantasies or action stimuli emerge?
- What are the principal clinically relevant conflicts within the family system?
- Is there a structural problem in the form of a lack of affect-marking on the part of the parents?
- What might the general therapeutic focus look like?
- How would one formulate the psychodynamic therapeutic focus in sentence form?

11.4 Case Report

11.4.1 Initial Contact

The mother of 18-month-old Mario initially contacted the Heidelberg parent–infant outpatient clinic by telephone. The secretary noted the following as the reason for presentation on the short registration form: "Mario wakes frequently at night (½ to 1 h or more). Is not able to settle back to sleep in his bed. Has always been like this. He has slept through the night for perhaps 3 weeks since birth." The registration sheet also provided information on the parents' age (both mid 30s) and profession (both physiotherapists). Mario was their first and only child.

All three family members attended the initial interview. Both parents came across as "convivial" and were keen to present themselves as being "on equal footing" in the hospital context, the father in particular creating a somewhat labored impression ("I'm not an expert, but …"). The mother, who appeared tired and strained, initially unburdened herself with much talking. She discussed little Mario's difficulties sleeping through the night and quickly came to the guilt-laden theme of her upcoming "separation" from her son. She was to resume work the next day and, in a parallel step, the father was to begin parental leave. This had produced in her a sense of "bereavement." In a tone mixed with anxiety and reproach, the mother spoke of what she anticipated: "Mario will just forget about me after tomorrow, once he's engrossed with his father." Although able to distance herself from such thoughts self-critically, the mother quickly broke into bitter tears. Her husband stood up and tended to his wife "as a matter of course," while at the same time appearing irritated and unwilling, as if to say: "Take her off my hands, I can't bear it any longer."

Mario occupied himself eagerly and age-appropriately with the toys that were available and climbed on his mother's lap when she began to cry. The parents confirmed that their son had a "strong antenna" for his mother's emotional state and would "come to her aid." Mario appeared "normal" and "inconspicuous," if perhaps a little too "reasonable" for his age. He approached the (male) therapist twice during the course of the interview and invited him to play. The father remained passive in the background. The therapist felt the urge to involve the father actively in the scene and became annoyed at the father's

"I'm-keeping-out-of-this-and-letting-my-wife-get-it-off-her-chest-to-someone" stance. This overall passive-aggressive relationship style between the parents prevailed for the entire interview. The therapist pondered whether making an interpretation to this effect might perhaps be "inflammatory" to the relationship, and thought: "In the best case, the two of them will do couples therapy." He decided against confrontation and instead for passive-aggressive adjustment.

He also became increasingly annoyed at the mother, who was making it unmistakably clear how much she needed her son, thereby binding him to her tightly.

It then became clear in the biographical history how anxiously preoccupied the mother (as well as the father) was with the threat of object loss and the fear of loneliness. The maternal grandmother had died of cancer when the mother was 12 years old. The mother was filled with recriminations: "She cleared off—that was her way of escaping my parents' perpetual fighting." The father had four siblings and had only ever known his parents as chronically overstrained and working. There had been no solidarity between the siblings, since they had all sought distance. By this point, both parents appeared to be more needy, the mother clinging almost desperately to the promise of help ("Give me lots of help, reduce my burden!").

The couple's relationship up to the time of birth was described as extremely limited. The husband's absence, often until late in the evening due to his work at the clinic (on his own treatment concept), was a recurrent issue. Although they had long wanted children, the mother in particular, by her own admission, had hesitated due to her dilemma about whether starting a family in view of her own family background was "reasonable," and whether the relationship could withstand children. Ultimately, it was a question of "child or separation."

11.4.2 Clinical Synopsis

This short excerpt from the session clearly highlights the significance of the theme "loss and separation." It is linked in a conflictual manner to dealing with needs for care, which strongly determine interpersonal relationships. At the same time, the mother's conflict-tinged and thus categorically distorted perception of her infant's behavior and experience also becomes apparent. However, there is no clear indication of a structural impairment to the parents' capacity for containment {XE "Containment"}. The significance of malfunctioning objects, of loss, jealousy, and dyadic relatedness with the lead affects of grief and aggression toward separation steer the conflict diagnosis in the direction of "need for care versus self-sufficiency" (according to OPD; see OPD Task Force 2008). Thus, the therapeutic focus is strongly conflict-centered.

Definition of conflict according to OPD-2: Need for care versus self-sufficiency

Dealing with need for care shapes object relations in such a way that experiencing and structuring of relationships in a conflictual way follows the wishes for care and security or their resistance. The associated lead affect is (prolonged) sadness and depression, since the significance of the malfunctioning object (fear) is constantly perceived. The themes of loss, failure, or jealousy are clinically relevant. The care theme in the early time with the infant can, for example, take the shape of altruistic cessation (resistance); alternatively, the partner, for his part, is coerced in a dependent and demanding manner to ensure security and care. The infant may also be drawn in to satisfy the "contact hunger." In the countertransference, feelings of worry and powerlessness become perceptible, as well as feelings of sadness or need for care in identification with a self-contribution of the parents.

From the mother's perspective, the focus could be formulated as follows: "If I leave Mario, it's as if I'm dead to him. He might get as sad, desperate, and angry as I was. That's why I have to bind him to me so tightly and am not able 'to bear' the third party that separates us." The assessment sheet on the following page (Fig. 11.1) illustrates the clinical synopsis in table form.

Child's name Mario	Age 18 months	Reason for presentation /symptoms Sleep maintenance disorder ICD -10 Diagnosis F43.2	
Dominant theme **Separation/loss**			
	Mother	**Father**	**Infant/toddler**
1. Level of relationship Current relationship reality (parents - infant) 2. Potential for transference (parent - therapist/infant - therapist) 3. Biographical aspects	1. Strong attachment, upcoming separation 2. "Give me lots of help, reduce my burden" 3. Sudden death of her mother (escape from perpetual crisis between her parents)	1. Is excluded, "handing over," makes an effort, strained by partnership 2. "Take her off my hands, I can't bear it any longer" 3. Close dyadic relationship	1. Helps the mother 2. Invites others to play
Level of defense 1. Resistance 2. Resisted 3. Fear	1. Strong attachment behavior 2. Sadness/anger 3. Abandonment/object loss	1. Adjusting, withdrawing 2. Anger 3. Object loss	1. Helping 2. Autonomy destroys the object 3. Object loss
Quality of triangulation	Dyadic relationships predominate ; triangulation difficult		
Level of enactment (including countertransference and action impulses)	Actively involve (against resistance) and encourage the father, in order to permit detachment from infant. Relieve mother's burden. Anger at mother.		
Conflict-centered therapeutic focus	Need for care versus self-sufficiency		
Structural level of mentalization	Good Moderate (distorted) X Low (absence of marking)		
Therapeutic orientation	Structure-centered Clear Primarily mixed Primarily clear X Conflict-centered		
Formulated focus	"If I leave Mario, it's as if I'm dead to him. He might get as sad, desperate, and angry as I was. That's why I have to bind him to me so tightly and am not able 'to bear' the third party that separates us."		

Fig. 11.1 Clinical synopsis

11.4.3 Course of Therapy

Altogether, therapy consisted of four 90-min sessions at 2-week intervals. Already in the first session, the dominant theme {XE "Dominant theme"} of loss and separation and the associated affects (see above) were actualized and enacted. Although the parents had long been suffering in a highly ambivalent oral-collusive atmosphere of tension and were able to identify these difficulties, the therapeutic process made them aware for the first time of the link between the theme of object loss and their son's sleeping problem as a reaction to the mother's "overprotection" and the resultant inhibition of his self-efficacy. Due to the parents' good capacity for self-reflection, it was not necessary to introduce a "practice" separation ritual; the mother, in particular, recognized the upcoming "separation" from Mario as a developmental task and understood her son's distressed crying and screaming as "mirroring herself." Supporting the father in his triangulating function was also a goal of the intervention; however, the comparatively virulent couples' conflict appeared to be a hindrance in this regard.

In the second session, the parents reported "first successes." The mother had consciously withdrawn herself as a "sleep-onset aid" and given the father more responsibility in this domain. Ultimately, both had been able to "bear" Mario's screaming for a certain length of time and noticed that their son needed less and less time to fall asleep alone in his bed. He still woke up and came into their bed, but this situation was seen more as a transitional solution. With astounding candidness, the mother talked about how jealous she was of her husband and son's "togetherness" once she had resumed work. It was possible to discuss the parents' rivalry about who was the "better mother," even though ultimately the father's silent triumph hung in the room.

Following the third session, the "separation was complete," and Mario was sleeping through the night in his own bed. As such, the infant was no longer a symptom carrier, and the "problems in the marital bed" came to the fore. After many months of abstinence, the husband was asking for "changes in the sexual sphere," which his wife was not prepared to make. After the deferment of conflict that had taken place as a result of parenthood, the couple's dispute had resurfaced with vigor; the possibility of inducing change with couples therapy was discussed and expressly recommended by the therapists. The parents said they would consider this option prior to the following session.

The fourth session was almost fully taken up with the couple's discord. They were nevertheless able to refrain from "resorting back" to the sleeping problems as an attempt at a solution. Mario continued to fall asleep alone and sleep through the night. In the meantime, the parents had seriously considered the possibility of a separation and had decided, in a first step, not to expend any more energy on their "problems as husband and wife," but to concentrate instead on their "duty as parents." They wanted to spare their infant a separation. This short-term therapy for an infant regulatory disorder, which proved to be a symptomatic solution to the parents' dysfunctional relationship, was concluded with an offer to the parents to come back at a later time for couples counseling. From a therapeutic perspective, this was possibly a disappointing decision, but one that could be respected. The family did not attend our outpatient clinic again.

11.5 Conclusion

Regulatory disorders in infants and toddlers occur in a complex relationship structure formed by the parents' relational experiences in their families of origin, with other partners, as a couple, and with their infant. The infant brings its intrinsic temperament- or constitution-related willingness to interact to the relationship, thereby forcing the parents to discard putatively successful coping processes (e.g., in the sense of collusively dealing with neurotic conflicts or compensating structural deficits) and to develop new, more adequate solutions.

Providing therapeutic support during this process requires profound diagnostic skill and a therapeutic concept that addresses the conflict- or structure-related vulnerabilities of the family system in an appropriate manner. The concept of focus-oriented therapy presented in this book attempts to meet this goal from a psychoanalytic, relational, and family-oriented perspective. For a more in-depth discussion, the reader is referred to the manual on which the present book is based (Cierpka and Windaus 2007).

References

Argelander H (1970) Überlegungen zum psychoanalytischen Konzept des Sprechstunden interviews. Psyche 27:1002–1011

Beavers WR (1982) Healthy, midrange, and severly dysfunctional families. In: Walsh F (ed) Normal family processes. Guilford Press, New York, pp 45–66

Cierpka M, Windaus E (Hrsg) (2007) Psychoanalytische Säuglings-Kleinkind-Eltern-Psychotherapie. Konzepte - Leitlinien - Manual. Brandes & Apsel, Frankfurt a.M.

Cierpka M, Hirschmüller B, Israel A, Jahn-Jokschies G, von Kalckreuth B, Knott M, Stasch M, Wiesler C, Windaus E (2007) Manual zur psychoanalytischen Behandlung von Regulationsstörungen, psychischen und psychosomatischen Störungen bei Säuglingen und Kleinkindern unter Verwendung des Fokuskonzeptes. In: Cierpka M, Windaus E (Hrsg) Psychoanalytische Säuglings-Kleinkind-Eltern-Psychotherapie. Konzepte - Leitlinien - Manual. Brandes & Apsel, Frankfurt a.M., pp 87–214

Fonagy P, Target M (2002) Neubewertung der Entwicklung der Affektregulation vor dem Hintergrund von Winnicotts Konzept des "falschen Selbst". Psyche (56):839–862

Gergely G, Fonagy P, Target M (2003) Bindung, Mentalisierung und die Ätiologie der Borderline-Persönlichkeitsstörung. In: Fonagy P, Target M (Hrsg) Frühe Bindung und psychische Entwicklung

OPD Task Force (ed) (2008) Operationalized psychodynamic diagnosis OPD-2. Manual of diagnosis and treatment planning. Hogrefe Verlag, Göttingen

Fraiberg S (1982) Pathological defenses in infancy. Psychoanal Q 51(4):612–635

Klüwer R (1983) Agieren und Mitagieren. Psyche 37:828–840

Lorenzer A (1970) Kritik des psychoanalytischen Symbolbegriffs. Suhrkamp, Frankfurt a. M

Malan DH (1965) Psychoanalytische Kurztherapie. Klett, Stuttgart

Menninger KA, Holzman PS (1977) Theorie der psychoanalytischen Technik. Frommann-Holzboog, Stuttgart

Rudolf G (2004) Strukturbezogene Psychotherapie. Leitfaden zur psychodynamischen Therapie struktureller Störungen. Schattauer, Stuttgart

Stern DN (1998) Die Mutterschaftskonstellation: Eine vergleichende Darstellung verschiedener Formen der Mutter-Kind-Psychotherapie. Klett-Cotta, Stuttgart

Windaus E (2007a) Konzepte der psychoanalytischen Säuglings-Kleinkind-Eltern-Psychotherapie. In: Cierpka M, Windaus E (Hrsg) Psychoanalytische Säuglings-Kleinkind-Eltern-Psychotherapie. Konzepte—Leitlinien—Manual. Brandes & Apsel, Frankfurt a. M., S11–S50

Windaus E (2007b) Behandlungskonzepte der tiefenpsychologisch fundierten und analytischen Psychotherapie im Säuglings- und Kleinkindalter. In: Hopf H, Windaus E (Hrsg) Lehrbuch der Psychotherapie, Bd. 5. CIP-Medien, München, S213–S230

Winnicott DW (1990) The maturational processes and the faciliating environment. Studies in the theory of emotional development. Karnac, London

Ziegenhain U (2004) Beziehungsorientierte Prävention und Intervention in der frühen Kindheit. Psychotherapeut 49(4):243–251

Index

M. Cierpka (ed.), *Regulatory Disorders in Infants*,
DOI 10.1007/978-3-319-43556-5

CPSIA information can be obtained
at www.ICGtesting.com
Printed in the USA
LVHW081813070419
613269LV00001B/101/P

9 783319 435541